Primary Management of Polytrauma

Suk-Kyung Hong • Dong Kwan Kim
Sang Ryong Jeon

Editors

Primary Management of Polytrauma

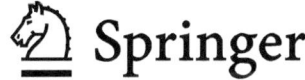 Springer

Editors
Suk-Kyung Hong
Department of Surgery
Asan Medical Center
Seoul
South Korea

Sang Ryong Jeon
Department of Neurosurgery
Asan Medical Center
Seoul
South Korea

Dong Kwan Kim
Department of Thoracic &
Cardiovascular
Asan Medical Center
Seoul
South Korea

ISBN 978-981-10-5528-7   ISBN 978-981-10-5529-4   (eBook)
https://doi.org/10.1007/978-981-10-5529-4

Library of Congress Control Number: 2019930574

This Springer imprint is published by the registered company Springer Nature Singapore Pte Ltd. The registered company address is: 152 Beach Road, #21-01/04 Gateway East, Singapore 189721, Singapore

Introduction

Trauma is an unexpected damage to the body by external forces such as traffic accident, fall, violence, and other causes. Every patient has a different injury mechanism, severity, and anatomic disruption. When the patients rush into emergency room in an accident, physician start to managing and treating under high-pressure scene. Even in the middle of chaos situation with anxiety, the professionals need to approach from the head to toe. However, injury which is more harm to patient should be managed with a priority to improve the patient's survival and reduce mortality and morbidity.

The primary approach to polytrauma patient is the most important step for successful treatment. The critical period immediately after injury, so called 'golden hour' is very essential. Initial rapid and systematic approach can result in better clinical outcomes and reduce preventable death rate.

This book deals with the primary management of polytrauma patients. With initial approach to identify life-threatening injury, specific organ injuries were reviewed, particularly brain, spine, chest, abdomen, musculoskeletal, and soft-tissue. Within these specialized areas, imaging, interventional radiology and inter-hospital transfer were reviewed comprehensively.

I believe this book will help the physicians who initially face polytrauma patients to approach systemically and comprehensively. This book will provide invaluable reference for physicians to take care of the poly-trauma patients primarily. We're grateful to the authors who contributed their knowledge, experience, writing, and valuable time.

Contents

1 Initial Assessment and Management   1
Dong-Woo Seo

2 Management of Shock   11
Nak-Jun Choi and Suk-Kyung Hong

3 Traumatic Brain Injury   19
Seungjoo Lee

4 Spinal Injury   33
Sang Ryong Jeon and Jin Hoon Park

5 Thoracic Injury   63
Dong Kwan Kim and Geun Dong Lee

6 Abdominal Injury   83
Suk-Kyung Hong

7 Musculoskeletal Injury   93
Ji Wan Kim

8 Soft-Tissue Injury 115
Young Chul Suh, Hyunsuk Peter Suh, and Joon Pio Hong

9 The Role of Radiology in Trauma Patients 133
Gil-Sun Hong and Choong Wook Lee

10 Interventional Radiology 149
Jong Woo Kim and Ji Hoon Shin

11 Interhospital Transfer 173
Yooun-Joong Jung

Initial Assessment and Management

Dong-Woo Seo

1.1 Introduction

Trauma is one of the major causes of death for relatively young age [1]. The primary causes of death following trauma are the head injury, chest injury, and major vascular injury. Up to 90% of patients who survive the initial trauma, the burden of ongoing morbidity from trauma, is even more significant.

The treatment of seriously injured patients requires the rapid assessment and treatment of injuries (Fig. 1.1). Because timing is critical, a speedy and accurate systematic approach is essential. A systematic approach to trauma care is organized according to the concepts of rapid assessment, triage, resuscitation, diagnosis, and therapeutic intervention [2].

1.2 Preparation and Triage

The trauma system can be very different by country or region. Proper transport standards are needed for each area [2]. During the prehospital phase, airway maintenance, control of external bleeding, spine immobilization, and immediate transport to the appropriate facility are necessary. Scene time should be minimized [3]. Obtaining information including time, related event, and mechanism of injury is an essential part of a prehospital phase. In trauma patients, predicting the damage through the injury mechanism is the most important. Before the arrival of injury patient at the hospital, EMS providers should inform the receiving ED (emergency department) about the information including time, related event, mechanism of injury, suspected injuries, vital signs, and treatments provided.

At the hospital phase, there should be a protocol prepared for trauma patients, which should include:

- Criteria for preparing for resuscitation
- Airway equipment (Make sure it works!)
- Warmed intravenous crystalloid solutions
- A protocol to summon additional people including laboratory and radiology person
- Standard protective equipment
- Periodic review protocol for quality improvement

D.-W. Seo (✉)
Department of Emergency Medicine,
University of Ulsan, College of Medicine,
Asan Medical Center, University of Ulsan
College of Medicine, Seoul, South Korea

© Springer Nature Singapore Pte Ltd. 2019
S.-K. Hong et al. (eds.), *Primary Management of Polytrauma*,
https://doi.org/10.1007/978-981-10-5529-4_1

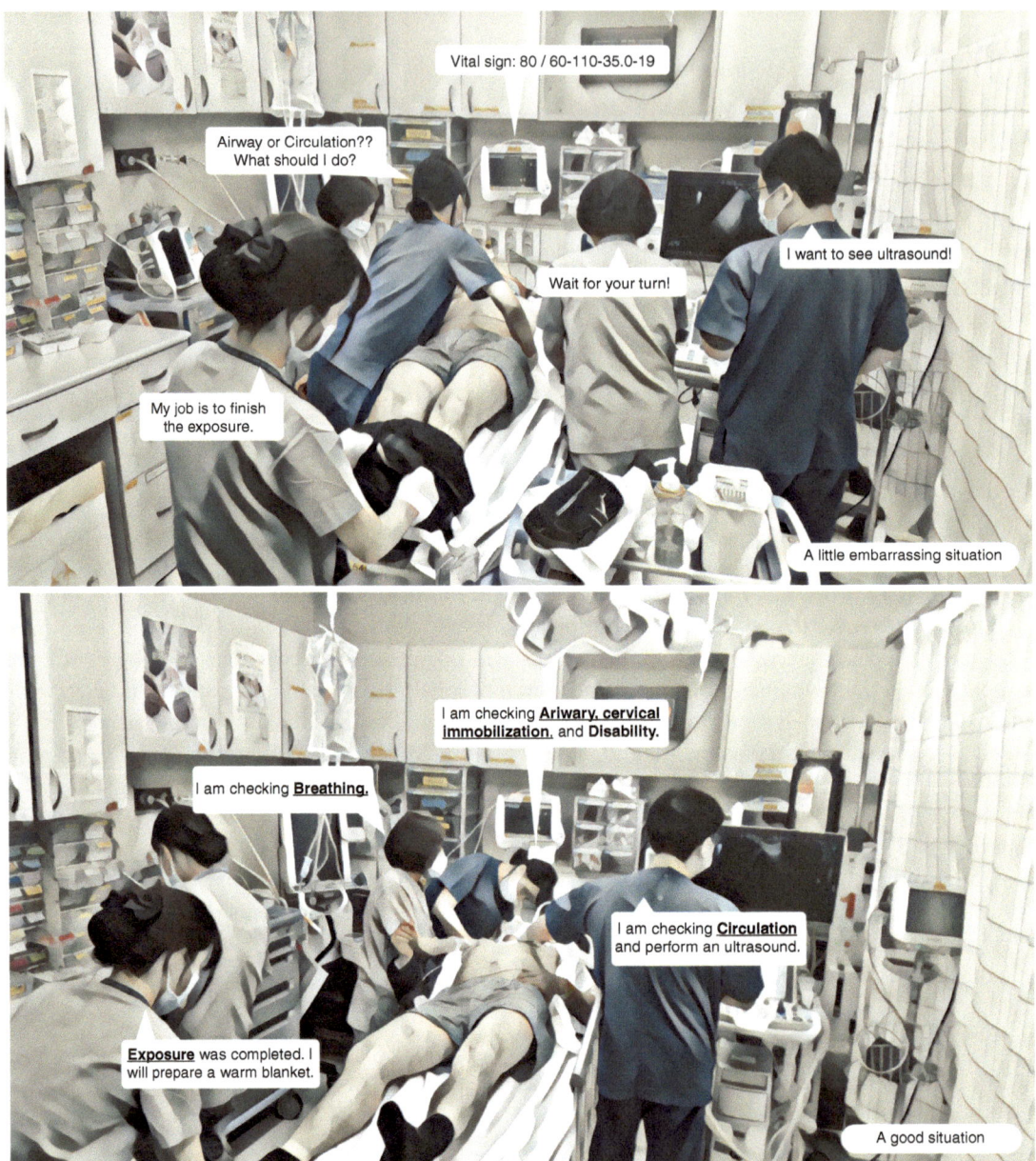

Fig. 1.1 The primary survey of a trauma patient

Because of concerns about communicable disease such as hepatitis and AIDS (acquired immunodeficiency syndrome), all provider who are likely to have contact with the patient must wear standard protective equipment including a face mask, eye protection, water impervious gown, and gloves (Fig. 1.2). In preparation for the patient's arrival, ED physician should assign tasks to team members, prepare resuscitation equipment, and check the presence of a surgeon. The team leader may need to consider the resources of the facility and determine which patients should be treated first. For patients transported to ED that is not trauma centers, consider an immediate transfer to a trauma center is appropriate.

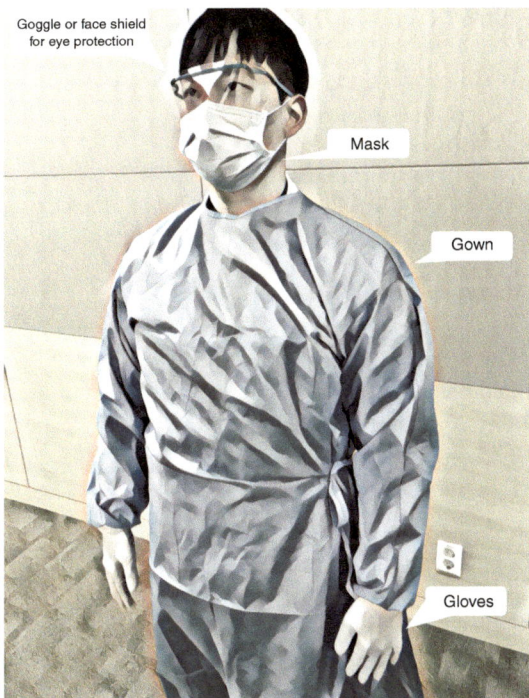

Goggle or face shield
for eye protection

Mask

Gown

Gloves

Fig. 1.2 Standard protective equipment

1.3 Primary Survey

1.3.1 Primary Survey Overview

A focused but as much information as possible history is obtained from the patient, caregiver, or EMS (emergency medical service) providers. Predicting the damage through the injury mechanism is very important. Information includes time, related event, mechanism of injury, intoxication, medication, and medical conditions. The primary survey consists of ABCDE (Fig. 1.1).

- A: Airway and cervical spine protection
- B: Breathing
- C: Circulation and hemorrhage control
- D: Disability
- E: Exposure

There are two things to keep in mind when conducting a primary survey. The first is that the primary survey is not necessarily in order. The second is that it can repeatedly be performed according to changes in the patient's condition. A quick assessment of the primary survey in a trauma patient can be done by identifying oneself and asking what happened. A proper answer can quickly measure the state of airway, breathing, and disability. On the contrary, if the patient does not answer correctly, you need quick assessment and management.

1.3.2 Airway and Cervical Spine Protection

1.3.2.1 Airway

In the initial evaluation of trauma patients, the airway should be assessed first. The quick assessment for signs of any airway obstruction should be performed. If there is foreign material in the airway, it should be removed immediately, and suction is often necessary. Facial bone fractures including maxilla and mandible can result in airway obstruction. The chin-lift or jaw-thrust maneuver is recommended to secure airway. Care should be taken to protect the cervical spine in all processes ensuring airway.

Although repeated tests are needed, if the patient can speak, it is a sign that airway patency is maintained. Orotracheal intubation may be necessary to achieve airway patency if the patient's Glasgow Coma Scale (GCS) is 8 or less points with head injuries. Nasopharyngeal intubation (including Levin tube) should be avoided in patients with a possible basal skull fracture.

While ensuring airway, it is recommended to use the two-person spinal stabilization technique (Fig. 1.3). In addition to one person securing the airway, the other focuses on cervical spine immobilization. If the patient is vomiting, the patient can be sideways and suctioned in a logroll fashion.

Trauma patients are frequently difficult to intubate because of a need for cervical spine immobilization, visual disturbance (blood or vomitus), upper airway injury, or concomitant facial injury. In this case, video laryngoscopy can be helpful, but practice is needed. Video laryngoscopy gives

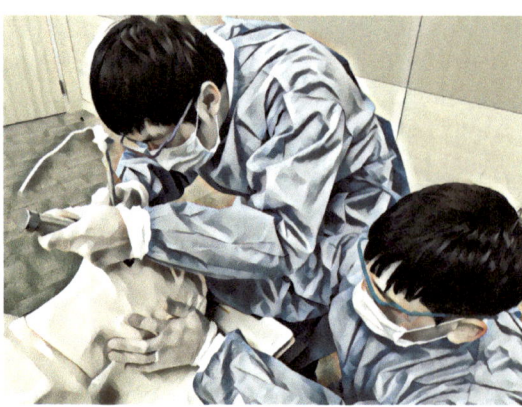

Fig. 1.3 Two-person spinal immobilization

less influence on cervical spine fixation. If endotracheal intubation fails, cricothyroidotomy may be necessary.

Securing an airway is critical, and it is vital to check whether it is always working. This can minimize mistakes by regularly administering the device and identifying the equipment immediately before the trauma patient visits. Sometimes, in a very difficult airway, a situation such as the power of the laryngoscopy is exhausted, or air leaks from the tube balloon arise. Make sure it works!

1.3.2.2 Cervical Spine Protection

If the patient's consciousness is impaired, assume a cervical spine injury until proven otherwise. Cervical spine protection should be performed throughout the treatment. Even when an x-ray or computed tomography (CT) of cervical spine shows normal findings, it is possible for a patient to have an unstable cervical spine injury. CT of cervical spine gives more information than x-ray, but it should not delay treatment because these images do not affect the decision on the emergency operation.

Detecting severe cervical spine injuries is not always clear. Careful clinical assessment is essential. Not all patients require cervical spine images. In alert patients, the National Emergency X-Radiography Utilization Study criteria (Table 1.1) {T5} is useful.

Table 1.1 NEXUS (National Emergency X-Radiography Utilization Study) Criteria for Cervical Spinal Imaging

No posterior midline cervical spine tenderness
No evidence of intoxication
Alert mental status
No focal neurologic deficits
No painful distracting injuries

1.3.3 Breathing

Once the airway is secured, inspect, auscultate, and palpate the thorax and neck to detect injuries. Physical signs do not always appear in patients with severe trauma. Hence, if in doubt, it is good to assume that there is an injury.

The injury requiring immediate treatment in the primary survey is as follows:

- Tension pneumothorax, hemothorax: deviated trachea, absent unilateral lung sound
- Flail chest: paradoxical chest wall movement
- Pneumomediastinum, airway rupture: crepitus
- Sucking chest wound

Any of these findings require immediate intervention. In particular, if tension pneumothorax is suspected, and if the chest tube cannot be inserted immediately, needle thoracostomy should be performed quickly and given time. A site for a needle thoracostomy is the second intercostal space in the midclavicular line. Delays including awaiting chest radiograph can result in cardiac arrest. Because procedures including intubation can aggravate a pneumothorax after procedure, radiographs and frequent reevaluation are needed. In case of a sucking chest wound, an occlusive dressing must be applied.

Trauma patients should receive supplemental oxygen. If not intubated, oxygen must be delivered through reservoir mask.

Table 1.2 Classification of hemorrhagic shock

	Class I	Class II	Class III	Class IV
Blood loss (mL) (%)	<750 (<15)	750–1500 (15–30)	>1500 (30–40)	>2000 (>40)
Hear rate (beats/min)	<100	>100	>120	>140
Systolic blood pressure	Normal	Normal	Decreased	Decreased
Pulse pressure	Normal	Decreased	Decreased	Decreased
Capillary refilling	Delayed	Delayed	Delayed	Delayed
Respiratory rate (beats/min)	14–20	20–30	30–40	>35
Urine output (mL/h)	>30	20–30	5–15	Minimal
Mental status	Slightly anxious	Anxious	Confused	Confused and lethargic

1.3.4 Circulation and Hemorrhage Control

1.3.4.1 Circulation and Hemorrhagic Shock

Hemorrhage is the leading cause of preventable deaths. Hemorrhage can cause shock, which can lead to patient death. It is important to predict and prevent hemorrhagic shock in advance. If a cardiac arrest occurs due to a hemorrhagic shock, it is challenging to reverse. At the initial evaluation, the hemorrhage status of the patient should be evaluated (Table 1.2). It is a widely used indicator, but there are many variations by the individual. Therefore, you should not trust it unconditionally. Repetitive and careful evaluation is required. Level of consciousness, skin color, and pulse are important indicators of hemorrhagic shock.

Level of Consciousness

Loss of consciousness may be due to a decrease in blood flow to the brain and may be an indicator of hemorrhagic shock. In particular, if a progressive loss of consciousness is accompanied by hypotension, the hemorrhagic shock should be suspected. The presence of intracranial lesions needs to be differentiated. However, in this case, blood pressure is usually normal or high at the beginning.

Skin Color

Skin color can be a helpful indicator. Patient with hemorrhagic shock may look pale. Determining skin color, however, can be difficult early because of lighting, temperature from the scene to the emergency room, and dirt.

Pulse

The pulse can be easily measured. However, the measurement results may vary considerably between clinicians. Tachycardia is usually accompanied by increased bleeding, but not at the last stage of hemorrhagic shock. Especially, children, pregnant women, older adults, or athletes require attention due to their different physiological responses. For example, in athletes, even if there is a lot of hemorrhages, there may be no tachycardia. For elderly patients, the possibility of taking a variety of medications should be kept in mind. Drugs such as beta-blockers can mask indicators of hemorrhagic shock. Think pessimistically and avoid profound shock.

1.3.4.2 Bleeding Control and Resuscitation

Direct Compression and Tourniquets

The source of bleeding should be identified as either external or internal. External bleeding control should be performed throughout the entire process of trauma patients, including prehospital stages. The most obvious way to control external bleeding is direct compression on the wound. Tourniquets and hemostatic dressing can also be used. Tourniquets are useful in massive exsanguination from an extremity. However, because of the risk of limb ischemia, a tourniquet can be used when direct compression is not possible.

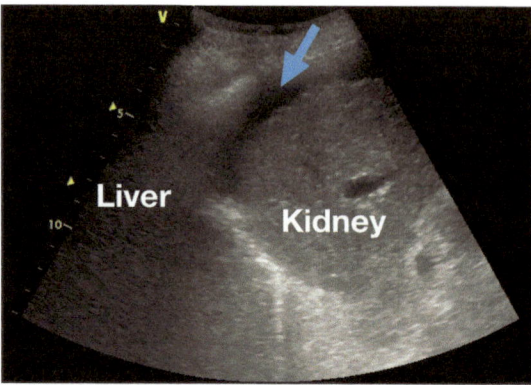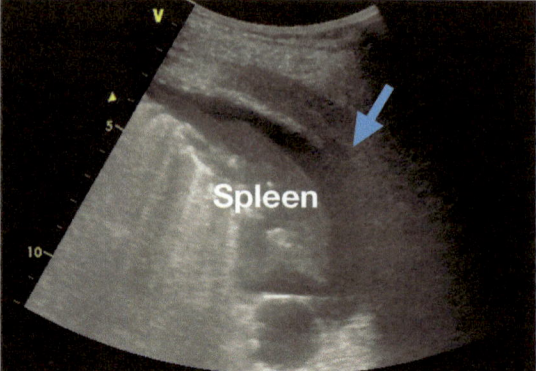

Fig. 1.4 Positive FAST exam with internal bleeding

In case of internal bleeding, the anatomical sites where massive bleeding can occur are the chest, abdomen, retroperitoneum, pelvis, long bone, and scalp. This type of bleeding can be identified by physical examination and imaging including FAST (focused assessment sonography in trauma). Repeated physical examination and FAST are needed because bleeding may not be detected when the amount is small. Figure showed the positive finding of FAST. Initial treatment includes pelvic binder in selected case and splint application. However, these patients need surgical intervention or radiological embolization (Fig. 1.4).

Resuscitation: Initial Fluid tx

In polytrauma patients, it is necessary to secure at least two large-bore peripheral IV lines (≥ 18 gauge). Obtain a blood sample for the blood type and screening test when securing the blood vessel. If a peripheral IV line cannot be obtained, consider central vein access (subclavian, internal jugular, or femoral vein). Rapid infusion pump use may be considered in unstable patients. In this case, large-bore central venous access is required to use the rapid infusion pump. In difficult situations, intraosseous access is also available.

Crystalloid (normal saline or lactated Ringer's solution) is the fluid of choice for initial resuscitation. A bolus of 1–2 L of a crystalloid solution may be required initially. Depending on the patient's response, additional dosing is determined. Aggressive volume resuscitation is not a substitute for definitive control of hemorrhage. Therefore, if ongoing bleeding is suspected, fluid therapy should be considered a temporary treatment for definitive control. If the patient is unresponsive to initial fluid therapy, consider transfusion. If massive bleeding is suspected in the initial evaluation, transfusion can be considered immediately without waiting for the response to the fluid therapy. Use a pressure bag to maximize the flow of fluid. The maximum rate of fluid infusion is determined by the internal diameter of the catheter and inversely by catheter length. And all fluid including blood product should be warmed (37–40 °C or 98.6–104 °F).

Resuscitation: Initial Transfusion

A major trauma patient is prone to bleeding diathesis. This may result in blood clotting and platelet dysfunction; then the patient's mortality rate increases. Study from both military and civilian experience reveals that trauma patients receiving more than ten units of packed red blood cells showed decreased mortality when they simultaneously receive fresh frozen plasma in a ratio of packed red blood cells to fresh frozen plasma of 1:1 rather than 1:4 (26% vs 87.5% mortality) [4]. Another study showed the administration of platelets in massive transfusion protocol in a 1:1:1 ratio with packed red blood cells and fresh frozen plasma. Because acidosis and hypothermia contribute to the bleeding diathesis, this status should be corrected as quickly as possible [5].

Table 1.3 Glasgow Coma Scale

	1	2	3	4	5	6
Eye	Does not open eyes	Opens eyes in response to painful stimuli	Opens eyes in response to voice	Opens eyes spontaneously		
Verbal	Makes no sounds	Incomprehensible sounds	Utters incoherent words	Confused, disoriented	Oriented, converses normally	
Motor	Makes no movements	Extension to painful stimuli (decerebrate response)	Abnormal flexion to painful stimuli (decorticate response)	Flexion/ withdrawal to painful stimuli	Localize to painful stimuli	Obeys commands

1.3.5 Disability

Perform a focused neurologic evaluation to assess level of consciousness, pupillary size and reaction, lateralizing sign, and spinal cord injury level. The GCS is a quick and straightforward method for assessing the level of consciousness (Table 1.3). If the GCS is 8 or less, it is advisable to assume that there is severe brain damage. It is recommended to secure a definitive airway to provide oxygenation and protect against aspiration. Perfusion state, oxygenation, and blood glucose levels should be assessed. If this test is abnormal, it should be treated as the cause of unconsciousness. In many trauma patients, drug and alcohol use is often accompanied, but if there is a declined consciousness, it should be assumed that there is a severe head injury. Prophylactic hyperventilation for maintaining intracranial pressure is not recommended [6]. The lucid interval associated with acute epidural hematoma is an example of a situation of rapidly progressive neurologic deterioration. Frequent reevaluation is needed.

1.3.6 Exposure and Environmental Control

The patient must be completely undressed for an accurate examination. The undressed examination should be performed promptly for preventing hypothermia. After the examination, the patient should be provided with warm blankets or other warming devices.

Due to the risk of worsening bleeding diathesis, hypothermia can be dangerous to trauma patients. Therefore, the medical staff should make efforts to prevent the patient from hypothermia. Transport environment, undressed examination, cold fluid, and emergency room temperature can make or exacerbate hypothermia. Efforts should be made to minimize body heat loss in the transport environment. The undressed examination should be performed promptly. Use warmed fluid. For crystalloids, microwave ovens can be utilized, and 39 °C is appropriate. For a blood product, use a warmer instead of microwave oven. It may be warm to the medical staff, but the temperature of the resuscitation room should be raised. If bleeding persists, hypothermia may occur despite all efforts because of massive transfusion and crystalloid infusion. In this case, the best treatment is early control of bleeding such as surgical intervention or embolization.

Objects impaled in the chest and abdomen should be left in place. The patient must be transported to the surgical field where the impaled object should be removed under direct visualization. The impaled object may be cut outside the skin to facilitate transport or prevent further injury [7].

1.4 Secondary Survey

If both primary surveillance and resuscitation are complete, a systemic examination from head to toe is required. This is called the secondary survey. Secondary surveys may take more time than primary surveys, but they should be done as quickly and accurately as possible. The important part of the secondary survey is to perform palpation by each site. If the patient status changes during secondary surveillance, primary survey and resuscitation may be necessary. Vital signs and consciousness should be continuously monitored during this period.

> Prevent hypothermia
>
> - Minimize body heat loss in the transport environment
> - Perform the undressed examination promptly
> - Use warmed fluid and blood product
> - Early control of bleeding such as surgical intervention or embolization

Head and neck
Scalp lacerations can result in hypovolemic shock. Because the hair can hide the wound, the head should be palpated to check for bleeding. Bleeding can be controlled staples that grasp the scalp. Inspect the tympanic membranes. When there is facial trauma, palpate all bony structures of the face. Sometimes it is hard to prevent bleeding of the maxillofacial fracture site. In such cases, surgical intervention or embolization should be considered. If there is evidence of basilar skull fracture, insert the gastric tube through the mouth rather than the nose. If neck laceration and vascular injury are suspected, avoid further exploration and immediately perform a surgical consultation.

Chest
Palpate entire chest cage including the clavicles, ribs, and sternum. Sternal tenderness may indicate a sternal fracture or myocardial injury. This injury may cause lethal arrhythmia. Distant heart sound and decreased pulse pressure can indicate cardiac tamponade. In chest x-ray, widened mediastinum or several signs can suggest an injury of the aorta.

Abdomen and pelvis
The abdomen and pelvis should be carefully examined because massive bleeding is possible and can be detected later. The most important aspect of abdominal screening is to find out if there is any damage that requires surgical treatment. A normal examination of the abdomen does not exclude an intraabdominal injury. Serial FAST can be helpful. Inspect the urinary meatus, scrotum, and perineum for the presence of any injury. Perform a rectal examination. However, the rectal examination is no longer routinely recommended in alert trauma patients without evidence of pelvic or spinal injury. Vaginal examination should be performed in patients who are at risk of vaginal injury.

Back and musculoskeletal system
Since the patient is in the supine position, it is easy to overlook the back injury. The patient's back should be examined using the log roll method. The most frequently missed conditions are the musculoskeletal injury. If the patient is unconscious, it is easy to miss the fracture of the extremity. Careful palpation should be performed to avoid missing the fracture. And if possible, check the motor and sensory function.

1.5 Initial Imaging and Laboratory Test

Essential x-ray includes the cervical spine, chest, and pelvis. The extended FAST examination is a rapid screening tool for the identification of significant bleeding in the abdomen, pericardial tamponade, pneumothorax, and hemothorax [8]. It can be performed to identify causes of shock during or immediately after the primary survey. If the vital sign is stable, CT can be taken. The whole body CT scan protocol has the advantage of being able to distinguish rapidly the whole body. The whole body CT scan protocol includes the brain, spine, chest, abdomen, pelvis, and extremity. However, CT should be performed selectively to reduce the radiation dose. Laboratory studies include blood type and screen, hemoglobin, glucose, cardiac marker, coagulation battery, blood gas, lactate, and pregnancy test.

Initial imaging and laboratory test

- Radiographs
  - Cervical spine
  - Chest x-ray
  - Pelvis x-ray
- Laboratory test
  - Blood type and screen
  - Hemoglobin
  - Glucose
  - Cardiac marker
  - Coagulation battery
  - Blood gas analysis
  - Lactate

References

1. Trauma Statistics & Facts – National Trauma Institute. https://www.nattrauma.org/what-is-trauma/trauma-statistics-facts/. Accessed 15 Sept 2017.
2. Rotondo MF, Cribari C, Smith RS. Resources for the optimal care of the injured patient. Chicago: American College of Surgeons; 2014.
3. Sasser SM, Hunt RC, Faul M, et al. Guidelines for field triage of injured patients: recommendations of the National Expert Panel on Field Triage, 2011. MMWR Recomm Rep. 2012;61(RR-1):1–20.
4. Duchesne JC, Hunt JP, Wahl G, et al. Review of current blood transfusions strategies in a mature level I trauma center: were we wrong for the last 60 years? J Trauma Acute Care Surg. 2008;65(2):272–8. https://doi.org/10.1097/TA.0b013e31817e5166.
5. Malone DL, Hess JR, Fingerhut A. Massive transfusion practices around the globe and a suggestion for a common massive transfusion protocol. J Trauma Acute Care Surg. 2006;60(6):S91–6. https://doi.org/10.1097/01.ta.0000199549.80731.e6.
6. Bratton SL, Chestnut RM, Ghajar J, et al. XIV. Hyperventilation. J Neurotrauma. 2007;24(supplement 1):S-87–90. https://doi.org/10.1089/neu.2007.9982.
7. Cartwright AJ, Taams KO, Unsworth-White MJ, Mahmood N, Murphy PM. Suicidal nonfatal impalement injury of the thorax. Ann Thorac Surg. 2001;72(4):1364–6. https://doi.org/10.1016/S0003-4975(00)02471-1.
8. Patel NY, Riherd JM. Focused assessment with sonography for trauma: methods, accuracy, and indications. Surg Clin N Am. 2011;91(1):195–207. https://doi.org/10.1016/j.suc.2010.10.008.

Nak-Jun Choi and Suk-Kyung Hong

Scenario

A 37-year-old female passenger was in a 60 km/h motor vehicle collision 30 min ago. She is drowsy but able to tell her name. The patient is complaining of abdominal discomfort. Her blood pressure is 80/65 mmHg, pulse 120, and respiratory rate 30.

Q: You are heard from ER, this patient has arrived. You have to go there as soon as possible. And next, what would you do in this situation?

A: First, you have to recognize that she is in shock and then assess the ABCDEs. If mental status is getting worse or the patient complains of dyspnea in shock state, do not hesitate to intubate. You must secure IV lines for hydration and can give 1 liter of crystalloid initially. After that, you must assess the responsiveness to initial fluid resuscitation. Therapeutic decisions are based on this response.

2.1 Introduction

Shock is defined as inadequate delivery of oxygen and nutrients necessary for normal tissue and cellular function. The initial cellular injury can be reversible. However, this injury will become irreversible if tissue hypoperfusion is prolonged or severe enough. Once shock is recognized, the correction of shock should begin immediately. Delay in restoration of the perfusion and cellular oxygen debt risks further cellular and organ damage and death [1, 2].

2.2 Evaluation of the Patient in Shock

The management of the patient in shock has been an integral component of primary approach of poly-trauma patients. All severely injured patients

N.-J. Choi (✉) · S.-K. Hong
Division of Acute Care Surgery, Department of Surgery, Asan Medical Center, University of Ulsan College of Medicine, Seoul, South Korea
e-mail: njchoi@amc.seoul.kr; skhong94@amc.seoul.kr

© Springer Nature Singapore Pte Ltd. 2019
S.-K. Hong et al. (eds.), *Primary Management of Polytrauma*,
https://doi.org/10.1007/978-981-10-5529-4_2

require assessment and treatment of life-threatening injuries. Logical treatment must be established, and priorities should be established. The patient's hemodynamics must be assessed quickly and efficiently. This process constitutes the ABCDEs to identify life-threatening conditions by the following sequences.

Table 2.1 provides general guidelines for establishing the amount of fluid and blood likely required [3]. We should reassess the volume status of the patient according to the response to fluid resuscitation and identify evidence of adequate end-organ perfusion and oxygenation (i.e., via urinary output, level of consciousness, and peripheral perfusion) [4, 5]. In cases of suspected bleeding, if the patient does not respond to volume loading and transfusions, we should go to the OR or angiography room immediately to stop the bleeding.

The patient's fluid responsiveness can be the key factor to determining the next step in managing trauma patients. The potential patterns of response to initial fluid administration can be divided into three groups: rapid response, transient response, and minimal or no response. Vital signs and management guidelines for patients in each of these categories are outlies in Table 2.2 [3]. Reassess patient response.

Organ failure due to hypoperfusion is the most common complication of hemorrhagic shock. This situation usually arises because adequate volume replacement is not achieved. Immediate, appropriate, and aggressive therapy that restores organ perfusion minimizes such complications.

If the hemorrhagic shock is obvious but does not respond to fluid resuscitation, immediate surgical intervention may be necessary. If the

Table 2.1 Estimated blood loss based on patient's initial presentation

	Class I	Class II	Class III	Class IV
Blood loss (mL) (%)	<750 (<15)	750–1500 (15–30)	>1500 (30–40)	>2000 (>40)
Heart rate (beats/min)	<100	>100	>120	>140
SBP	Normal	Normal	Decreased	Decreased
Pulse pressure	Normal	Decreased	Decreased	Decreased
Capillary refilling	Delayed	Delayed	Delayed	Delayed
RR (beats/min)	14–20	20–30	30–40	>35
Urine output (mL/h)	>30	20–30	5–15	Minimal
Mental status	Slightly anxious	Anxious	Confused	Confused and lethargic

Table 2.2 Response to initial fluid resuscitation

	Rapid response	Transient response	Minimal or no response
Vital signs	Return to normal	Transient improvement, recurrence of decreased blood pressure and increased heart rate	Remain abnormal
Estimated blood loss	Minimal (10–20%)	Moderate and ongoing (20–40%)	Severe (>40%)
Need for more crystalloid	Low	Low to moderate	Moderate as a bridge to transfusion
Need for blood	Low	Moderate to high	Immediate
Blood preparation	Type and crossmatch	Type-specific	Emergency blood release
Need for operative intervention	Possibly	Likely	Highly likely
Early presence of surgeon	Yes	Yes	Yes

patient has stabilized somewhat after initial resuscitation, the risk of fluid overload is minimized by careful monitoring [6]. Remember, the goal of therapy is restoration of organ perfusion and adequate tissue oxygenation, not normalizing blood pressure. If the patient has no fluid responsiveness and evidence of bleeding is not clear, other causes such as neurogenic shock or obstructive shock should be sought. Constant reevaluation, especially when patients' conditions deviate from expected patterns, is the key to recognizing such problems as early as possible.

2.3 Resuscitation Strategy

2.3.1 Vascular Access

Vascular access should be performed initially to provide sufficient volume. A short, large-bore catheter is used to supply large volumes of fluid in a short time. So, in patients suspected of hemorrhagic shock, two large-caliber (16 gauge or larger) peripheral venous catheters must be obtained first [3].

The most commonly used peripheral veins are the forearms and antecubital veins. If it is difficult to obtain a peripheral vein, a central venous catheter can be inserted, or saphenous vein cutdown can be performed, depending on the clinician's skill and experience.

Subclavian and internal jugular catheterization is not commonly used in trauma patients with hemorrhagic shock. The vein is collapsed due to volume depletion and is prone to complications such as pneumothorax during catheterization. Although ultrasound-guided internal jugular vein catheterization has been widely used in many situations, this is unusual in trauma patients because of the possibility of cervical trauma and the need for cervical collar immobilization. In this situation, femoral vein is a good alternative for catheterization [7].

Since the aseptic technique during catheterization is not likely to be retained at an urgent moment, the unnecessary line should be removed as soon as the patient's condition stabilizes.

Pitfalls
Vascular access should be avoided at the site of injured limb.

Intraosseous access can be an effective alternative for children with IV access difficulties.

2.3.2 Initial Fluid Therapy

The most common causes of shock in trauma patients are hypovolemia due to massive bleeding [8]. The most important things are to find the source of bleeding and stop it. During that process, initial fluid therapy is important enough to determine the patient's outcome. Among various types of fluids, such as crystalloid, colloid, and blood components, warmed isotonic solutions, such as lactated Ringer's and normal saline, are used commonly for initial resuscitation [9–11]. If bleeding is highly suspected through physical examination or FAST, blood components, especially packed RBCs, should be administered as soon as possible to prevent volume overloading [12–14].

For initial fluid resuscitation, it starts with the dose of 1–2 L for adults and 20 mL/kg for pediatric patients. While administrating the fluid, you should think about the additional fluid supply or the next treatment based on the patient's response [3].

The initial fluid therapy of traumatic shock is directed toward restoring cellular and organ perfusion with adequately oxygenated blood. The goal is perfusion not normotensive blood pressure. If blood pressure is raised rapidly before the bleeder stops, bleeding can last. So, use of vasopressin to raise blood pressure is not recommended for hemorrhagic shock. Furthermore, it can worsen tissue perfusion.

Pitfalls
Massive hydration of normal saline may cause hyperchloremic metabolic acidosis.

In case of patients with chronic kidney disease or AKI, lactated Ringer's solution may cause serum K+ level to go up.

Q: The patient's blood pressure does not increase. What's the most probable cause of shock? What can you do for further management?

A: Hemorrhage is the most common cause of shock in trauma. In this case, the patient shows transient response to fluid resuscitation that means ongoing bleeding might exist. You must order RBC transfusion. FAST can be helpful to identify the source of bleeding during primary survey. If there is no abnormality in FAST, you must find other focus of bleeding through secondary survey. It is important that secondary survey should not disrupt resuscitation. Check the patient's body temperature, coagulopathy, and acid-base balance.

2.3.3 Hemostatic Resuscitation

The main concepts of hemostatic resuscitation are using a balanced combination of blood products including packed RBCs, FFP, and platelets and rapid correction of hemostasis impairing factors such as coagulopathy, hypothermia, and acidosis, what we call lethal triad. FFP is utilized for its clotting factor content in trauma resuscitation [15]. Administration of FFP should be guided by serial measurement of clotting times, fibrinogen levels, prothrombin time (PT), and activated partial thromboplastin time (aPTT).

Massive transfusion is generally defined as >10 units of packed RBCs within the first 24 h or more than 4 units of packed RBC in the first 1 h

of admission. The massive transfusion protocol including early administration of packed RBCs, FFP, and platelets can reduce excessive crystalloid administration, thus improving mortality in trauma patients [16–18]. Current data support a target ratio of plasma: red blood cell: platelet transfusions of 1:1:1 [19–21].

Coagulopathy may be the result of physiologic derangements such as acidosis, hypothermia, or hemodilution related to fluid or blood administration in trauma patients. Classically, resuscitation-associated causes of coagulopathic bleeding after traumatic injury, of which hypothermia, metabolic acidosis, and dilutional coagulopathy were recognized as key factors of bleeding with trauma [22–24]. However, endogenous acute coagulopathy, which occurs within several minutes following trauma, before and independent of iatrogenic factors, is clearly recognized as the primary cause of coagulation after trauma. The coagulation process is a complex enzyme reaction that depends on patient's body temperature and pH as described below [25].

Hypothermia can be caused by a variety of factors such as hemorrhagic shock, traumatic brain injury, and so on. The most effective way to prevent hypothermia is to use warm fluids.

Acidosis can occur in a variety of situations, and it reflects tissue hypoperfusion in trauma patients. Sometimes massive resuscitation with normal saline can results in hyperchloremic metabolic acidosis.

Pitfalls
During ABCDEs in primary survey, patients can easily undergo hypothermia. The physician should be aware of it.

2.3.4 Hypotensive Resuscitation

The aim of permissive hypotension is to decrease rate of blood loss in the early period after trauma while maintaining adequate organ perfusion.

In the past, the management of patients in shock has been focused on administrating aggressive fluid with crystalloid to restore circulating blood volume rapidly and thus maintaining organ perfusion. However, this management can potentially increase bleeding by elevating the blood pressure and dislodging established blood clots [26]. Furthermore excessive fluid resuscitation can dilute coagulation factors and increase tissue edema, which may play a role in the occurrence of abdominal compartment syndrome and multiple organ failure.

Permissive hypotension is the method of maintaining the minimum blood pressure to maintain only organ perfusion in order to minimize further bleeding. Numerous animal models of uncontrolled hemorrhage have demonstrated a significant reduction in mortality when maintaining a lower blood pressure than normal with fluid restriction [27, 28]. Although, this method may avoid the adverse effects of excessive fluid administration, it has the potential risk of hypoperfusion. In setting the target blood pressure for permissive hypotension, we should consider the patient's perfusion status such as mental status, urinary output, serum lactate level, and other parameters.

It is important to keep in mind that permissive hypotension is a temporary method until the bleeder stops. We should avoid prolonged permissive hypotension that can cause aggravated coagulopathy, tissue ischemia, and lactic acidosis.

2.3.5 Reevaluation of Fluid Resuscitation

The most important aspect of fluid resuscitation is the assessment of the patient's volume status via various parameters, and you can predict whether the patient has fluid responsiveness or recovered from the shock by monitoring those parameters [29]. When the patient's volume status is depleted, fluid administration can be beneficial for it increases stroke volume. Wherever, if the patient's volume is not depleted, stroke volume will not repond to fluid administration. The aim of fluid resuscitation is to administer fluid until the stroke volume of the patient responds to fluid bolus, as shown in the Frank-Starling curve (Fig. 2.1) [30].

As mentioned earlier, various parameters are used to evaluate the patient's volume status and fluid responsiveness. The passive leg raise (PLR) test is a noninvasive method that can be easily performed by the bedside (Fig. 2.2). The PLR has the effect of temporarily increasing preload by increasing the venous return by lifting the lower limbs [31]. Traditionally, CVP has been used to assess the patient's volume status, but the use of CVP at one moment has recently been limited due to various biases, and there is a limit to correlating pressure and volume status [32–34]. However monitoring continuously changing CVP can help to assess fluid responsiveness.

The urinary output reflects the renal blood flow and is one of the prime monitors of resuscitation

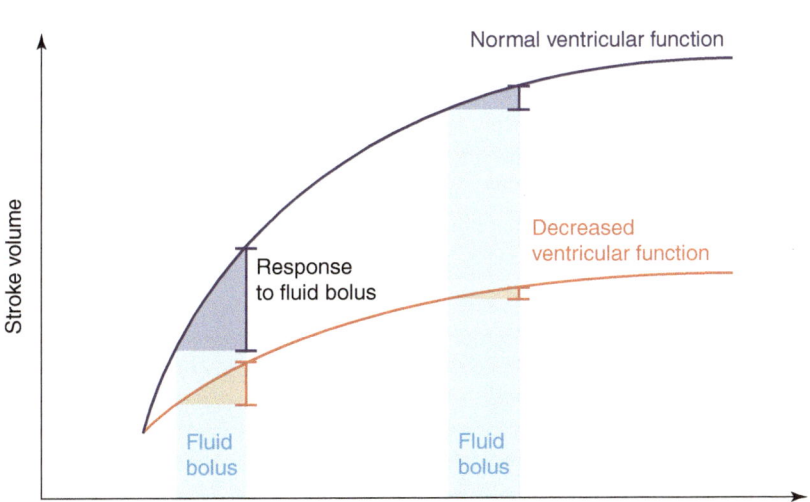

Fig. 2.1 Frank-Starling curve for fluid administration

Fig. 2.2 Passive leg
raise test

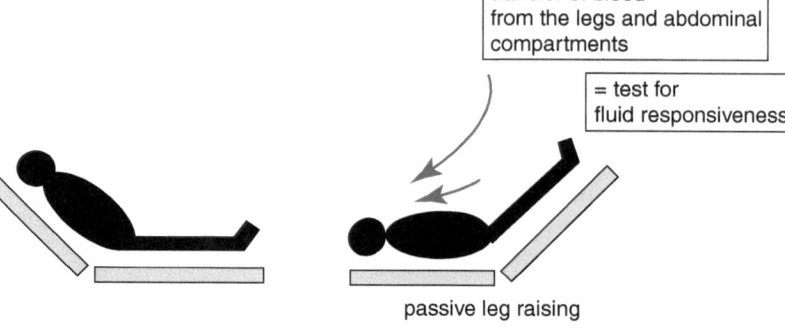

transfer of blood
from the legs and abdominal
compartments

= test for
fluid responsiveness

passive leg raising

and patient response [35]. Adequate resuscitation volume replacement should produce a urinary output of approximately 0.5 mL/kg/h in adults, whereas 1 mL/kg/h is an adequate urinary output for pediatric patients. If the urine output is less than this standard, it means that perfusion is not yet sufficient, and additional resuscitation is needed.

Metabolic acidosis is caused by anaerobic mechanism, which results from tissue hypoperfusion and production of lactic acid in traumatic shock. We can assess fluid responsiveness by continuously monitoring BD or lactic acid during fluid resuscitation. If acidosis becomes worse during fluid resuscitation, it should be treated with fluids, blood, and consideration of operative intervention to control hemorrhage [36].

Recently, the use of ultrasound for trauma patient is increasing through FAST. You can also measure volume status by measuring the IVC in the subxiphoid view with ultrasound [37]. The normal range is about 1.5–2.5 cm. It should be taken into account that the preload may be reduced due to positive pressure in patients with a mechanical ventilator [38].

Functional hemodynamic monitoring such as stroke volume variation (SVV) and pulse pressure variation (PPV) has shown clinical usefulness to predicting fluid responsiveness in many clinical trials [39–41].

Pitfalls
Sodium bicarbonate should not be used to treat metabolic acidosis secondary to hypovolemic shock. It can promote CO_2 retention and make acidosis worse.

Scenario: Continued
The patient reveals no abnormality in external appearance. Her chest X-ray and pelvic X-ray are normal. FAST exam shows fluid collection in Morrison's pouch and pelvic cavity.

Q: What's the diagnosis you can speculate? What's the next step for proper management?

A: You might regard hemoperitoneum such as liver laceration, mesentery contusion, or vessel injury as a cause of shock. If the patient's vital sign is stable, you can consider CT scan to identify more accurate bleeding focus and embolization through angiography. But in this situation, if the patient has no response to initial fluid resuscitation, you have to guess bleeding focus roughly and immediate surgical intervention is preferred.

Scenario: Continued
Blood and plasma are given immediately, and the patient is taken to the operating room for operative control of hemorrhage.

References

1. Bereiter DA, Zaid AM, Gann DS. Adrenocorticotropin response to graded blood loss in the cat. Am J Physiol. 1984;247:E398–404.
2. Bond RF, Manley ES Jr, Green HD. Cutaneous and skeletal muscle vascular responses to hemorrhage and irreversible shock. Am J Physiol. 1967;212:488.
3. American College of Surgeons Committee in Trauma. Advanced Trauma Life Support for Doctors. Chicago: American College of Surgeons; 2009.
4. Revell M, Greaves I, Porter K, et al. Endpoints for fluid resuscitation in hemorrhagic shock. J Trauma. 2003;54(5 Suppl):S63–7.
5. Hoyt DB. Fluid resuscitation: the target from an analysis of trauma systems and patient survival. J Trauma. 2003;54(5 Suppl):S31–5.
6. Mizushima Y, Tohira H, Mizobata Y, et al. Fluid resuscitation of trauma patients: how fast is the optimal rate? Am J Emerg Med. 2005;23(7):833–7.
7. Wiiliams JF, Seneff MG, Frideman BC, et al. Use of femoral venous catheters in critically ill adults: prospective study. Crit Care Med. 1991;19:550–3.
8. Sauaia A, Moore FA, Moore EE, et al. Epidemiology of trauma deaths: a reassessment. J Trauma. 1995;38:185–93.
9. Shires T, Coln D, Carrico J, et al. Fluid therapy in hemorrhagic shock. Arch Surg. 1964;88:688–93.
10. Alam HB, Rhee P. New development in fluid resuscitation. Surg Clin North Am. 2007;87(1):55–72. vi
11. Carrico GJ, Canizaro PC, Shires GT, et al. Fluid resuscitation following injury: rationale for the use of balanced salt solutions. Crit Care Med. 1976;4(2):46–54.
12. Cotton BA, Guy JS, Morris JA Jr, et al. The cellular, metabolic, and systemic consequences of aggressive fluid resuscitation strategies. Shock. 2006;26:115–21.
13. Holcomb JB, Jenkins D, Rhee P, et al. Damage control resuscitation: directly addressing the early coagulopathy of trauma. J Trauma. 2007;62:307–10.
14. Cotton BA, Gunster OL, Isbell J, et al. Damage control hematology: the impact of a trauma exsanguination protocol on survival and blood product utilization. J Trauma. 2008;64:1177–82.
15. Gonzalez EA, Moore FA, Holcomb JB, et al. Fresh frozen plasma should be given earlier to patients requiring massive transfusion. J Trauma. 2007;62:112–9.
16. Nunez TC, Yoing PP, Holocomb JB, et al. Creation, implementation, and maturation of a massive transfusion protocol for the exsanguinating trauma patient. J Trauma. 2010;68(6):1498–505.
17. Cotton BA, Au BK, Nunez TC, et al. Predefined massive transfusion protocols are associated with a reduction in organ failure and post injury complications. J Trauma. 2009;66:41–8.
18. Riskin DJ, Tsai TC, Riskin L, et al. Massive transfusion protocols: the role of aggressive resuscitation versus product ratio in mortality reduction. J Am Coll Surg. 2009;2:198–205.
19. Borgman MA, Spinella PC, Perkins JG, et al. The ratio of blood products transfused affects mortality in patients receiving massive transfusion at a combat support hospital. J Trauma. 2007;63:805–13.
20. Holcomb JB, Wade CE, Michalek JE, et al. Increased plasma and platelet to red blood cell ratios improves outcome in 466 massively transfused civilian trauma patients. Ann Surg. 2008;248:447–58.
21. Shaz BH, Dente CJ, Nicholas J, et al. Increased number of coagulation products in relationship to red blood cell products transfused improves mortality in trauma patients. Transfusion. 2010;50:493–500.
22. Kashuk JL, Moore EE, Milikan JS, et al. Major abdominal vascular trauma-a unified approach. J Trauma. 1982;22:672–9.
23. Harrigan C, Lucas CE, Ledgerwood AM. The effect of hemorrhagic shock on the clotting cascade in injured patients. J Trauma. 1989;29:1416–21.
24. Phillips TF, Soulier G, Wilson RF. Outcome of massive transfusion exceeding tow blood volumes in trauma and emergency surgery. J Trauma. 1987;27:903–10.
25. Brohi K, Cohen MJ, Ganter MT, et al. Acute traumatic coagulopathy: initiated by hypoperfusion: modulated through the protein C pathway? Ann Surg. 2007;245:812–8.
26. Pepe PE, Dutton RP, Fowler RL. Preoperative resuscitation of the trauma patient. Curr Opin Anesthesiol. 2008;21:216–21.
27. Bickell WH, Bruttig SP, Millnamow GA, et al. The detrimental effects of intravenous crystalloid after aortotomy in swine. Surgery. 1991;110:529–36
28. Owens TM, Watson WC, Prough DS, et al. Limiting initial resuscitation of uncontrolled hemorrhage reduces internal bleeding and subsequent volume requirements. J trauma. 1995;39:200–7.
29. Revell M, Greaves I, Porter K, et al. Endpoints for fluid resuscitation in hemorrhagic shock. J Trauma. 2003;54(5 suppl):S63–7.
30. Sarnoff SJ. Myocardial contractility as described by ventricular function curves: observations on Starling's law of the heart. Physiol Rev. 1988;35:107–22.
31. Cherpanath TG, Hirsch A, Geerts BF, et al. Predicting fluid responsiveness by passive leg raising: a systematic review and meta-analysis of 23 clinical trials. Crit Care Med. 2016;44(5):981–91.
32. Dellinger RP, Carlet JM, Masur H, et al. Surviving Sepsis Campaign guidelines for management of severe sepsis and septic shock. Crit Care Med. 2004;32:858–73.
33. Rivers E, Nguyen B, Havstad S, et al. Early goal-directed therapy in the treatment of severe sepsis and septic shock. N Engl J Med. 2001;345-1368-77.
34. Marik PE, Baram M, Vahid B. Does central venous pressure predict fluid responsiveness? A systematic review of the literature and the tale of seven mares. Chest. 2008;134:172–8.
35. Lucae CE, Ledgerwood AM. Cardiovascular and renal response to hemorrhagic and septic shock. In: Clowes Jr CHA, editor. Trauma, sepsis and shock:

the physiological basis of therapy. New York: Marcel Dekker; 1988. p. 87–215.

36. Cohn SM, Nathens AB, Moore FA, et al. Tissue oxygen saturation predicts the development of organ dysfunction during traumatic shock resuscitation. J Trauma Inj Infect Crit Care. 2007;62:44–54.

37. Prekker ME, Scott NL, Hart D, et al. Point-of-care ultrasound to estimate central venous pressure: a comparison of three techniques. Crit Care Med. 2013;41:833–41.

38. Barbier C, Loubières Y, Schmit C, et al. Respiratory changes in inferior vena cava diameter are helpful in predicting fluid responsiveness in ventilated septic patients. Intensive Care Med. 2004;30(9):1740–6.

39. Marik PE, Cavallazzi R, Vasu T, et al. Dynamic changes in arterial waveform derived variables and fluid responsiveness in mechanically ventilated patients: a systematic review of the literature. Crit Care Med. 2009;37:2642–7.

40. Pinsky MR. Functional haemodynamic monitoring. Curr Opin Crit Care. 2014;20(3):288–93.

41. Hofer CK, Müller SM, Furrer L, et al. Stroke volume and pulse pressure variation for prediction of fluid responsiveness in patients undergoing off-pump coronary artery bypass grafting. Chest;128:848–54.

Traumatic Brain Injury

3

Seungjoo Lee

3.1 Initial Diagnostic Approach

3.1.1 When Do We Need a Brain CT Scan in Head-Injured Patients?

Indications of brain CT scan

GCS ≤ 14
Unresponsiveness
Focal neurologic deficits
Amnesia for injury
Altered mental status
Progressive neurologic deficits
Signs of basal or calvarial skull fracture
Prior to general anesthesia (in case of neurologic exam cannot be followed)

3.1.2 What Is Radiologic Diagnosis of Head-Injured Patients?

3.1.3 Need an ICP Monitoring?

Indications of ICP Monitoring

GCS < 8 + abnormal brain CT
GCS < 8 + normal brain CT if two of the following are present:
(1) Age > 40
(2) SBP < 90 mmHg
(3) Abnormal motor posturing

S. Lee (✉)
Department of Neurosurgery and Critical care medicine, Asan Medical Center, University of Ulsan College of Medicine, Seoul, South Korea
e-mail: rghree@amc.seoul.kr

© Springer Nature Singapore Pte Ltd. 2019
S.-K. Hong et al. (eds.), *Primary Management of Polytrauma*,
https://doi.org/10.1007/978-981-10-5529-4_3

3.2 Classification of Traumatic Brain Injury

3.2.1 Primary Injury

3.2.1.1 Cerebral Concussion

Cerebral concussion is the most common form (80~90%) of traumatic brain injury (TBI) and has also been referred to as mild traumatic brain injury (MTBI). It might underestimate the true incidence because most patients do not receive hospital treatment.

The definition of concussion is rapid onset of impairment of neurologic function, which most often and typically resolves spontaneously over short time frame. It is a clinical diagnosis based on the combination of injury mechanism and acute symptoms and signs [1].

Pathogenesis
Concussion occurs when linear and/or rotational forces are transmitted to the brain. A concussive injury is caused by a complex cascade of ionic, metabolic, and pathophysiological events that is accompanied by microscopic axonal injury. This disruption of ionic balance and normal metabolism requires energy to re-establish homeostasis [2–4].

Clinical Symptoms and Course
The symptom of concussion is characterized by a common set of physical, cognitive, behavioral, and other symptoms. Headache and dizziness are

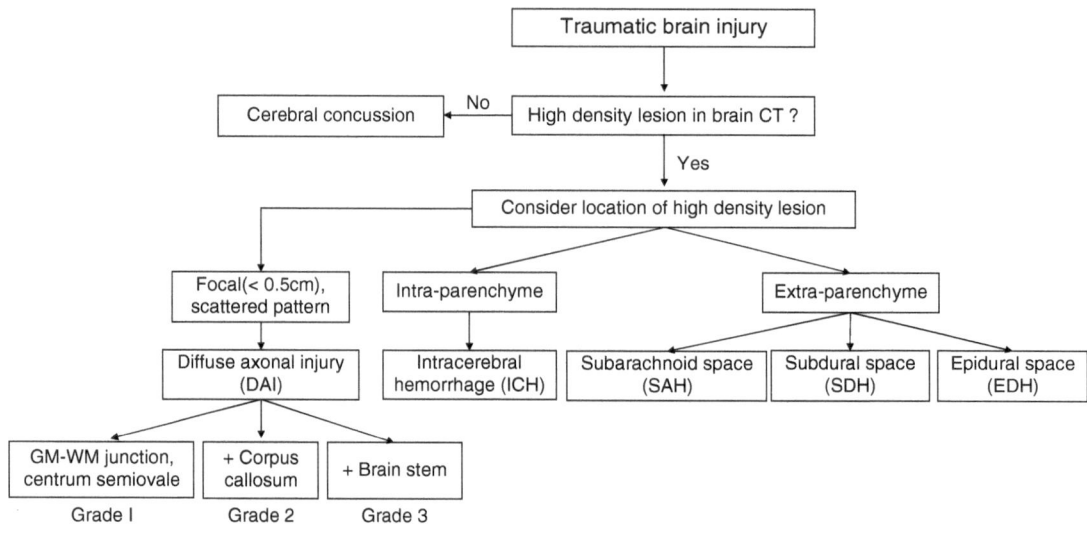

the most common symptoms of a concussion. Several symptoms of concussion are considered nonspecific and overlap with other disorders such as sleep disturbance, depression, and other medical disorders [5].

The 80–90% of concussion patient shows symptom resolution by 7 days following their injury, although symptom resolution may not always indicate a complete cognitive recovery as persistent deficits may be present on neuropsychological (NP) testing (Table 3.1).

Treatment and Outcomes

The emergency department is typically the first and only point of medical contact of concussion patients. About 90% of patients are treated and released without hospital admission. Most individuals with concussion do not require or undergo neuroimaging studies.

If indicated, CT is the preferred technology to rule out structural or more severe underlying brain injury (e.g., skull fracture, intracranial bleed, contusion, cerebral swelling, brainstem herniation).

The Canadian CT Head Rule is useful for this purpose and includes the following high-risk factors and two additional medium-risk factors.

High-Risk Factors

- Failure to reach GCS score of 15 within 2 h
- Suspected open skull fracture
- Any sign of basal skull fracture (e.g., Battle's sign, periorbital ecchymosis, cranial nerve palsy, hemotympanum)
- More than two episodes of vomiting
- Age older than 65 years

Medium-Risk Factors

- Amnesia after impact for longer than 30 min
- Dangerous mechanism of injury

The treatment of a concussion consists of physical and cognitive rest. In the immediate period after concussion, drugs that could alter mental status, such as benzodiazepines, should be avoided. After this acute phase, medications may be considered for symptomatic relief, although those that affect the CNS, such as stimulants, certain antiemetic medications, and antidepressants, should be used with caution. Treatment is based on common approaches to each specific symptom.

Most patients achieve a complete recovery in symptoms, cognitive functioning, postural stability, and other functional impairments over a period of 1–3 weeks following concussion. The rate of recovery varies across patients [5].

3.2.1.2 Diffuse Axonal Injury (DAI)

DAI describes a process of widespread axonal damage in the aftermath of acute or repetitive TBI, leading to deficits in cerebral connectivity that may or may not recover over time. It is a component of injury in 40% to 50% of hospital admissions for traumatic brain injury (TBI). DAI is typically characterized by coma without focal lesion [6].

Pathophysiology

DAI results from severe angular and rotational acceleration and deceleration that delivers shear and tensile forces to axons. It may result in severe neurological impairment despite lack of gross cerebral parenchymal contusions, lacerations, or hematomas. The histologic findings of DAI have been well documented and include disruption and swelling of axons, "retraction balls" (swollen proximal ends of injured axons), and punctate hemorrhages in the pons, midbrain, and corpus callosum. DAI is often associated with punctate hemorrhages, termed *Strich hemorrhages*, which represent bleeding from small cerebral vessels [7].

The location and severity of axonal injuries are important determinants of functional recovery. The Adams classification is used to grade DAI from a pathology standpoint [8] (Table 3.2).

Grading (Figs. 3.1 and 3.2)

Symptoms and Course

Some degree of DAI is likely in patients suffering moderate to severe TBI with loss of consciousness, with initial Glasgow Coma Scale (GCS) assessment perhaps reflecting functional impairment of the brainstem and the reticular activating system within the midbrain. Recovery of responsiveness and alertness may develop slowly a protracted course over weeks to months.

With regard to functional outcome, DAI is likely the most common cause of severe impairment after TBI. Disruptions in consciousness were initially attributed specifically to brainstem injury; however, coma after DAI is also frequently associated with axonal damage in cerebral white matter as well. Persistent cognitive and memory deficits, seen in TBI in general, are prominent in these patients with deficits in information processing.

Table 3.1 Signs and symptoms of a concussion

Physical
Headache
Nausea/vomiting
Balance problems
Dizziness
Visual disturbance
Fatigue
Sensitivity to light
Sensitivity to noise
Numbness and tingling
Dazed
Stunned
Cognitive
Feeling mentally "foggy"
Feeling slowed down
Difficulty concentrating
Difficulty remembering
Forgetful of recent information and conversations
Confused about recent events
Answers questions slowly
Repeats questions
Emotional
Irritable
Sadness
More emotional
Nervousness
Sleep
Drowsiness
Sleep more/less than usual
Difficulty falling asleep

Harmon et al. [5]

Table 3.2 Adams classification of diffuse axonal injury

Grade I (mild DAI)	Microscopic changes in white matter of cerebral cortex, corpus callosum, brainstem, and occasionally the cerebellum
Grade II (moderate DAI)	Grossly evident focal lesions in the corpus callosum
Grade III (severe DAI)	Additional focal lesions in the dorsolateral quadrants of the rostral brainstem (involving superior cerebellar peduncle)

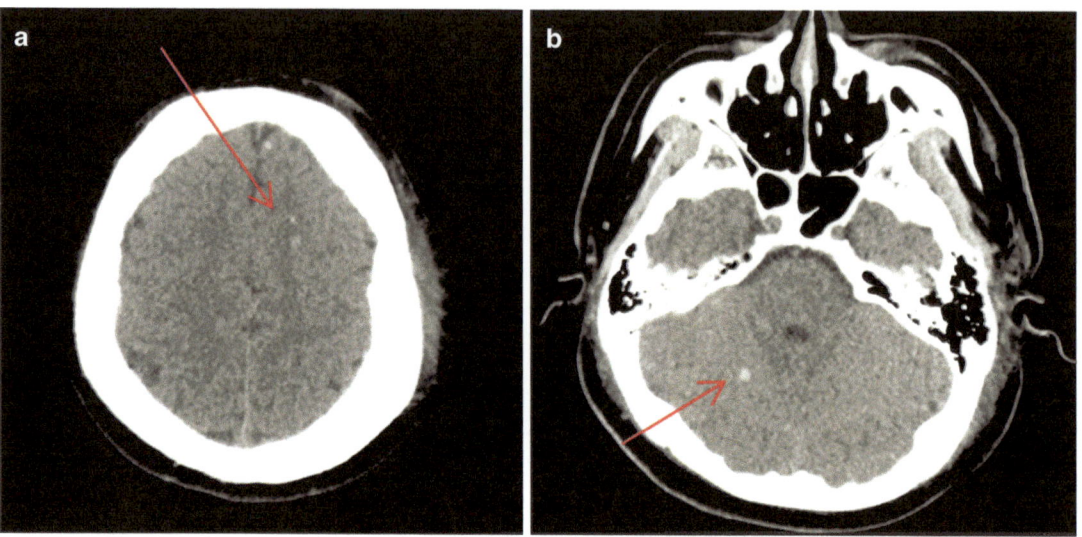

Fig. 3.1 Grade I DAI. (**a**, **b**) Small petechial hemorrhages of cerebellar hemisphere and frontal lobe on brain CT scan

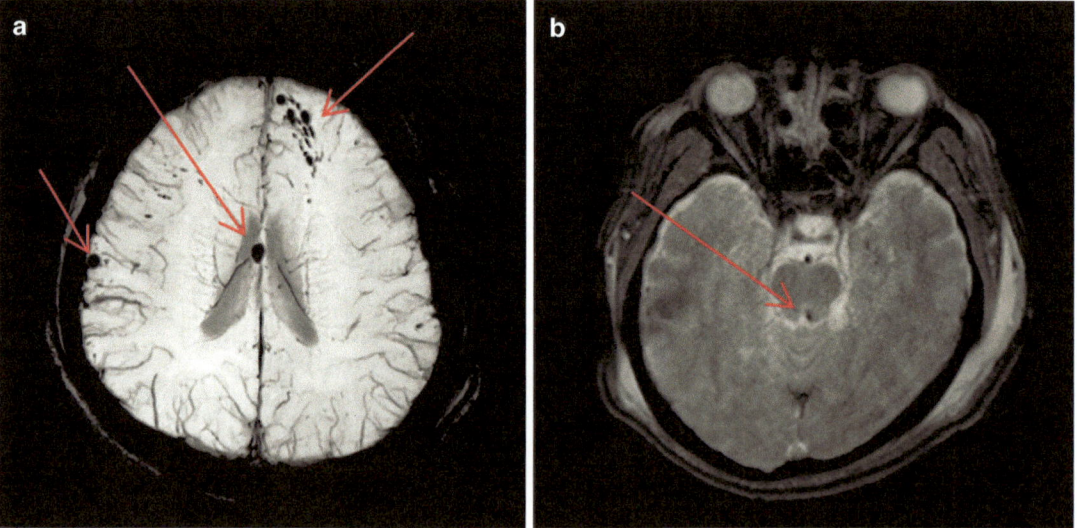

Fig. 3.2 Grade II and III DAI. (**a**) DAI grade II. Small hemorrhagic lesion of frontal lobe and corpus callosum was presented on susceptibility-weighted MR image. (**b**) DAI grade III. Small petechial hemorrhage of dorsolateral pons was seen on gradient echo MR image

Hypothalamic injury and panhypopituitarism have been associated with DAI, possibly due to shear injury across the pituitary stalk from the same high kinetic energy forces that cause DAI. Additionally dopaminergic pathways in the anteroventral third ventricular region mediate arginine vasopressin release and may be disrupted in DAI. This may contribute to sodium and free water derangements seen complicating post-TBI management [6].

Treatment

There are no established specific standard treatments for diffuse axonal injury. Close observation in intensive care units should be employed, and cares should be taken for preventing to develop other neurological and medical complications. The development of more sensitive diagnostic tools and targeted therapeutic interventions for DAI is needed.

As intracellular calcium accumulates, calcium-induced failure of the mitochondrial respiratory chain leads intact axons to undergo secondary axotomy. Dosage of cyclosporine (CsA) is effective in attenuating secondary progression to axotomy in the injured axon. Both CsA and FK506 could reduce progressive cytoskeletal damage and inhibit secondary axotomy. The weak regenerative capacity of CNS axons has been partially attributed to the activity of myelin-derived axon outgrowth inhibitors, which includes Nogo-A, oligodendrocyte-myelin glycoprotein (Omgp), and myelin-associated protein (MAP). Erythropoietin (EPO) is another neuroprotective agent under investigation. Some TBI models show benefit from calpain or caspase inhibitors [9].

3.2.1.3 Epidural Hematoma (EDH) and Subdural Hematoma (SDH)

Acute EDH

Pathogenesis
Traffic-related accidents (TA), falls, and assaults account for 53%, 30%, and 8%, respectively, of all EDH. In pediatric patients, falls are the leading cause of EDH in 49% of cases, and TAs are responsible for 34% of all EDH [10].

EDH can result from injury to the middle meningeal artery, the middle meningeal vein, the diploic veins, or the venous sinuses (Fig. 3.3).

Clinical Presentation
In patients with EDH, 22–56% are comatose on admission or immediately before surgery. The classically described "lucid interval" (a patient who is initially unconscious, then wakes up, and secondarily deteriorates) was observed in 47% undergoing surgery for EDH. Between 12% and 42% of patients remained conscious throughout the time between trauma and surgery. Pupillary

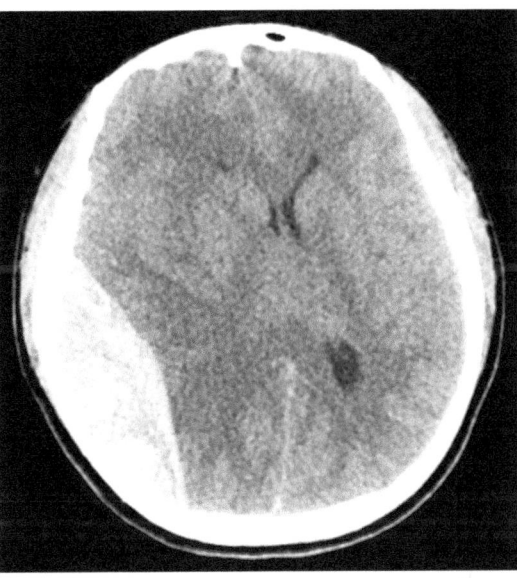

Fig. 3.3 Brain CT scan of acute epidural hematoma, lens (biconvex)-shaped high-density lesion along the right temporoparietal convexity, and midline shifting were seen

abnormalities are observed in between 18% and 44% of patients, and up to 27% of patients are neurologically intact [10].

Other presenting symptoms include focal deficits, such as hemiparesis, decerebration, and seizures. Early seizures are noted in 8% of pediatric patients presenting with EDH.

EDHs in the posterior fossa are a rare finding, accounting for approximately 5% of all posttraumatic intracranial mass lesions. These EDHs are particularly challenging to manage because these patients may remain conscious until late in the evolution of the hematoma, when they may suddenly lose consciousness, become apneic, and respiratory arrest [7].

Surgical Indications [10]
- An epidural hematoma (EDH) greater than 30 cm^3 should be surgically evacuated regardless of the patient's Glasgow Coma Scale (GCS) score.
- An EDH less than 30 cm^3 *and* with less than a 15-mm thickness *and* with less than a 5-mm midline shift (MLS) in patients with a GCS score greater than 8 *without* focal deficit can be managed non-operatively with serial

computed tomographic (CT) scanning and close neurological observation in a neurosurgical center.

A large frontotemporoparietal craniotomy provides the best access for surgical management of EDH. However, with improved preoperative localization by CT and earlier detection of smaller EDHs, it is possible to perform a more targeted craniotomy through a limited "slash" incision for evacuation of EDHs.

If neurological deterioration has been rapid or herniation is present, an initial burr hole is placed over the thickest part of the clot as seen on CT, and the clot is promptly removed to reduce ICP.

After evacuation of the extradural hematoma, if the underlying dura becomes tense, a limited opening should be made in the dura, and any hematoma is removed with gentle suction and irrigation [11].

There remain significant variations in the application of craniotomy versus craniectomy for the treatment of traumatic mass lesions. The decision is dependent on preoperative radiographic findings, intraoperative assessment of cerebral edema, and surgeon preferences.

Prognosis
The mortality in patients in all age groups and GCS scores undergoing surgery for evacuation of EDH is approximately 10%. Mortality in comparable pediatric case series is approximately 5% [10].

Acute SDH [7, 11, 12]
Pathogenesis
The incidence of acute SDH is between 12% and 29% in patients admitted with severe TBI. Most SDH are caused by TAs, falls, and assaults [12]. SDHs are located between the dura and arachnoid layer and may result from arterial or venous hemorrhage. Classically, SDHs are caused by tearing of bridging veins that span the subdural space to drain cortical blood directly into dural sinuses. However, many SDHs result from bleeding from other structures adjacent to the subdural space, such as superficial cortical vessels.

Most acute SDHs result from venous vascular injury at the brain surface, resulting in two distinct pathologies. The first type of hematoma, produced by contact forces and associated with contusions or lacerations, results from cortical bleeding into the adjacent subdural space and is most common at the temporal pole. This complex of SDH and damaged and necrotic brain is termed *burst lobe*. The second type of SDH is located over the cerebral convexity and is produced by inertial forces that tear bridging veins. The underlying brain damage in this type of injury is usually milder and primarily caused by local ischemia from mass effect or compromised venous outflow. Rapid deterioration, as in the case of classic EDH, may accompany these lesions, especially if cortical arteries are ruptured [7].

Clinical Presentation
Between 37% and 80% of patients with acute SDH present with initial GCS scores of 8 or less. A lucid interval has been described in 12 to 38% of patients before admission. The pupillary abnormalities are observed in 30–50% of patients on admission or before surgery [12] (Fig. 3.4).

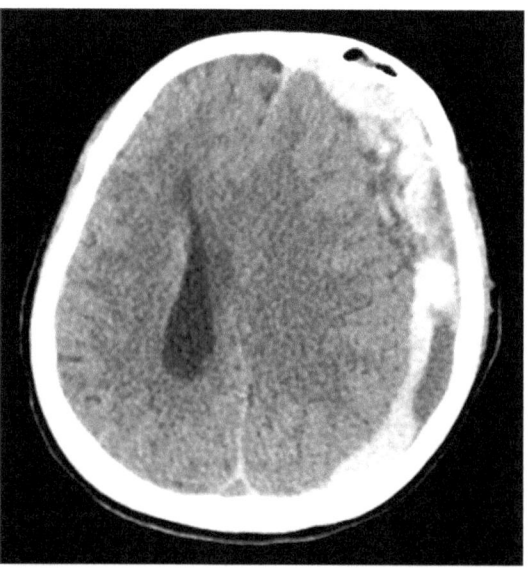

Fig. 3.4 Brain CT scan of acute subdural hematoma. Large crescentic shape high-density lesion covers left frontotemporoparietal convexity. Lateral ventricle is compressed and midline shifting is existed due to mass effect of hematoma

Surgical Indications [12]

- An acute subdural hematoma (SDH) with a thickness greater than 10 mm *or* a midline shift greater than 5 mm on computed tomographic (CT) scan should be surgically evacuated, regardless of the patient's Glasgow Coma Scale (GCS) score.
- All patients with acute SDH in coma (GCS score less than 9) should undergo intracranial pressure (ICP) monitoring.
- A comatose patient (GCS score less than 9) with an SDH less than 10-mm thick and a midline shift less than 5 mm should undergo surgical evacuation of the lesion if the GCS score decreased between the time of injury and hospital admission by 2 or more points on the GCS and/or the patient presents with asymmetric or fixed and dilated pupils and/or the ICP exceeds 20 mm Hg.

The most commonly used surgical techniques are:

- Burr hole trephination
- Craniotomy with or without dural grafting
- Large decompressive hemicraniectomy, with or without dural grafting

The choice of operative technique is influenced by the surgeon's expertise, training, and evaluation of the particular situation. Some centers treat all SDH with decompressive craniectomies, whereas other centers used solely osteoplastic craniotomies.

Prognosis

The prognosis of SDH is still poor in many cases. It is thought that the coexisting brain damage (DAI, contusion, laceration) is responsible for poor neurological function after injury. In some patients, compression of the microcirculation and resultant low CBF may explain the poor clinical condition and outcome. All age groups with GCS scores between 3 and 15 with SDH requiring surgery quote mortality rates between 40% and 60%. Mortality among patients presenting to the hospital in coma with subsequent surgical evacuation is between 57% and 68% [12].

Comparisons of EDH vs SDH

	Acute EDH	Acute SDH
Cause	Injury of middle meningeal artery/vein, diploic veins, venous sinuses	Injury of bridging veins, dural sinuses, cortical laceration, cortical vessels
Mechanism	Contact forces	Contact forces Inertial loading
Computed tomography findings	Biconvex (lens-shape) shape	Crescentic shape
Lucid interval	47%	12 to 38%
Surgery	Craniotomy or craniectomy	Craniotomy or craniectomy
Mortality	10%	40 to 60%

3.2.1.4 Traumatic Parenchymal Lesions

Pathogenesis

Brain contusions represent focal regions of subpial hemorrhage and swelling. Contusions are most common in regions that contact bony surfaces in the cranial vault during trauma: frontal and temporal poles, orbitofrontal gyri, and inferolateral temporal lobe surfaces.

Contusions can be characterized by mechanism, anatomic location, or adjacent injuries. For example, *fracture contusions* result from direct contact injuries and occur immediately adjacent to a skull fracture. *Coup contusions* refer to those that occur at the site of impact in the absence of a fracture, whereas *contrecoup contusions* are those that are diametrically opposite to the point of impact. *Gliding contusions* are focal hemorrhages involving the cortex and adjacent white matter of the superior margins of the cerebral hemispheres; they are caused by rotational mechanisms rather than contact forces. *Intermediary contusions* are lesions that affect deep brain structures, such as the corpus callosum, basal ganglia, hypothalamus, and brainstem [7].

Contusions can cause significant mass effect owing to surrounding edema or hemorrhagic progression to an intracerebral hematoma. Contusions also represent a significant source of secondary injury to adjacent tissue via release of neurotransmitter and local biochemical changes.

Contusions are more severe when associated with a skull fracture, less severe in patients with DAI, and more severe in patients who do not experience a lucid interval.

Intracerebral hematomas (ICH) account for 20–30% of all traumatic intracranial hematomas. ICHs are associated with extensive lobar contusions, from which are often difficult to distinguish. Generally, an ICH is a parenchymal lesion composed of at least two thirds blood. Multiple ICHs are found in approximately 20% of TBI patients. ICHs often arise from cerebral contusions. As a result, most traumatic ICHs occur in the orbitofrontal and temporal lobes, as do most cerebral contusions. Deeper ICHs, such as those occurring in the basal ganglia and internal capsule, are less common and found in approximately 2% of TBI patients [7].

Patients on chronic anticoagulation therapy are at increased risk of developing ICH, even after mild head injury.

ICHs have been shown to evolve over time. The entity of delayed-traumatic ICH (DTICH) is a lesion of increased attenuation developing after admission to hospital, in a part of the brain which the admission CT scan had suggested was normal [13].

The incidence of DTICH ranges from 3.3% to 7.4% in patients with moderate to severe TBI. Evacuated DTICH represent approximately 1.6% of all evacuated traumatic ICH, and mortality ranges from 16 to 72%. Therefore, the importance of careful monitoring and of serial CT scanning cannot be overemphasized. Approximately 70% of clinically significant DTICH presented within 48 h of injury [14] (Fig. 3.5).

Surgical Indications [14]

- Patients with parenchymal mass lesions and signs of progressive neurological deterioration referable to the lesion, medically refractory intracranial hypertension, or signs of mass effect on computed tomographic (CT) scan should be treated operatively.

- Patients with Glasgow Coma Scale (GCS) scores of 6 to 8 with frontal or temporal contusions greater than 20 cm^3 in volume with midline shift of at least 5 mm and/or cisternal compression on CT scan and patients with any lesion greater than 50 cm^3 in volume should be treated operatively.

- Patients with parenchymal mass lesions who do not show evidence for neurological compromise,

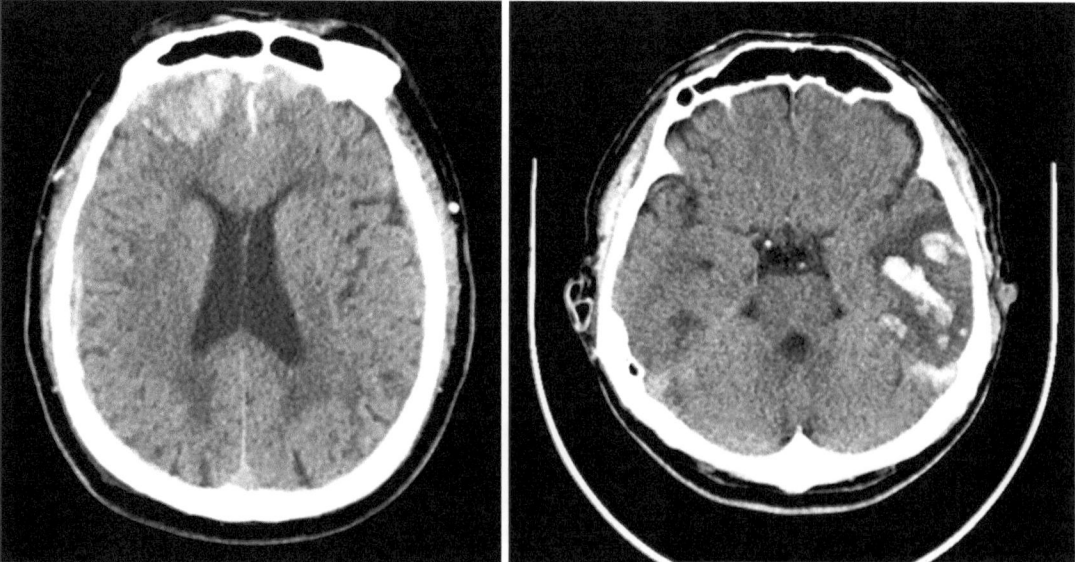

Fig. 3.5 Brain contusion. High-density parenchymal lesion on the frontal and temporal lobe. Contusion frequently occurred on the frontal pole and temporal pole because of direct bony contact of brain parenchyma

have controlled intracranial pressure (ICP), and no significant signs of mass effect on CT scan may be managed non-operatively with intensive monitoring and serial imaging.

Surgical Methods [14]

The standard surgical treatment of focal lesions, such as intracerebral hemorrhages or contusions, is craniotomy with evacuation of the lesion.

Evacuation of traumatic mass lesions is often effective in amelioration of brain shift and reduction of ICP and can decrease the requirement for intensive medical treatment.

Other methods, such as stereotactic evacuation of focal mass lesions, have also been used, although much less commonly. These procedures, however, become less effective when the patient's intracranial pathology is diffuse and involves intracranial hypertension as a result of posttraumatic edema or hemispheric swelling.

Outcome

The outcomes of traumatic intraparenchymal lesion are varied. 40–57% of patients those who treated for traumatic ICH showed good outcome or functional independence [15, 16].

3.2.1.5 Skull Fracture

The presence of a skull fracture is associated with a higher incidence of intracranial lesions, neurological deficit, and poorer outcome. Skull fractures are indicators of clinically significant injuries, as well as the importance of CT scans in evaluation of all patients with known or clinically suspected cranial fractures.

Simple Linear Fracture

Linear skull fracture is commonly diagnosed by plain skull radiographs. If patients are indicated, brain CT scan should be done to exclude other intracranial pathology. Most of linear skull fracture do not need any treatment. It is important to distinguish from cranial suture lines or vessel grooves (Fig. 3.6 and Table 3.3).

Depressed Cranial Fractures

Simple Depressed Skull Fractures

There is no difference in outcome (seizures, neurologic deficits, or cosmetic appearance) in surgical and nonsurgical management. In young age, skull bony remodeling can make the deformity smoothly.

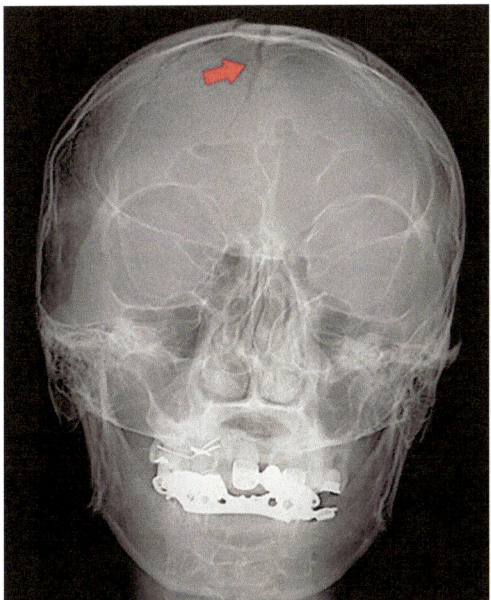
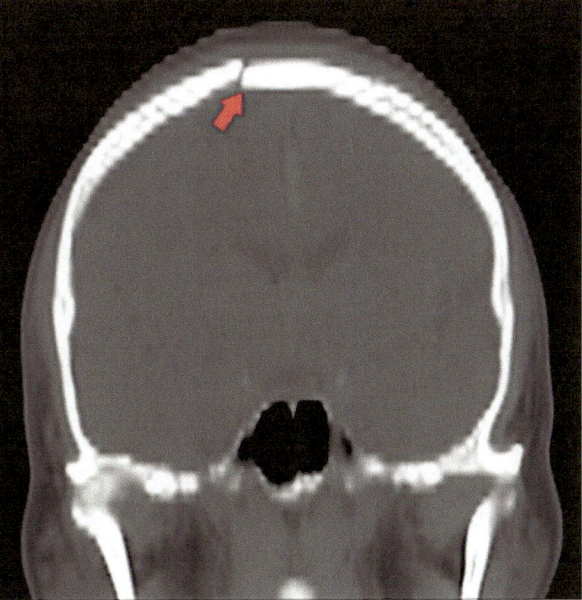

Fig. 3.6 Linear skull fracture. Linear fracture lines in simple skull X-ray and CT scan

Table 3.3 Differential diagnosis point of linear skull fracture

Feature	Linear skull fracture	Vessel groove	Suture line
Density	Dark black	Gray	Gray
Course	Straight	Curving	Follows course of known suture lines
Branching	Usually none	Often branching	Joins other suture lines
Width	Very thin	Thicker than fracture	Jagged, wide

Mark. S. Greenberg, *Handbook of Neurosurgery*, 7th editions

Surgical management is needed when extent of depression is greater than the full thickness of the adjacent calvarium, with the benefits of better cosmesis, a diminution in late-onset posttraumatic epilepsy, and a reduction in the incidence of persistent neurological deficit [17].

Compound Comminuted Depressed Skull Fractures (FCCD)

Depressed cranial fractures (Fig. 3.7) may complicate up to 6% of head injuries and account for significant morbidity and mortality. FCCDs account for up to 90% of these injuries and are associated with an infection rate of 1.9–10.6%, an average neurological morbidity of approximately 11%, an incidence of late epilepsy of up to 15%, and a mortality rate of 1.4–19% [18].

Traditionally, FCCDs are treated surgically, with debridement and elevation, primarily to attempt to decrease the incidence of infection. Closed ("simple") depressed cranial fractures undergo operative repair if the depressed bone fragments violate into the brain parenchyma.

Treatment
Surgical Indication [18]
- Patients with open (compound) cranial fractures depressed greater than the thickness of the cranium should undergo operative intervention to prevent infection.
- Patients with open (compound) depressed cranial fractures may be treated non-operatively if there is no clinical or radiographic evidence of dural penetration, significant intracranial hematoma, depression greater than 1 cm, frontal sinus involvement, gross

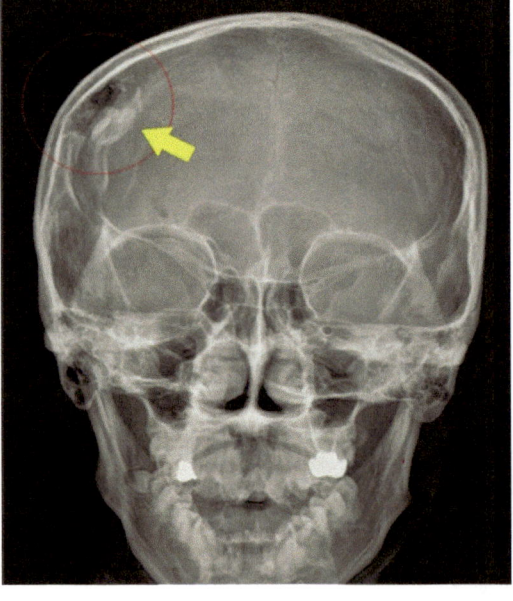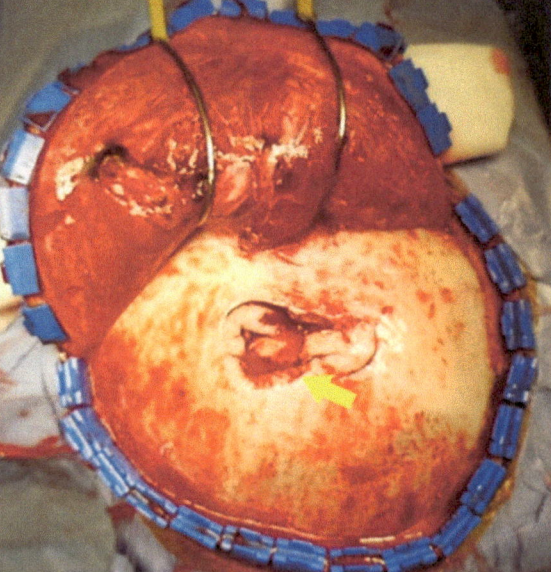

Fig. 3.7 FCCD. Compound skull fractures in simple skull X-ray and intraoperative pictures

cosmetic deformity, wound infection, pneumocephalus, or gross wound contamination.

- Non-operative management of closed (simple) depressed cranial fractures is a treatment option.

The recommended surgical method is "elevation and debridement." Primary bone flap replacement is a good surgical option in the absence of wound infection. In highly suspicious wound infection, staged surgery of cranioplasty is recommended. In every treatment of FCCD patients, antibiotics should be included [11, 17–19] (Figs. 3.8 and 3.9).

Basal Skull Fracture (BSF)

Most BSF are extensions of fractures through the cranial vault. 6–12% of adult patients with head injuries have a skull fracture, with 20% of skull fractures involving the skull base.

The common causes of BSF are TA, falls, and industrial accidents. BSF more frequently occur in young age group and male. The risk of CSF leak after a BSF is 10–30% for adult patients [20].

The symptoms or signs of basal skull fractures include:

1. CSF rhinorrhea
2. CSF otorrhea, hemotympanum, or laceration of external auditory canal
3. Raccoon's eye sign (periorbital ecchymoses) or Battle's sign (postauricular ecchymoses)
4. Cranial nerve injury (facial nerve, vestibulocochlear nerve, temporal bone fracture; olfactory nerve, cribriform plate fracture; abducens nerve, clival fracture).

Treatment

Most of BSF do not require specific treatment. However, combined trauma-related lesions such as pseudoaneurysm, carotid-cavernous fistula, or persistent CSF fistula may require specific treatment (Table 3.4).

Temporal bone fracture

	Longitudinal fracture	Transverse fracture
Incidence	More common	Less common
Relationship of direction with EAC	Parallel	Perpendicular
Ossicular chain	Often disrupt	Less disrupt
Cranial nerve VII, VIII	More spare	Less spare

3.2.2 Secondary Brain Injury: Brain Swelling and Herniation

3.2.2.1 Herniation Syndrome
(Table 3.5)

Uncal Herniation

Uncal herniation is caused by mass lesions in the middle fossa or temporal lobe that displace the medial edge of the uncus and hippocampal gyrus medially over the ipsilateral edge of the tentorium cerebelli.

This results in compression of the midbrain, ipsilateral cerebral peduncle, and oculomotor nerve and leads to contralateral hemiparesis, ipsilateral pupillary dilation, and decreased level of consciousness.

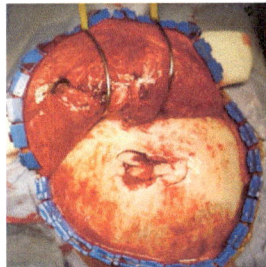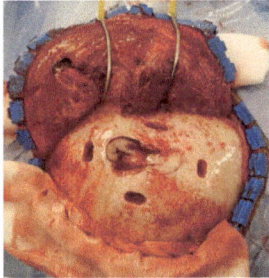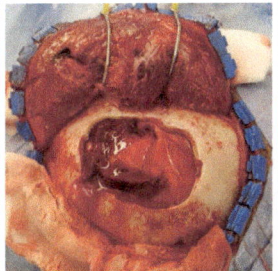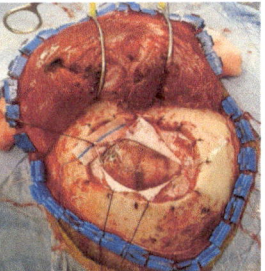

Fig. 3.8 Operative procedures for repair of FCCD

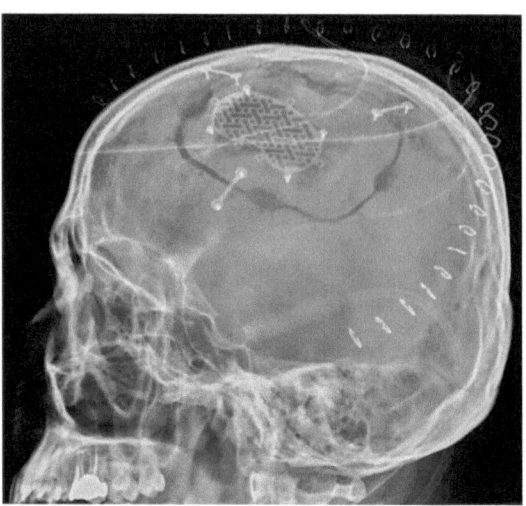

Fig. 3.9 Postoperative simple skull X-ray of reconstruction of FCCD

Sometimes, the herniation may cause stretching of the contralateral oculomotor nerve and compression of the contralateral cerebral peduncle against the tentorium, resulting in ipsilateral hemiparesis (Kernohan's notch phenomenon). Pupillary asymmetry after TBI is often an indicator of neurological deterioration that should prompt immediate therapeutic intervention.

Tonsillar Herniation

Herniation of the cerebral tonsils through the foramen magnum may occur with either supratentorial or infratentorial. This herniation causes obliteration of the cisterna magna and compression of the medulla oblongata, the latter resulting in sudden apnea or respiratory arrest.

Subfalcine Herniation

Lesions in the anterior or middle fossa may result in herniation of the cingulate gyrus under the free edge of the falx cerebri. Pericallosal arteries can be compressed, resulting in unilateral or bilateral frontal cerebral infarctions; it may result in lower extremity monoparesis or paraparesis.

Table 3.4 Treatment options for traumatic intracranial hemorrhage

Condition	Management
Subdural hematoma	
>10 mm thick and >5 mm midline shift	Surgical evacuation
<10 mm thick and <5 mm midline shift, *and* GCS score <9 with ≥2 point decrease, *and/or* pupillary dysfunction, *and/or* ICP >20 mm Hg	Surgical evacuation
GCS score <9	ICP monitoring
Epidural hematoma	
>30 mL volume, regardless of GCS score	Surgical evacuation
<30 mL volume, *and* <15 mm thickness, *and* <5 mm midline shift, *and* GCS score >8 without focal neurological deficit	Conservative management with intensive monitoring and serial imaging
Intrafarenchymal hematoma	
Progressive neurological deterioration referable to lesion, medically refractory intracranial hypertension, or mass effect on CT	Surgical evacuation
Any lesion >50 mL	Surgical evacuation
Frontal or temporal contusions >20 mL, *and* GCS score = 6–8, *and* ≥5 mm midline shift, *and/or* cisternal compression on CT	Surgical evacuation
No evidence of neurological compromise, *and* controlled ICP, *and* no significant signs of mass effect on CT	Conservative management with intensive monitoring and serial imaging

Huang [11]
CT computed tomography, *GCS* Glasgow Coma Scale, *ICP* intracranial pressure

Central Herniation

Central herniation is defined as a downward shift of the brainstem toward the foramen magnum. This can result in brainstem ischemia and hemorrhage, the latter occasionally resulting from reversal of the displacement by operative decompression. Clinically, central herniation results in impaired consciousness and a Cushing response

Table 3.5 Herniation syndromes

Type of herniation	Associated structures	Symptoms or signs
Uncal herniation	Oculomotor nerve Cerebral peduncle Posterior cerebral artery	Ptosis, ipsilateral mydriasis Contralateral hemiparesis Decreased consciousness
Tonsillar herniation	Medulla	Sudden apnea, respiratory arrest
Subfalcine herniation	Cingulate gyrus Pericallosal arteries	Leg weakness
Central herniation	Basilar perforating branches Brainstem (midbrain, pons, medulla) Reticular formation	Depressed consciousness Apnea, respiratory irregularity Hypertension, bradycardia

Shahlaie et al. [7]

to brainstem ischemia (arterial hypertension, bradycardia, and respiratory irregularity).

References

1. McCrea MA, Nelson LD, Guskiewicz K. Diagnosis and management of acute concussion. Phys Med Rehabil Clin N Am. 2017;28:271–86.
2. Barkhoudarian G, Hovda DA, Giza CC. The molecular pathophysiology of concussive brain injury-an update. Phys Med Rehabil Clin N Am. 2016;27(2):373–93.
3. Prins ML, Hales A, Reger M, Giza CC, Hovda DA. Repeat traumatic brain injury in the juvenile rat is associated with increased axonal injury and cognitive impairments. Dev Neurosci. 2010;32:510–8.
4. Vagnozzi R, Tavazzi B, Signoretti S, Amorini AM, Belli A, Climatti M, et al. Temporal window of metabolic brain vulnerability to concussions: mitochondrial-related impairment-part I. Neurosurgery. 2007;61:379–89.
5. Harmon KG, Drezner JA, Gammons M, Guskiewicz KM, Halstead M, Herring SA, et al. American Medical Society for Sports Medicine position statement: concussion in sport. Br J Sports Med. 2013;47:15–26.
6. Su E, Bell M. Diffuse axonal injury. In: Laskowitz D, Grant G, editors. Translational research in traumatic brain injury. Boca Raton: Taylor and Francis Group, LLC; 2016.
7. Shahlaie K, Zwienenberg-Lee M, Muizelaar JP. Clinical pathophysiology of traumatic brain injury. In: Winn HR, editor. Youmans and Winn neurological surgery, vol. 4. 7th ed: New York:Elsevier; 2016.
8. Adams HU, Mitchell DE, Graham DI, Doyle DA. Diffuse brain damage of immediate impact type. Its relationship to 'primary brain stem damage' in head injury. Brain. 1977;100(3):489–502.
9. Li X-Y, Feng D-F. Diffuse axonal injury: novel insights into detection and treatment. J Clin Neurosci. 2009;16:614–9.
10. Bullock MR, Chesnut R, Ghajar J, Gordon D, Hartl R, Newell DW, et al. Surgical management of acute epidural hematomas. Neurosurgery. 2006;58(3):7–15.
11. Huang MC. Surgical management of traumatic brain injury. In: Winn HR, editor. Youmans and Winn neurological surgery. 7th ed: New York:Elsevier; 2016.
12. Bullock MR, Chesnut R, Ghajar J, Gordon D, Hartl R, Newell DW, et al. Surgical management of acute subdural hematomas. Neurosurgery. 2006;58(3):16–24.
13. Gentleman D, Nath F, Macpherson P. Diagnosis and management of delayed traumatic intracerebral haematomas. Br J Neurosurg. 1989;3:367–72.
14. Bullock MR, Chesnut R, Ghajar J, Gordon D, Hartl R, Newell DW, et al. Surgical management of traumatic parenchymal lesions. Neurosurgery. 2006;58(3):25–46.
15. Kunze E, Meixensberger J, Janka M, Sörensen N, Roosen K. Decompressive craniectomy in patients with uncontrollable intracranial hypertension. Acta Neurochir (Wien). 1998;71:16–8.
16. Nussbaum ES, Wolf AL, Sebring L, Mirvis S. Complete temporal lobectomy for surgical resuscitation of patients with transtentorial herniation secondary to unilateral hemispheric swelling. Neurosurgery. 1991;29:62–6.
17. Greenberg MS. Head trauma. In: Greenberg MS, editor. Handbook of neurosurgery. 7th ed. New york: Thieme; 2010.
18. Bullock MR, Chesnut R, Ghajar J, Gordon D, Hartl R, Newell DW, et al. Surgical management of depressed cranial fractures. Neurosurgery. 2006;58:56–60.
19. AbdelRahman MAF. Management of bone fragments in nonmissile compound depressed skull fractures. Acta Neurochir. 2016;158:2341–5.
20. Phang SY, Whitehouse K, Lee L, Khalil H, McArdle P, Whitfield P. Management of CSF leak in base of skull fractures in adults. Br J Neurosurg. 2016;30(6):596–604.

Spinal Injury

Sang Ryong Jeon and Jin Hoon Park

Fig. 4.1
Multidisciplinary
approach to multiple
traumatic patient

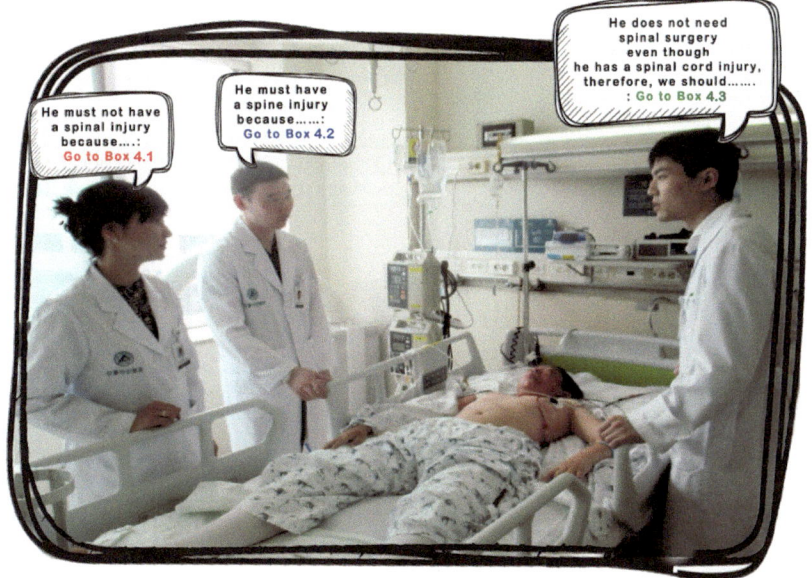

Box 4.1 When Polytrauma Patient Is Alert Without Neurologic Deficit and Shows the Findings from ① to ③, We Can Speculate the Patient Has No Spinal Injury (Fig. 4.1)

① No pain in motion and no tenderness
② No painful distracting injury
③ No pain in motion, no tenderness even without neck color or brace

S. R. Jeon (✉) · J. H. Park
Department of Neurological Surgery, ASAN Medical
Center, University of Ulsan College of Medicine,
Seoul, South Korea
e-mail: srjeon@amc.seoul.kr; jhpark@amc.seoul.kr

© Springer Nature Singapore Pte Ltd. 2019
S.-K. Hong et al. (eds.), *Primary Management of Polytrauma*,
https://doi.org/10.1007/978-981-10-5529-4_4

However, if the patient shows pain in motion or tenderness after the removal of a brace, start immobilization again and study further. A flow diagram is in Fig. 4.2a.

NEXUS *(National Emergency X-Radiography Utilization Study) criteria to assess spinal clearance* [1]:

- No posterior midline cervical spine tenderness.
- No evidence of intoxication.
- A normal level alertness.
- No focal neurologic deficit.
- No painful distracting injury.
- If patients meet all the listed criteria, then cervical radiography is not necessary.

Fig. 4.2 (**a**) Radiological diagnostic algorithm in alert multi-traumatic patients. (**b**) Radiological diagnostic algorithm in multi-traumatic patients with altered consciousness

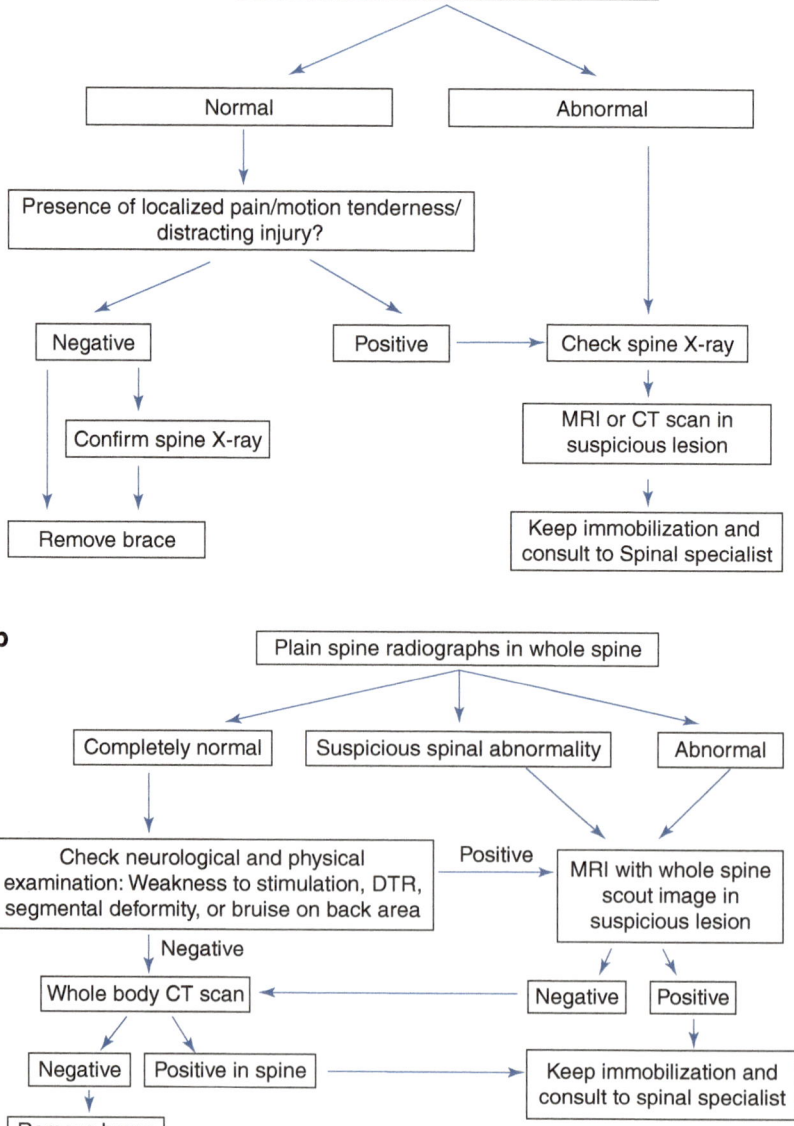

Box 4.2 We Should Expect Spinal Injury When the Patient Shows the Findings from ①, ②, ③ or ④ (Fig. 4.1)

① Alert with neurological deficit or pain on spinal area
② Poor conscious and abnormal X-ray findings
③ Poor conscious and increased DTR, suspicious weakness responding to painful stimulation
④ Poor conscious and trauma in back or neck

Even though the poor conscious patient does not show definite abnormal neurological change or abnormal X-ray findings, we should be more careful, because the assessment of the spinal injury might be more difficult. Therefore, we should manage this patient under the suspicion of spinal injury until we excluded a spinal injury from the final diagnosis.

In alert patient with suspicious spinal injury, management should be followed as given below:

Start immobilization
⇒ Check subluxation in simple spine X-ray.
⇒ Further study with CT and /or MRI.
In all poor consciousness patients:
Check X-ray in whole spine and CT evaluation in suspicious area:
Neurological examination is most important key to rule out spinal injury.
A flow diagram is in Fig. 4.2b.

Box 4.3 Medical Management in Acute Cervical SCI [2] (Fig. 4.1)

① Use of cardiac, hemodynamic, and respiratory monitoring device should be recommended, because life-threatening cardiovascular or respiratory insufficiency may occur or be recurrent.
② Correction of hypotension in SCI: keep systolic BP over 90 mmHg, ASAP.
③ Maintain mean arterial blood pressure between 85 and 90 mmHg for the first 7 days.

In multiple injury patients, we have to suspect combined spinal injury. When we met spinal injury first, we also have to suspect combined other sites spinal injury. We should consider that spinal cord injury would be accompanied by the 5–10% of traumatic brain injury, 10–30% of multiple traumas, and up to 30% of abdominal and thoracic trauma. In this reason, we should keep in mind the possibility of spinal injury should be excluded through the multidisciplinary discussion when we met a polytrauma patient.

Case Scenario: Patient 1

A 33-year-old male patient visited the emergency center with driver traffic accident without consciousness before 1 hour. His face showed multiple abrasion and laceration. His right knee was lacerated, and the tendon around the knee was exposed. An abnormal eyeball deviation was absent, and light reflexes in both pupils were normal. Several bruises in abdomen and chest were seen, and vital sign was unstable. Although there was no abnormal neurological deficit such as an increased DTR and localized weakness, multiple and severe facial lacerations surrounding the neck gave us a suspicion that the patient might have encountered a high-energy extension or flexion force to the cervical spine during the accident.

In addition, degloving injury of knee also gave us a suspicion of combined high-energy seat belt injury at the T-L spine (Fig. 4.3).

Because there were hypotension (90/50 mmHg) and tachycardia (92 pulses/minutes) indicating hypovolemic shock, volume replacement was done after achieving intravascular access.

Because of the possibility of spinal injury, a neck brace was kept, and he was transferred carefully using a hardback board for radiological examination. Although there was no abnormality in brain computed tomography (CT), there was liver and spleen laceration on abdominal CT. In addition to the combined ankle and hand fracture, there was C2 spinal burst fracture with kyphotic angulation (Fig. 4.4) on the plain radiography and CT scan.

After emergent abdominal surgery including splenectomy and bleeding control of lacerated liver, the vital sign became stable, and patient' consciousness showed clearance without any extremity weakness. After identifying a cervical magnetic resonance image (MRI) showing no cord compression, cervical spinal (C2-3) posterior fusion surgery for stabilization was done followed by hand and ankle surgery at the same day. There was no sequela after all treatments above (Fig. 4.5).

Fig. 4.3 Multiple injury patient

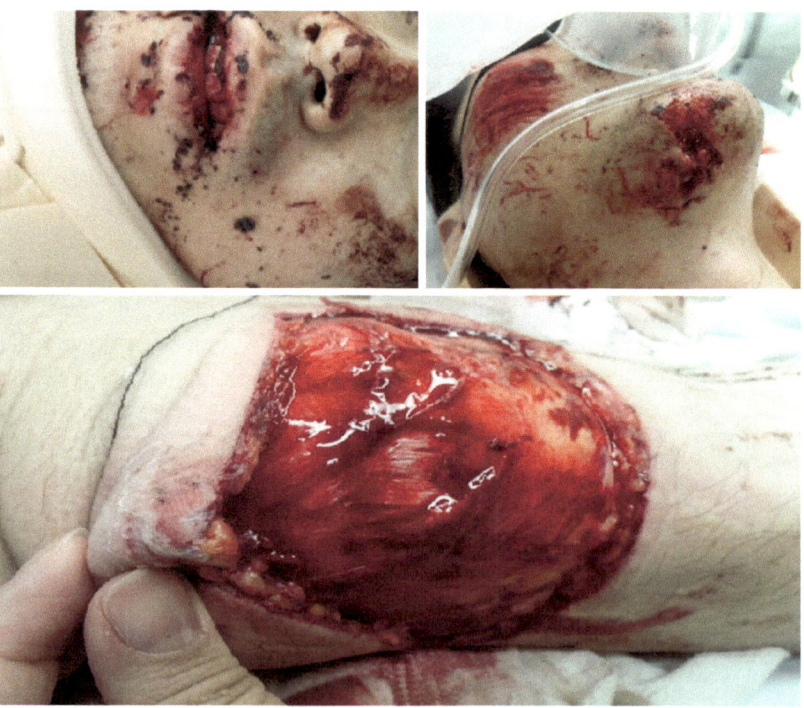

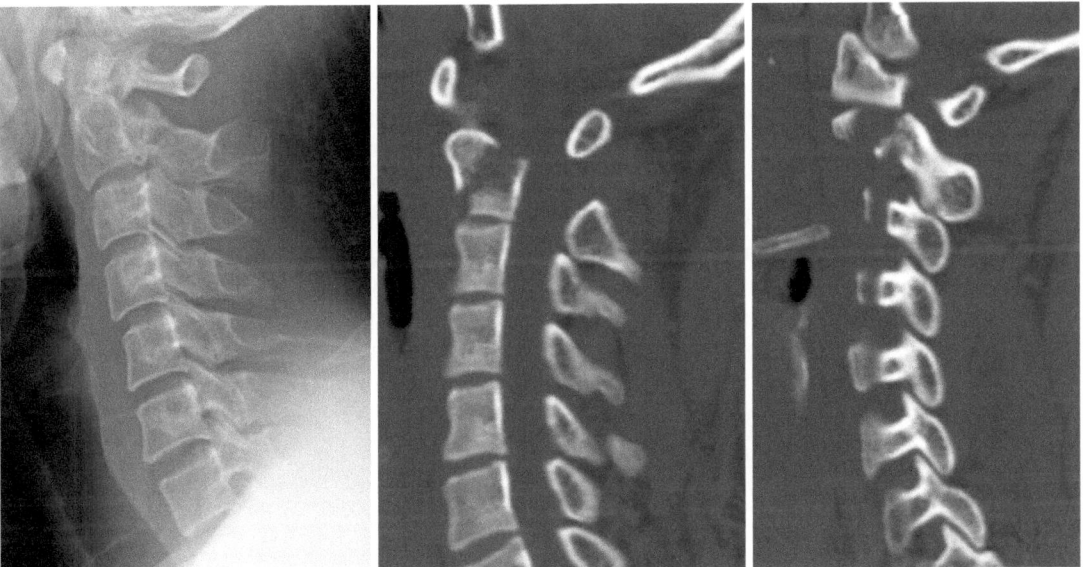

Fig. 4.4 CT scan of multiple injury patient

Fig. 4.5 X-ray after surgical reduction and stabilization of spinal fracture

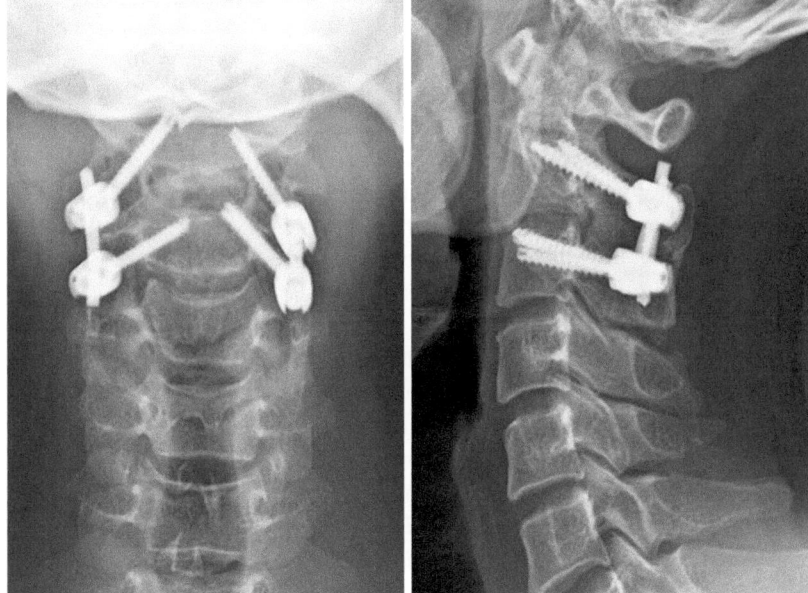

4.1 Approach to Spine in Multiple Traumas

Spinal injuries are reported in up to 46% among patients experiencing major trauma. This spinal injury means trauma-related spinal anatomical abnormality with or without spinal cord injury. These include spinal bone fracture, dislocation, disc injury, paraspinal ligament, or muscle injury. When we first met the polytraumatic patient in the emergency setting, the possibility of spinal injury should be considered. Undetected spinal injury may result in serious neurologic disability or paresis of extremities. Trauma including motor vehicle collisions or falls may be primary cause of spinal cord injury (SCI), but spinal injury without neurological deficit may deteriorate into SCI during transfer or position change [3]. Although the cervical spine has been reported prone to injury and highly associated with neurological deficit after high-energy trauma, failure to diagnose cervical spine injuries occurs with a frequency of 5–20%, and this is similar in the thoracic or lumbar spine.

Thus, the immobilized transfer of this multi-traumatic patient is as important as securing the airway and vascular access from the first scene. Neutral spine position during transport by using a rigid cervical collar, sandbags on either side of the head, and rigid backboard with straps should be maintained. The pads or inflatable beanbag boards can be utilized to reduce pressure on the occiput and sacrum [4].

After safe transfer of the multi-traumatic patient to the emergency medical center, the role of first physician is important for a correct clinical and radiological assessment. After identifying secure airway and vascular access, physical and neurological examination should be done following imaging studies. A spinal imaging process for the multi-traumatic patient in the emergency center can be recommended as given in Fig. 4.2 [5].

In conclusion, the top priority problem among multiple traumas in one patient should be decided according to the vital sign, the progression of physical and neurological deterioration, and all kinds of organ dysfunction or destruction amount including spinal instability assessment which is the most important criteria necessary for spinal reconstruction surgery. Because described patient 1 showed stable neurological sign despite of an evidence of instability (i.e., more than kyphosis 10 degree), we decided intraperitoneal bleeding control to achieve the stable vital sign as first priority followed by delayed spinal surgery. However, excessive motion of cervical spine should be avoided to prevent neurological deterioration during prior surgery.

In an emergency room without spine specialist, transportation to level 1 trauma center (definitive spine care center) should occur within 24 h of injury. It is associated with patient's outcomes.

Summary
1. The immobilized transfer of this multi-traumatic patient is as important as securing the airway and vascular access from the first scene.
2. The different radiological assessments should be considered according to the presence of consciousness when we first met the multi-traumatic patient.
3. The top priority problem among multiple traumas in one patient should be decided according to the vital sign, the progression of physical and neurological deterioration, and all kinds of organ dysfunction or destruction amount including spinal instability assessment.

4.2 The Neurological Evaluation of Acute Spinal Cord Injury

A standardized examination for spinal cord injury (SCI) is conducted according to the methods described in the *International Standards for Neurological Classification of Spinal Cord Injury* [6], which is the gold standard for classification of SCI. The neurological assessment for traumatic SCI involves three parts: the sensory, motor, and sacral sparing examinations.

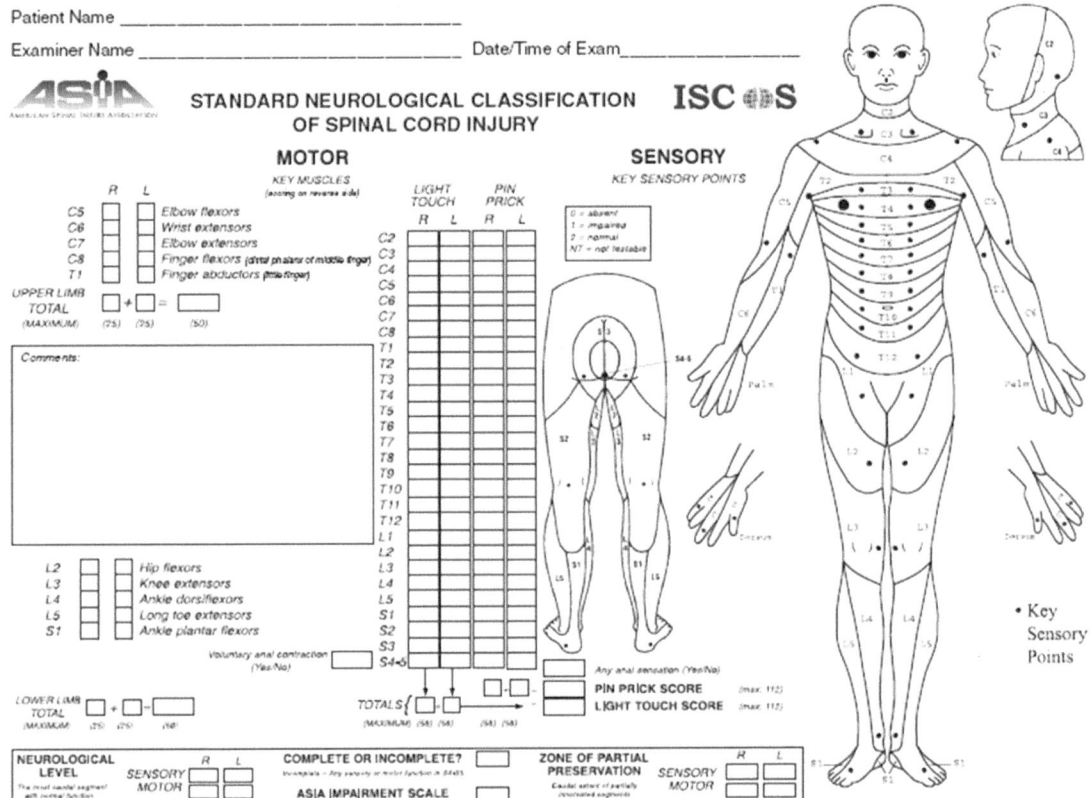

Fig. 4.6 American Spinal Injury Association scoring worksheet for the evaluation of spinal cord injury (From American Spinal Injury Association. Standard for neurological classification of spinal injured patient, IL: American Spinal Injury Association, 1982, Revised 2002)

As the worksheet suggested, a sensory function is assessed by testing light-touch and pinprick sensation for 28 dermatomes, graded on a 3-point scale, with 0 for absent, 1 for impaired, and 2 for normal. The motor examination involves manual strength testing of 5 key muscles in each extremity, graded on a 6-point scale from 0 to 5. Sacral sparing is assessed by the presence of any of the following: pinprick or light-touch sensation, deep anal sensation, and the ability to voluntarily contract the anal sphincter or the presence or absence of the bulbocavernosus reflexes [6].

The severity of injury is graded by the ASIA Impairment Scale (AIS), a 5-point ordinal scale from A to E. An AIS grade of A represents a complete injury, and grade E represents normal status. A complete injury is defined by the absence of motor and sensation without sacral sparing (Fig. 4.6 and Table 4.1).

Table 4.1 American Spinal Injury Association

Grade	
A	Complete. No sensory or motor function is preserved in the sacral segments S4-S5.
B	Incomplete. Sensory but not motor function is preserved below the neurological level and includes the sacral segments S4-5.
C	Incomplete. Motor function is preserved below the neurological level, and more than half of the key muscles below the neurological level have a muscle grade < 3 (grades 0–2).
D	Incomplete. Motor function is preserved below the neurological level, and at least half of the key muscles below the neurological level have a muscle grade ≥ 3.
E	Normal. Sensory and motor functions are normal.

Reference Manual for the International Standards for Neurological Classification of Spinal Cord Injury. Chicago: American Spinal Injury Association; 2003

4.3   Initial Management

4.3.1   Cardiovascular and Pulmonary Resuscitation

In vehicle crashes, falls, or sports-related injuries, all patients should be assumed to have an unstable spine until radiological proving. The possibility of an unstable spine must be considered as well as airway, breathing, and circulation when transferring the patient. Commonly, airway obstruction after trauma is caused by the tongue, blood, secretions, or foreign body. This airway can be managed using the chin lift and jaw-thrust technique and the removal of obstructed material. In a patient with decreased consciousness, an oropharyngeal or nasopharyngeal airway should be inserted gently. Use of fiber-optic laryngoscopes is associated with increased motion of the cervical spine compared to fiber-optic bronchoscopic intubation. The method "manual in-line stabilization" can be performed for intubation in the field with assistant paramedics: the head of the patient should always be supported by both hands or both knees on each side of the head to maintain adequate stabilization, from the side or from behind during intubation.

If a satisfactory airway or adequate ventilation cannot be achieved with the above methods, gentle endotracheal intubation is required. Care should be taken to avoid excessive movement and extension of neck. A video-assisted endotracheal or nasotracheal intubation can be helpful to avoid extension of the neck. Respiratory insufficiency should be suspected in all patients with cervical cord injuries. Hypoventilation with slow respiration can result from paralysis of the intercostal muscles and spinal shock. High cervical cord injury which may affect phrenic nerve (C3-5) dysfunction results in the paralysis of diaphragm as well as the intercostal muscles dysfunction. Thus the patients with respiratory dysfunction and quadriplegia or quadriparesis are the indication of early intubation. Hypoxia is an important cause of secondary SCI and must be avoided.

Assessment of circulation is equally important in the acute spinal cord injury because hypotension also highly contribute secondary SCI [7].

Although the cause of hypotension can be confused among hypovolemia, cardiac dysfunction, or decreased sympathetic tone in the traumatic setting, two types of shock deserve special consideration in the SCI condition. First, neurogenic shock caused by loss of sympathetic tone is typically seen with lesions above the T6-T8 spinal level and can be characterized by hypotension, hypothermia, and bradycardia. Second, spinal shock is characterized by loss of reflex, sensation, and motor function below injured level. Despite any cause of hypotension, intravascular volume expansion through the intravenous access should be considered for the initial management. Fluid resuscitation and vasoactive agent is generally recommended unless contraindicated. Although both α- and ß-adrenergic medications including dopamine, norepinephrine, and epinephrine are useful in SCI condition, phenylephrine should be avoided because of its exclusive α-adrenergic receptor activity and reflex bradycardia. It is recommended that mean arterial pressure should be maintained higher than 85 mm Hg for the initial 7 days after SCI as well as systolic blood pressure higher than 90 mm Hg [7, 8].

After securing airway, breathing, and circulation, spinal immobilization should be recommended. In cervical facet dislocation or malalignment seen in a radiographic image, Gardner-Wells tongs or Halo ring traction can be under consideration for rapid closed reduction. However, this traction should not be performed in a patient who is incorporative or unconscious [9]. Initial cervical traction in cervical fracture-dislocation is safe and effective. Reduction rate is 80%, but permanent neurological complication rate is only 1% and safer than manual reduction under anesthesia.

4.3.2   Pharmaceutical Agents

4.3.2.1 Steroids

For the treatment of traumatic SCI, high-dose corticosteroids have been widely used for decades. Their pharmacological mechanisms for neuroprotection are antioxidant properties, enhancement of spinal cord blood flow, reduced calcium influx, reduced axonal death, and attenuated lipid peroxidation. However, the efficacy of this treatment has been questioned currently, since three landmark National Acute Spinal Cord Injury Study (NASCIS) trials began [10]. Recently, steroid use for spinal cord injury is not recommended according to the AANS/CNS medical evidence-based guidelines on the management of acute cervical spine and spinal cord injuries [11].

4.3.2.2 The Other Agents

Many diverse clinical trials using a gangliosides, thyrotropin-releasing hormone, or gacyclidine, etc. were performed, previously. However, there has been no agent which gave us the definite evidence for clinical improvement to the spinal cord injured patient [12–14].

Skill I

Gardner-Wells tongs traction (Fig. 4.7)

Preparation: placed with patient supine on a bed. Option: shave hair around proposed pin sites. Betadine skin preparation, then infiltrate local anesthetic.

Pin sites: the pins are placed in the temporal ridge (above the temporalis muscle),

2–3 fingerbreadths (3–4 cm) above pinna. Place directly above external acoustic meatus for neutral position traction; 2–3 cm posterior for flexion (e.g., for locked facets); 2–3 cm anterior for extension. One pin has a central spring-loaded force indicator. Tighten pins until the indicator protrudes 1 mm beyond the flat surface. Retighten the pins daily until indicator protrudes 1 mm for 3 days only, then stop.

Initial weight in lbs. ≈ 3lbs*cervical vertebrae level, increase in 5–10 lbs increments usually at 10–15 minutes intervals until desired alignment is attained (as sees neurological examination and lateral X-ray after each △ to avoid over-distraction). Under most circumstances, do not exceed 10 lbs per vertebrae level (some say 5 lbs/level). Stop if occipito-cervical instability is demonstrated or if any disc space height exceeds 10 mm (over-distraction) or if any neurological deterioration. Once the facets are perched or distracted, gradual reduction of the weight will usually result in reduction. After reduction, maintenance weight should be kept at 10 lbs.

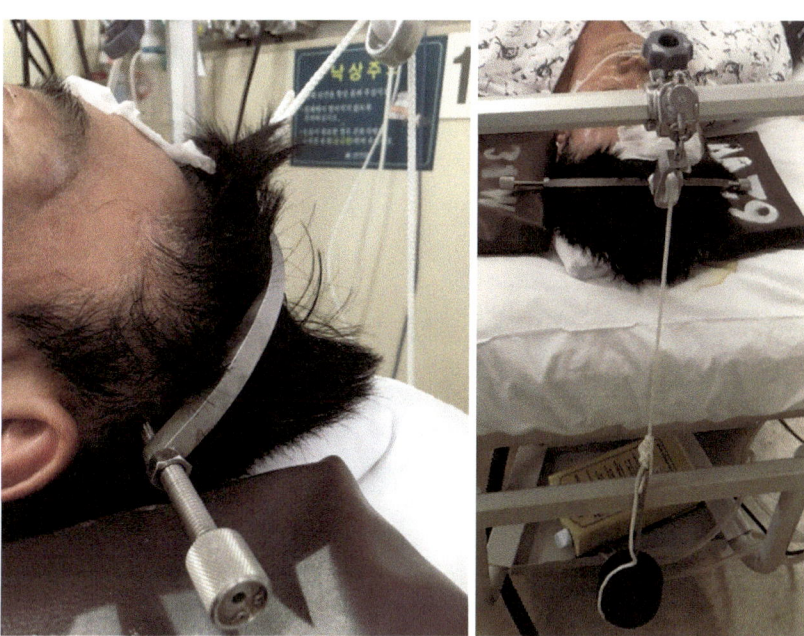

Fig. 4.7 Gardner-Wells tongs traction

Case Scenario: Patient 2

A 36-year-old male patient visited the emergency center after an industrial accident 12 hours before. His consciousness was alert but complained of severe back pain and paralysis of his lower extremities (Grade II, AIS C) as well as open fractures in both arms. Because his back abnormally bended forward showing deformation, he could not lay down flat. Although our imaging process recommended dynamic X-ray, CT, and MRI according to above image process guideline, only simple X-ray was possible due to abnormal position of this patient (Fig. 4.8).

After an emergency manual, closed reduction, was attempted to pull the shoulder and pelvis, dislocation was successfully reduced. CT scan showed L3 and L5 body burst fracture, widened right-side sacroiliac joint. MRI showed L2-3 and L5-S1 level disc injuries resulting in serious neural compression and interspinous ligament injuries at same levels (Fig. 4.9)

Emergency lumbosacral decompression and stabilization surgery following open fracture surgery of both arms were done. For the 2-year follow-up, this patient can ambulate without any assistance, but there was mild abnormal sensation on both legs (Fig. 4.10) (AISA D)

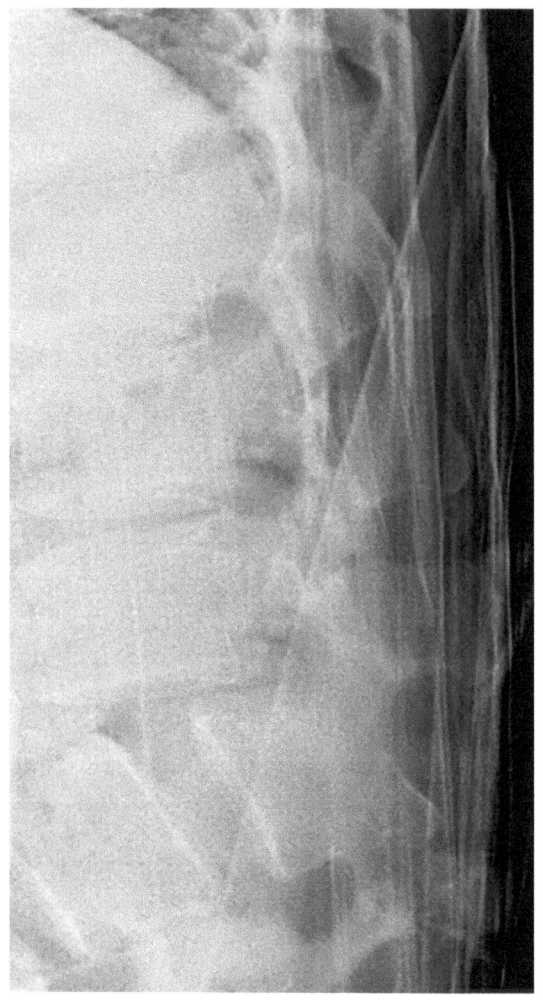

Fig. 4.8 X-ray of lumar spinal dislocation

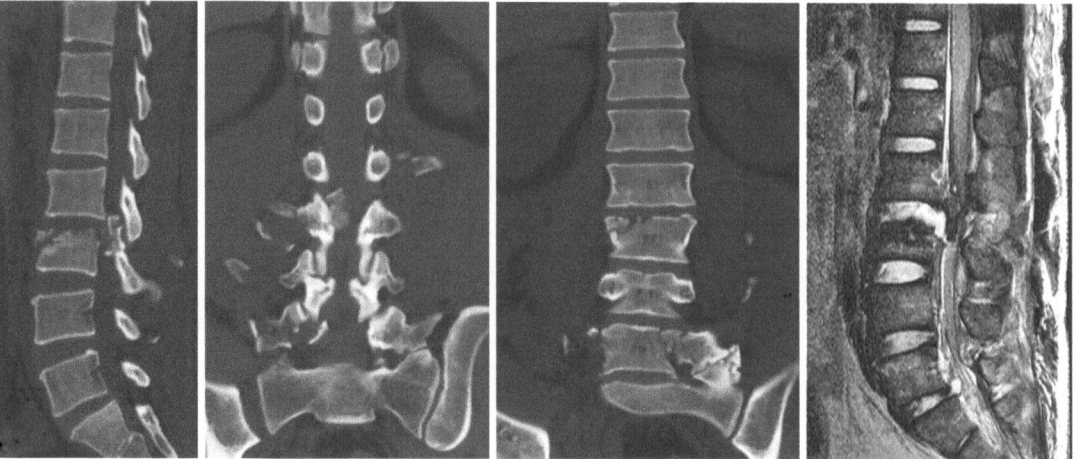

Fig. 4.9 CT scan and MRI of closed reduction

Fig. 4.10 Standing X-ray of surgical stabilization

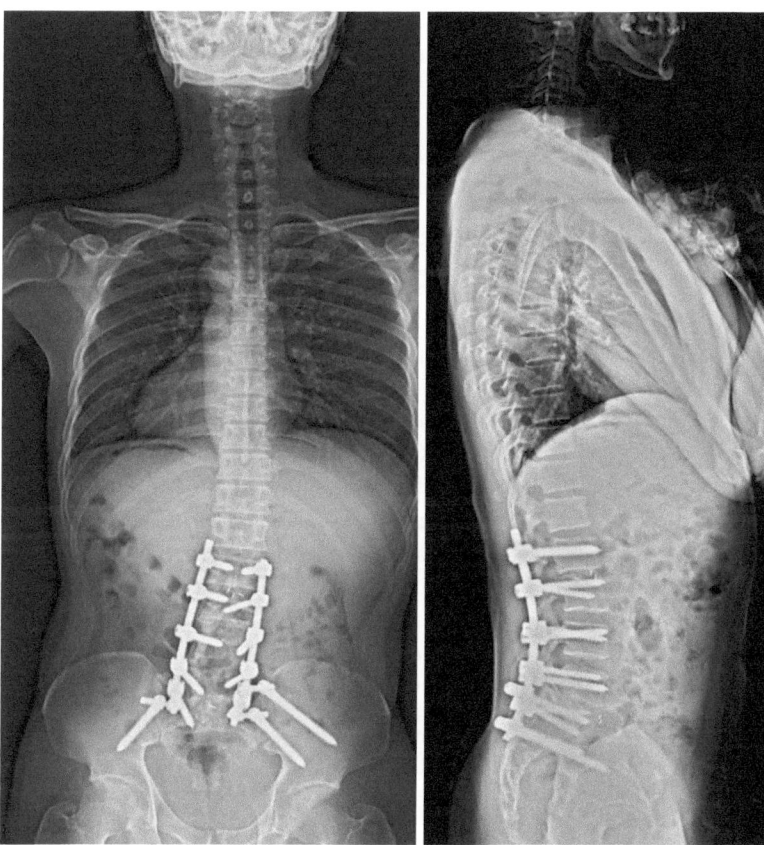

4.4 Spinal Imaging in the Emergency Setting

After the neurological and physical examination, the next step is identifying imaging studies including plain radiographs, computed tomography (CT) with multi-planar reconstruction, and magnetic resonance image (MRI). Specific image choices depend on patient's condition and different protocol at each center. The CT and MRI with angiography can be possibly included in the traumatic SCI setting.

4.4.1 Plain Radiography

A spinal plain X-ray can be performed in patients with localized pain, deformity, edema, neurological dysfunction, etc. In addition to standard anterior-posterior and lateral images, special images including an oblique view, an open-mouth view, and a swimmer's view can be included in the traumatic SCI patients. Although flexion-extension images are frequently advocated to assess ligament injury by some authors, it is contraindicated in a patient with a neurological deficit like case 2. And flexion-extension movement should be done voluntarily. Because MRI is increasingly popular in trauma settings, ligamentous integrity can be easily assessed by this means [15, 16].

Sometimes, this plain X-ray is only possible because of patient's poor condition in the emergency setting like case 2. Proper and rapid managements only with this simple X-ray could be necessary following further imaging studies.

4.4.2 Computed Tomography (CT)

In the present, CT is the method of choice for the evaluation of acute spinal trauma [17–20].

This provides us high-quality three-dimensional anatomical information including fracture and its fragment, facet dislocation, neural compression, or ligamentous integrity. A CT with an angiography can give us additional information about special arterial anatomy surrounding the spine-like vertebral artery.

This CT is particularly helpful for high cervical spinal (C1-C2) fracture, because the precise fracture subtype is often difficult to discern with plain radiography [17, 18]. The sensitivity of CT for the detection of cervical spine injuries (98%) is significantly better than that of plain radiography (52%). In the era of CT screening, no study has demonstrated that plain radiography adds clinically relevant information [17, 18].

CT scan gives us detailed information about the bony injury like fracture, dislocation, or joint subluxation more than MRI as easily seen in patient 2. Nowadays, whole-body CT at emergency room for multiple trauma patient is available, which provides many information very quickly.

4.4.3 Magnetic Resonance Imaging (MRI)

Technical improvements of imaging quality as well as decreased scan time lead us to use popularly for the traumatic spinal injury work-up. Because it can provide good visualization of the spinal cord and surrounding structures noninvasively, its popularity increases gradually. MRI can show epi- and subdural hematoma, cord contusion, cord edema, disc injury, and ligament disruption [15, 21, 22]. In addition, it can also provide a little information of surrounding vertebral arterial injury. If an angiographic technique is supported (i.e., MR angiography), more extensive information about the vessel injury can be obtained. A recent prospective analysis of the accuracy of MRI for diagnosis of posterior ligamentous complex injuries reported overall sensitivity and specificity rates of 91% and 100%, respectively, and 100% accuracy in diagnosis of unstable fractures [21].

Although there are some controversies in the timing or indication of MRI, this can be indicated in patients who show neurological deficit with or without radiographic abnormality (SCIWORA) on plain radiography or CT for detecting spinal problem and determining the management plan. MRI has an advantage to visualize soft tissue injuries like disc, ligament, or neural compression more than other imaging methods as easily seen in patient 2.

4.4.4 Whole-Body CT Scan

Integration of whole-body CT into early trauma care significantly increased the probability of survival in patients with polytrauma. Whole-body CT is recommended as a standard diagnostic method during the early resuscitation phase for patients with polytrauma. An increasing number of trauma centers are using it during the early resuscitation phase, even in hemodynamically unstable patients, because it is thought to be an effective method [5]. In our center, this scan method has been routinely used for the initial assessment of polytrauma patient.

> **Tips and Pitfalls**
> Because of the possibility of multiple spinal fractures, a patient with cervical spine injury should be evaluated with whole spine images. Sometimes, a simple X-ray cannot show the lower-level cervical trauma, such as C6-7 fracture and dislocation, due to shoulder shadow. Thus, the CT scan should be done in this situation. And sometimes, fracture-dislocation can make spontaneous reduction during transportation. This situation can be considered in the emergency room.
>
> ① *Should not miss C6-7 fracture-dislocation hidden by shoulder* (Fig. 4.11)
>
> Simple X-ray looks normal except soft tissue swelling. However, C6-7 fracture-dislocation can be detected on CT.
>
> ② *Should not miss spontaneous reduction with SCI*

In initial X-ray, C5-6 fracture-dislocation is found (Fig. 4.12).

It seems to be reduced during transfer to hospital. Therefore, C5-6 fracture-dislocation cannot be detected on simple X-ray at transferred hospital (Fig. 4.13).

If doctors did not check initial X-ray in the unconscious patient, SCI might be neglected. After reduction, only MRI shows the injury of spine and spinal cord.

4.5   Management According to Specific Spinal Trauma

The possible spinal problem after trauma is depicted in Fig. 4.14.

4.5.1   Injuries of the Occipuit-C1-C2 Region (Upper Cervical Lesion)

The craniovertebral junction (CVJ) is formed by three main bony structures: the occiput, the first (C1) and second cervical vertebrae (C2), and

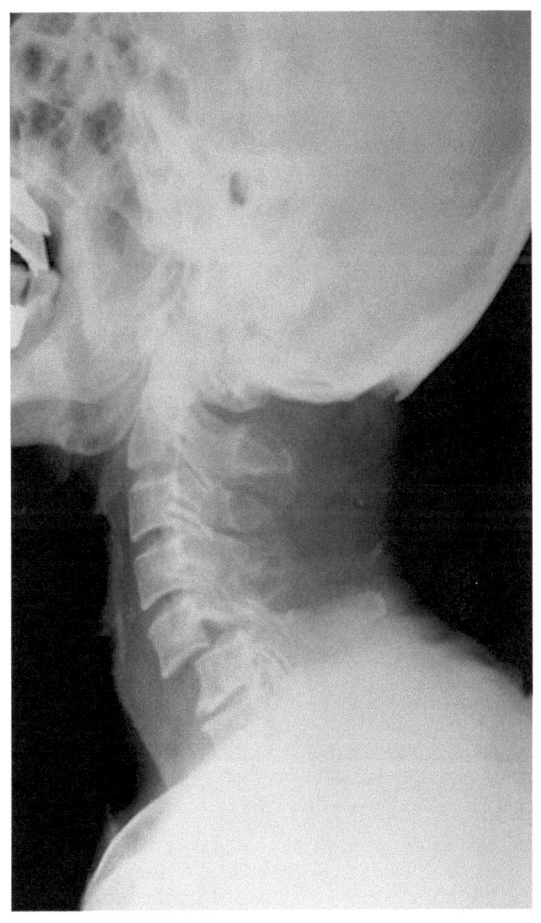

Fig. 4.12 An initial X-ray

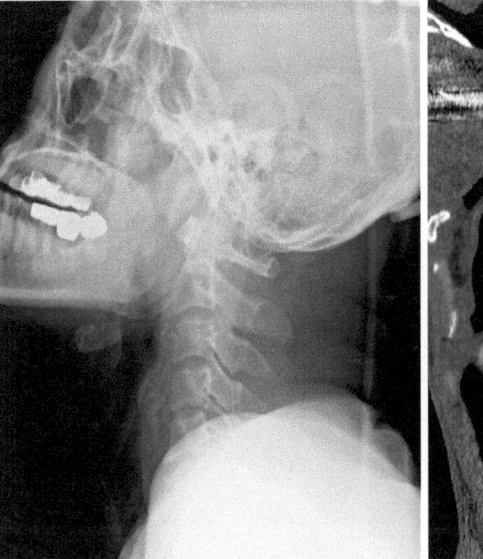
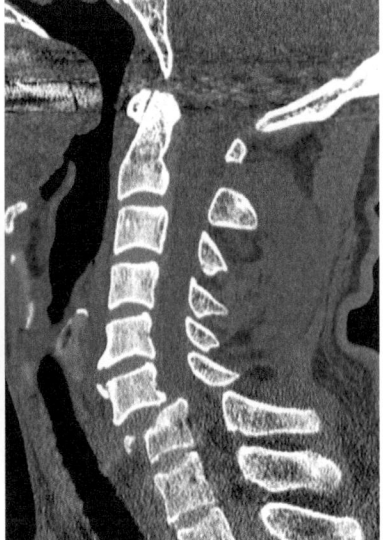

Fig. 4.11 X-ray and CT scan of C6-7 fracture and dislocated patient

Fig. 4.13 Follow up X-ray and MRI after closed reduction

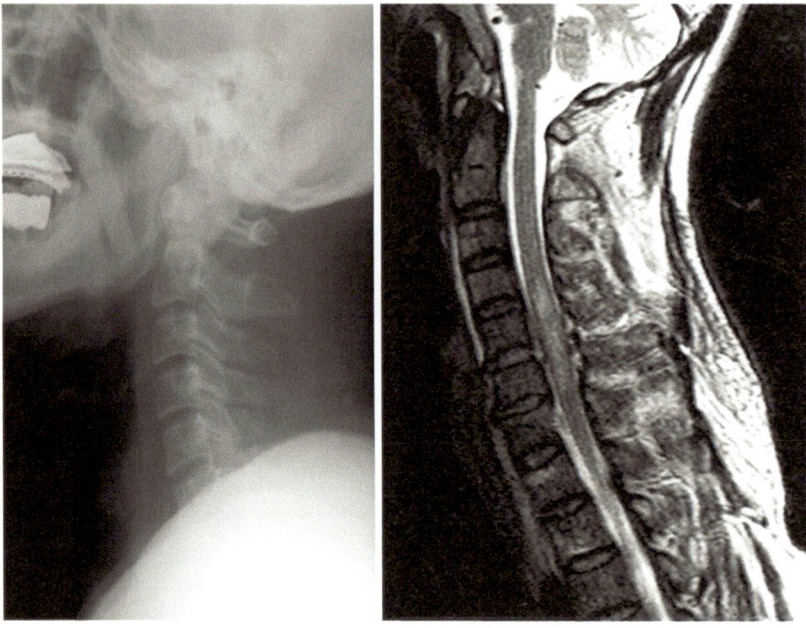

Fig. 4.14 Spinal traumatic lesions according to the location

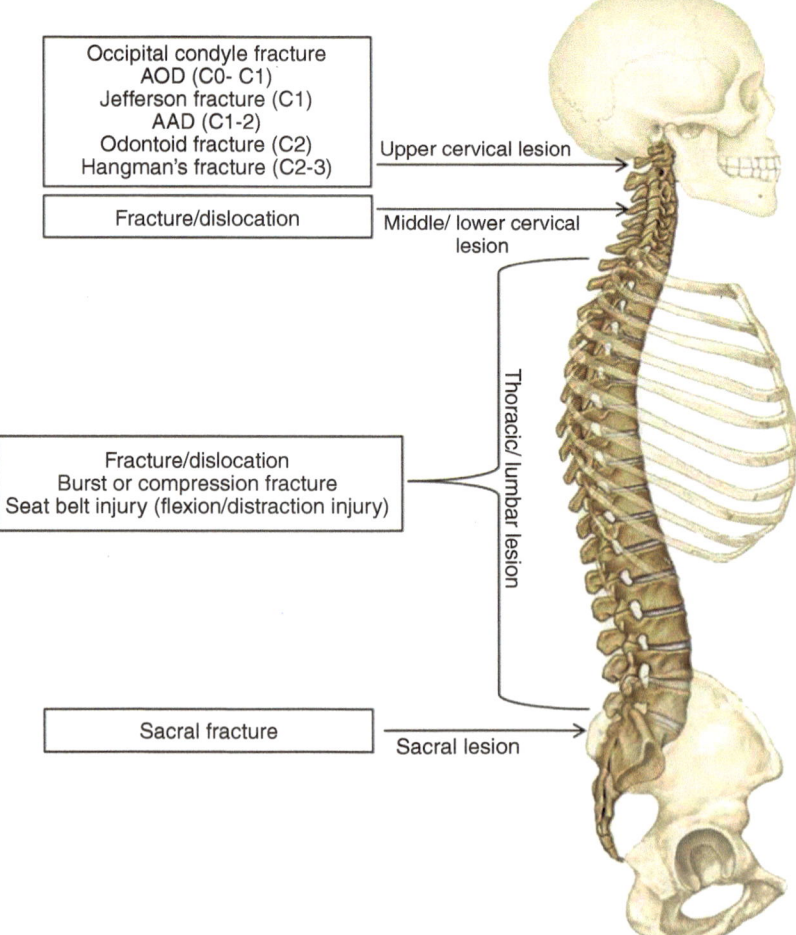

multiple ligaments and membranes that facilitate an extensive range of motion, protection for the neurovascular structures which it contains. Specific traumatic injury in this region should be considered according to the ligament injury, bone fracture, or a combination of the two.

The traumatic conditions in this region are occipital condyle fractures, atlanto-occipital dislocation (AOD), atlantoaxial dislocation (AAD), Jefferson fracture, odontoid fracture, and hangman's fracture (Fig. 4.14). The former three traumas are rare, but may be fatal, while the latter three traumatic conditions are more popular. Early diagnosis, sometimes prompt intubation, and early immobilization of the neck and head appear to improve survival in young patients who suffer a traumatic injury this upper cervical lesion. Sometimes, these life-saving procedures should be necessary before the patient arrives at the trauma center, increasing the chance for survival. A delay in the diagnosis of AOD is associated with an increased likelihood of neurological deterioration [23, 24].

Case Scenario: Patient 3

A 63-year-old male patient visited the emergency center who fell from a height of 3 m 1 day before. His consciousness was alert but complained of severe neck pain and paralysis in all extremities (Grade IV in upper extremities and Grade III in lower extremities, AIS C). Cervical spinal cord injury was highly suspected; thus, cervical spinal imaging work-up including X-ray, CT scan, and MRI was performed. On X-ray lateral image, lower cervical spinal fracture could not be found due to shoulder shadow (Fig. 4.15).

A left-side sagittal CT scan showed C2 body and C6 inferior articular process fractures, and mid-sagittal CT scan also showed C7 body fracture and displaced bony fragment into spinal canal (Figs 4.16 and 4.17).

Axial CT scan showed Jefferson fracture at C1 level.

T2-weighted sagittal MRI showed prevertebral hematoma, C7 burst fracture, spinal cord compression, and cord signal change. T2-weighted axial MRI also showed Jefferson fracture at C1 level, but intact transverse ligament (Fig. 4.18) (red arrow).

Because this fracture gap of Jefferson fracture at C1 level was 6 mm (less than 7 mm), nonsurgical treatment was done. Burst fracture on C7 level was surgically treated with C6-7-T1 fusion and decompression (Fig. 4.19).

For the 2-year follow-up, this patient can ambulate without any assistance and showed normal muscular power and sensation (ASIA E).

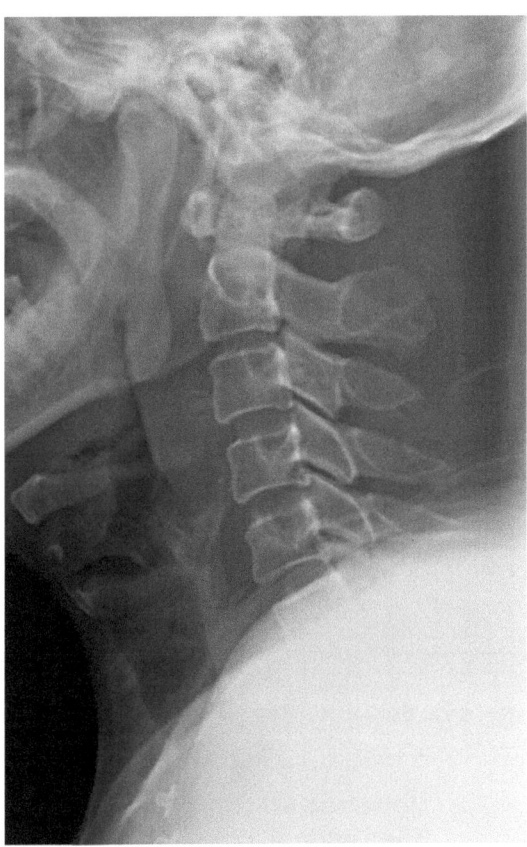

Fig. 4.15 X-ray of patient

Fig. 4.16 Sagittal CT scan of patient

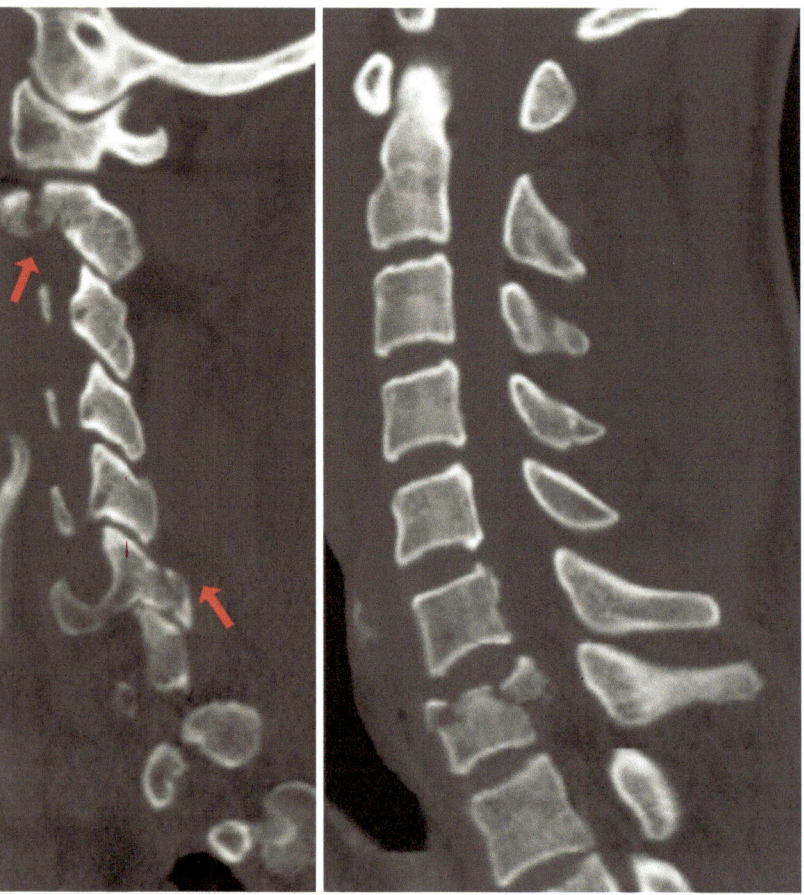

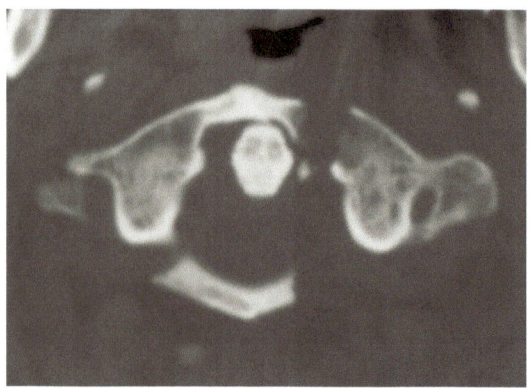

Fig. 4.17 Patient's Axial CT scan of C1 (Atlas)

4.5.2 Jefferson Fracture (See Patient 3)

A Jefferson fracture (JF) is created by sudden and direct axial loading on the vertex. The lateral artic-

ular masses of the atlas (C1) become compressed between the occipital condyles and the superior articular facets of the axis. By its nature, this is a decompressive injury because the bony fragments are displaced radially away from the neural structures shown in patient 3. Although the typical JF is regarded stable which could be managed with brace, surgery can be considered when following condition combined. First, the transverse ligament is disrupted; second, fracture displacement is more than 7 mm; and third, atlantoaxial distance on sagittal X-ray image is more than 3 mm [25].

Previously described patient 3 was not indicated C1-2 fusion surgery. However, the different 74-year-old male patient also showed Jefferson fracture with 7 mm displacement on CT scan and definite transverse ligament disruption (red arrow) on MRI was indicated C1-2 fusion surgery according to above criteria (Figs. 4.20 and 4.21).

Fig. 4.18 MRI of patient

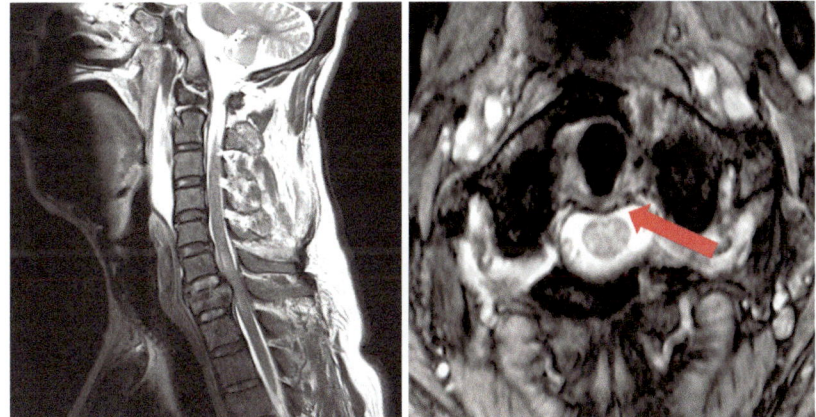

Fig. 4.19 Postoperative X-ray after surgical stabilization

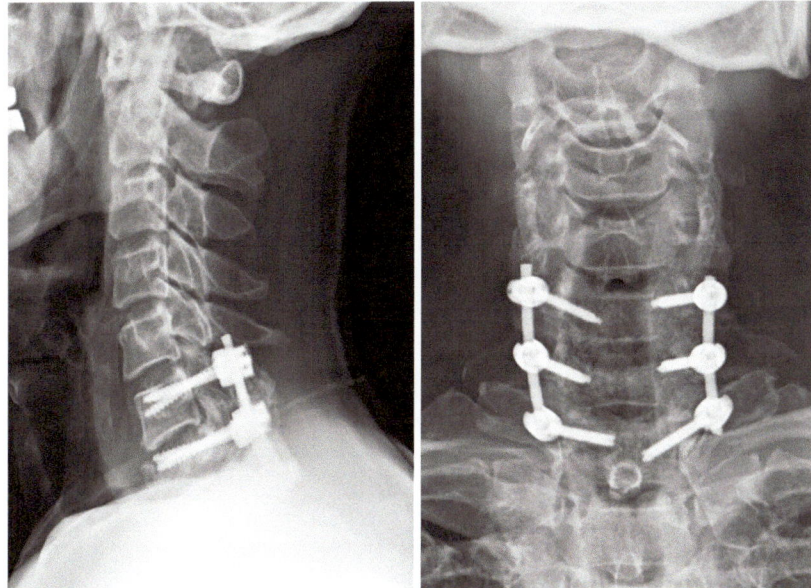

Fig. 4.20 CT scan and MRI of patient with Unstable Jefferson fracture

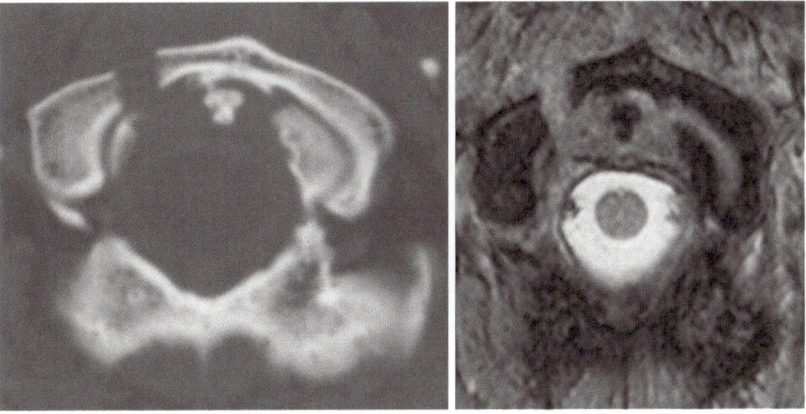

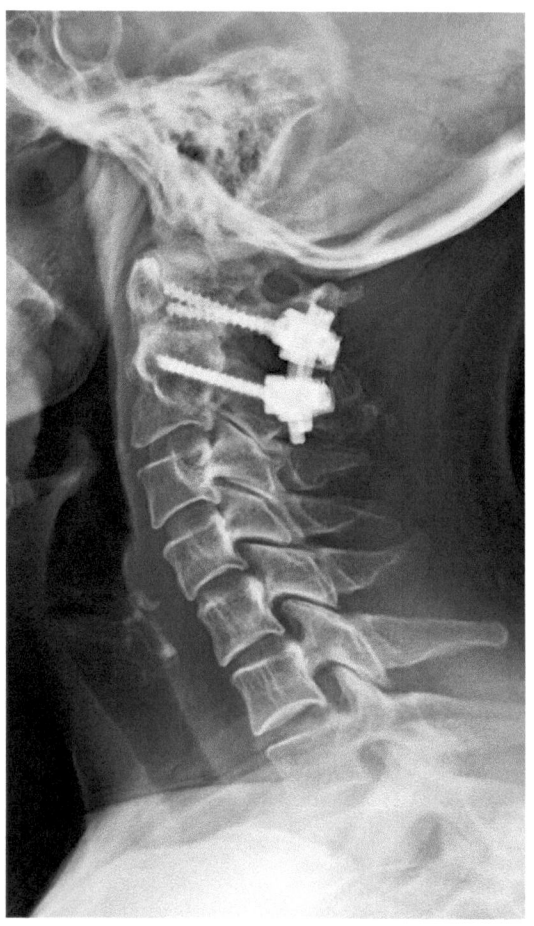

Case Scenario: Patient 4

A 53-year-old female patient visited the emergency center who fell down during golf play 1 hour before. Her consciousness was alert, but complained neck pain, right toe pain, and eyebrow laceration. Her neurological examination was normal. Although eyebrow laceration was sutured in the emergency room, her imaging examinations showed right first toe fracture, type 2 spinal odontoid fracture, and left-side unilateral C5-6 facet dislocation (Fig. 4.22)

Because there was a concern of odontoid fracture gap distraction, closed reduction using Gardner-Wells tongs traction could not be done. Through single incisional approach, anterior odontoid screw fixation, and simultaneous C5-6 level open reduction and fusion surgery were planned as well as right first toe pinning. If she had only odontoid fracture which is type III without prominent displacement, conservative management could be considered (Fig. 4.23)

Fig. 4.21 Postoperative X-ray after surgical stabilization in patient with Unstable Jefferson fracture

Fig. 4.22 Sagittal CT scan of patient

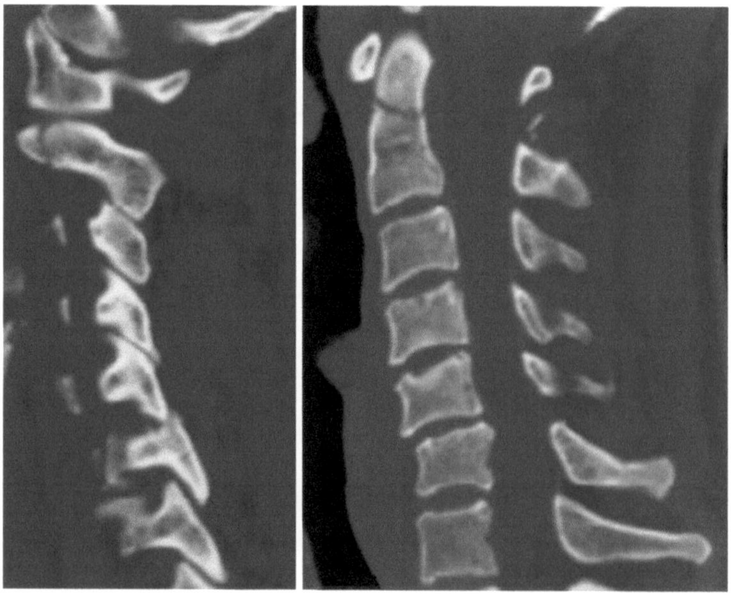

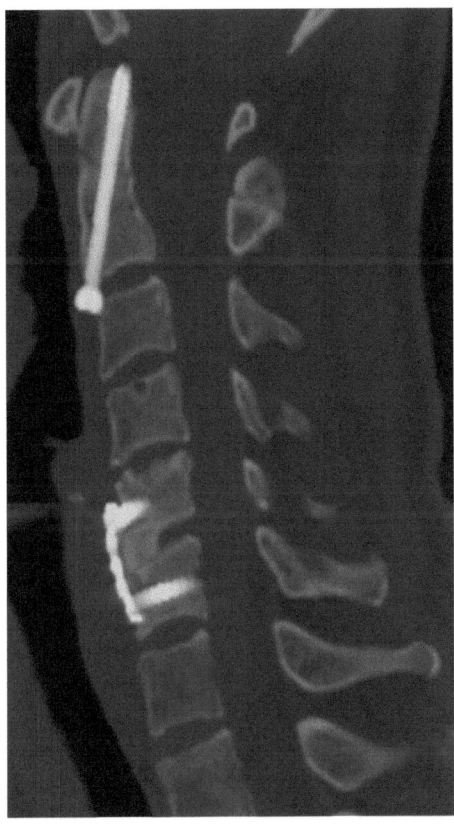

Fig. 4.23 Postoperative sagittal CT scan of patient

4.5.3 Odontoid Fractures (See Patient 4)

Odontoid fractures represent the most common fracture of the axis. They account for 50% to 60% of all axis fractures and are associated with other spine injuries in 34% of patients. The most commonly used classification scheme was developed by Anderson and D'Alonzo [26]. They classified odontoid fractures into three types based on the anatomic location of the fracture (Fig. 4.24).

Among them, type I and almost type III odontoid fractures can be treated nonsurgically. A cervical collar is generally considered sufficient. However, most type II and a shallow type III fracture should be considered as a surgical candidate.

Surgical management of these fractures can be approached either anteriorly or posteriorly. Anterior screw fixation has become increasingly popular owing to the potential morbidity and loss of motion associated with posterior C1-2 fusions [27]. For a patient with severely comminuted fractures or whose transverse ligament is disrupted, a posterior approach is recommended.

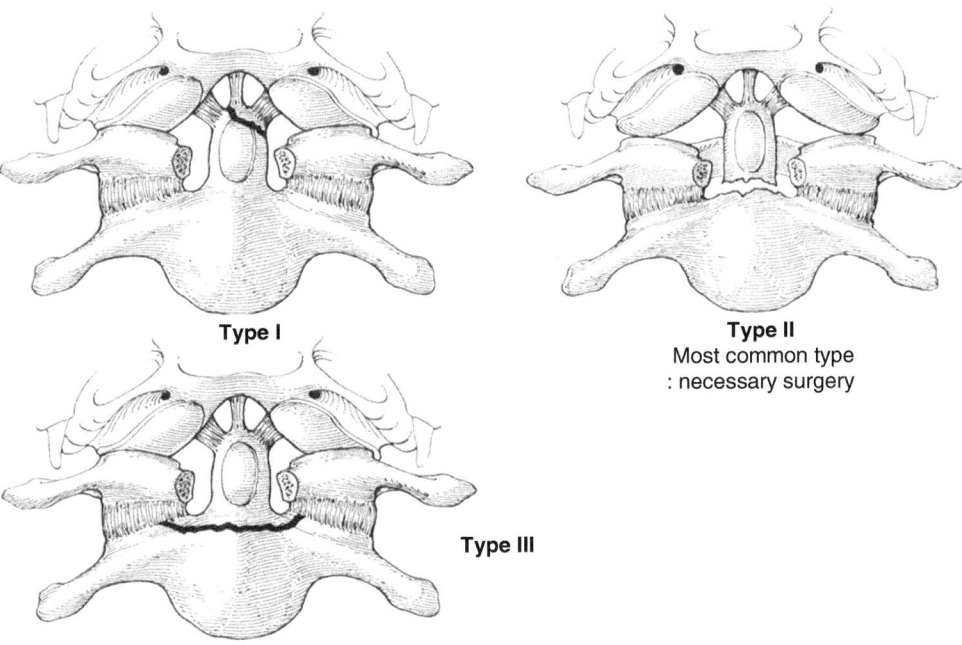

Fig. 4.24 Classification of odontoid fracture

4.5.4 Hangman's Fracture (See Patient 1)

Hangman fracture, or traumatic spondylolisthesis of the axis, is the second most common type of axis fracture involving bilateral fractures of the pars interarticularis. This injury typically involves hyperextension and axial loading, and most patients with this injury present with neck pain and are neurologically intact because the bilateral fracture tends to widen the spinal canal.

Radiographic evaluation includes plain radiographs, CT scans, and MRI to evaluate for ligamentous injury and neural compression. CT angiography should be done to evaluate for VAI.

For fractures with more than 5 mm of subluxation or at least 30 degrees of angulation, surgical fixation should be strongly considered. Although C2-3 fusion surgery through anterior approach may be easier and possible, the complication including esophagus, vessel, and nerve injuries is critical. Posterior C2-3 fusion and the connection between pedicle fracture gaps using longer C2 screw can be feasible like patient 1. There are various surgical methods in hangman's fracture.

If C2-3 disc and facet are intact, C1-2 posterior fixation or screw fixation through C2 pedicle only could be considered. But, if C2-3 disc and facet are not intact, C1, C 2, and C3 posterior fixation or C2-3 fixation with long pedicle screws of C2 could be considered.

4.5.5 Subaxial Cervical Spine Injury and Treatment Guideline According to SLICS System

Subaxial spinal injury includes compression fracture, burst fracture, laminar fracture, teardrop fracture, uni- or bilateral facet dislocation, or combinations of those. For the assessment of spinal stability and surgical necessity, subaxial injury classification and severity score (SLICS) system is popularly used [28] (Table 4.2).

This is described under the three core mechanisms and assigned 1–4 points reflecting severity. Patients with a score sum of 3 or less are considered acutely stable and therefore candidates for nonoperative management with brace immobilization and rapid ambulation.

Table 4.2 Subaxial injury classification severity score (SLICS)

Injury Parameter	Points
Morphology	
No abnormality	0
Compression fracture	1
Burst fracture	2
Distraction (perched facets, hyperextension)	3
Rotation or translation (e.g., facet dislocation, teardrop fracture)	4
Discoligamentous complex	
Intact	0
Indeterminate (isolated interspinous widening or MRI signal change)	1
Disrupted (widening of disc space, facet perch, or dislocation)	2
Neurological status	
Intact	0
Root injury	1
Complete spinal cord injury (ASIA A)	2
Incomplete spinal cord injury (ASIA B or better)	3
Neurological deficit in the setting of continued spinal cord compression	+1' (modifier)

ASIA American Spinal Injury Association International Standards for Neurological Classification of Spinal Cord Injury Impairment Scale grade, *MRI* magnetic resonance imaging, *PLC* posterior ligamentous complex

Patients with a score sum of 5 or greater are considered acutely unstable and thus recommended for operative intervention for acute spinal stabilization, deformity correction, and neurological decompression if necessary. A patient with a score sum equal to 4 points can be considered for either operative or nonoperative treatment.

According to above criteria, 80-year-old female patient with C5 and C6 burst fracture, but no neurological deficit and no ligament injury on MRI, indicated 2 points on SLCIS system was treated nonsurgically and kept Philadelphia brace for 2 months (Fig. 4.25).

The other two patients, 62/M patient with burst fracture on C7 level and 40/M patient with teardrop fracture on C5 level indicated also SLCIS 2 and SLICS 4 points and were treated with only Philadelphia brace for 2 months (Fig. 4.26)

However, 60-year-old male patient showed ASIA A neurogical status after trauma developed 1 day before. A CT scan showed C7-T1 complete dislocation (spondyloptosis) and C7 burst fracture and bilateral pedicle fracture. Disc at C7-T1 level and posterior ligament injury was seen. On SLICS system, facet dislocation (4 points), disrupted disc and posterior ligaments (2 points), and AISA A (2 points) led us to do a surgical treatment (total 8 points). Open reduction and stabilization with pedicle screw fixation were done through posterior approach, and patient improved into ASIA C (Fig. 4.27).

The other a 43-year-old male patient with ankylosing spondylitis visited our emergency center due to paralysis following a trauma (ASIA B). CT scan showed a C5 oblique burst fracture, and the bilateral pedicles were separated superiorly and inferiorly. The sagittal reconstructed CT

Fig. 4.25 CT scan and MRI of stable fracture in SLICS (2 points)

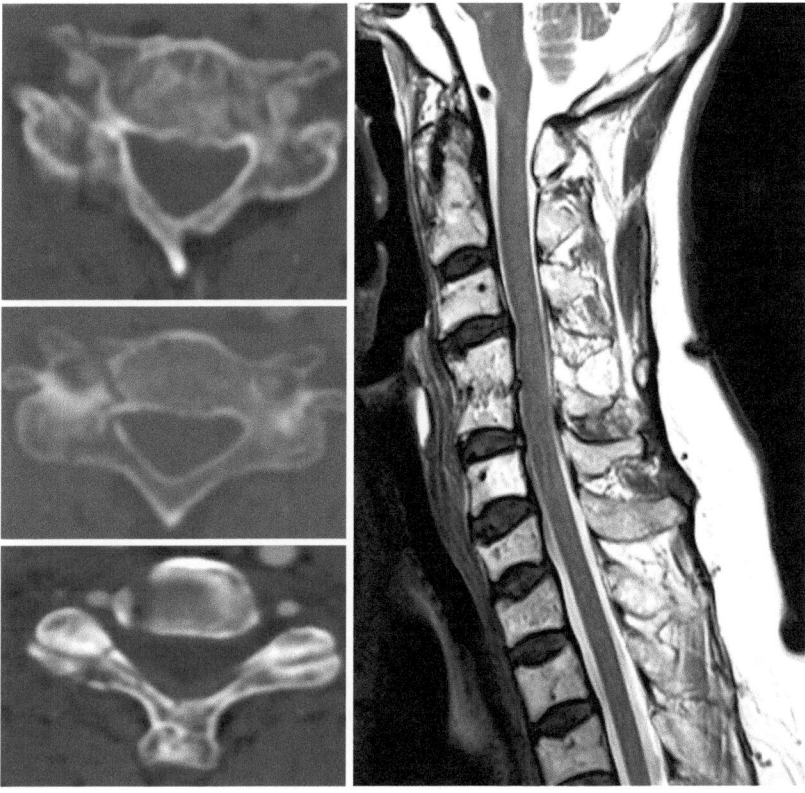

Fig. 4.26 CT scan of stable fracture in SLICS (4 points)

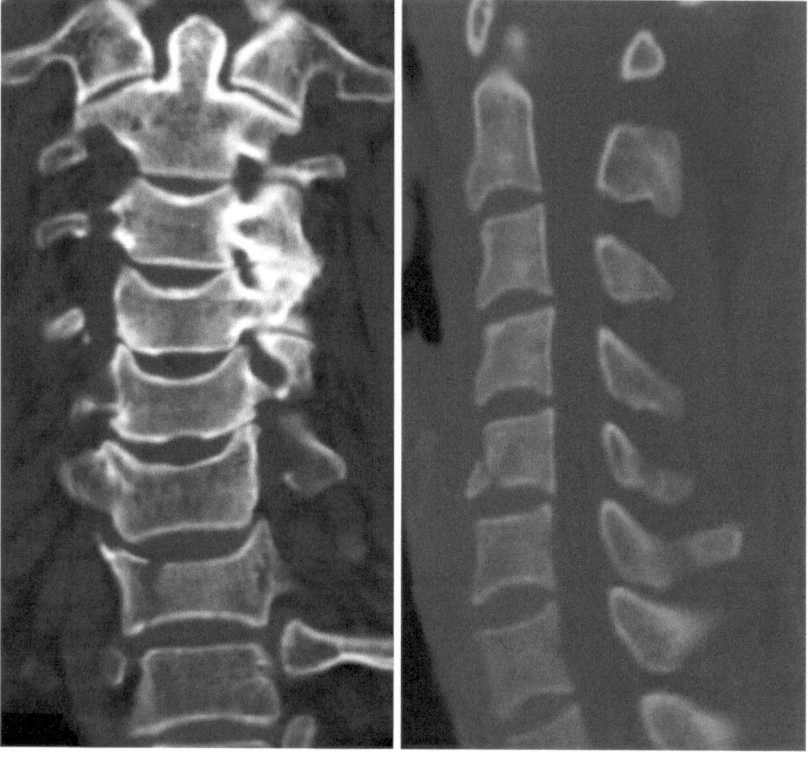

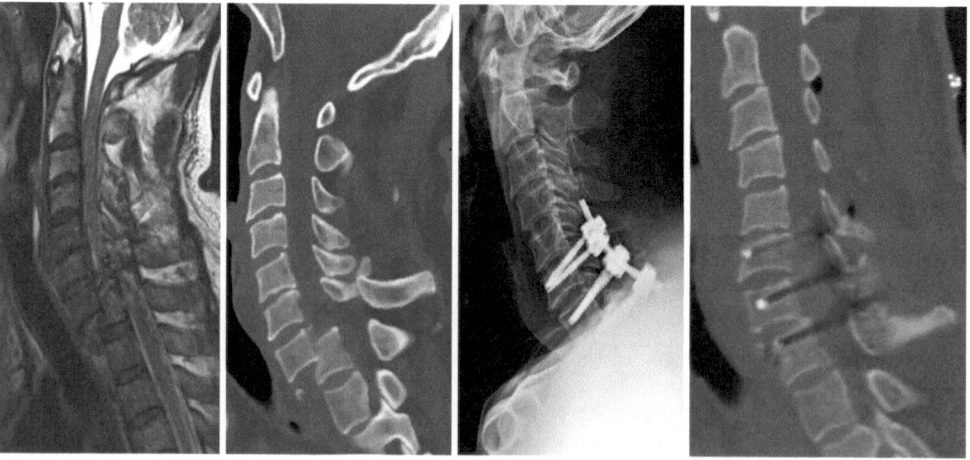

Fig. 4.27 MRI and CT scan of unstable fracture in SLICS (8 points)

image revealed bamboo spine and C5 vertebrae body fracture. Hyperextension between the fractured segments of the C5 body was noted because the fracture gap was anteriorly open. Magnetic resonance imaging (MRI) showed cord compression and injury at the C4-5 level. On SLICS system, distraction due to hyperextension (3 points), no discoligamentous injury due to ankylosing spondylitis (0 points), and AISA B (3 points) led us to do a surgical treatment (total 6 points). Open reduction and stabilization with pedicle screw fixation were done through posterior approach patient improved into ASIA D (Figs. 4.28 and 4.29)

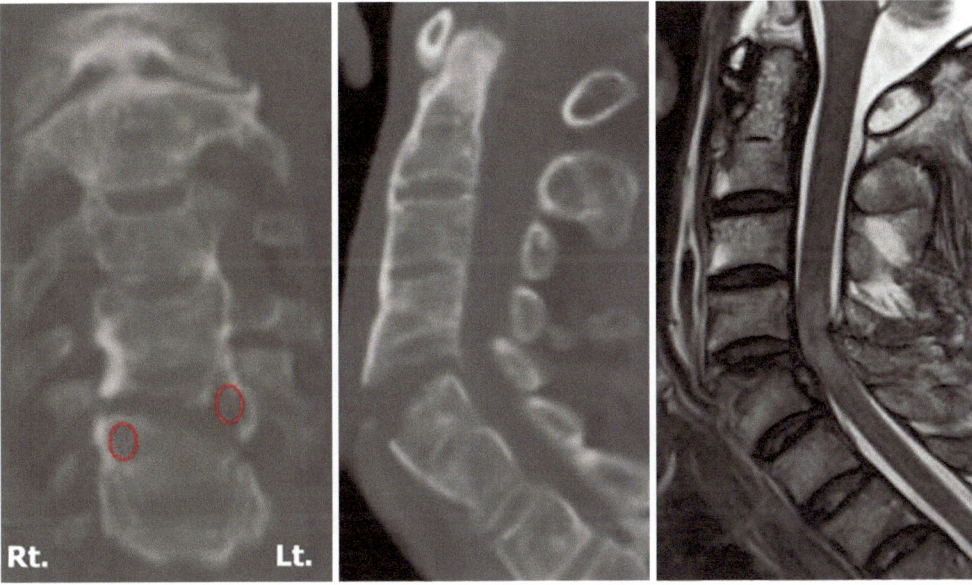

Fig. 4.28 CT scan and MRI of unstable fracture in SLICS (6 points)

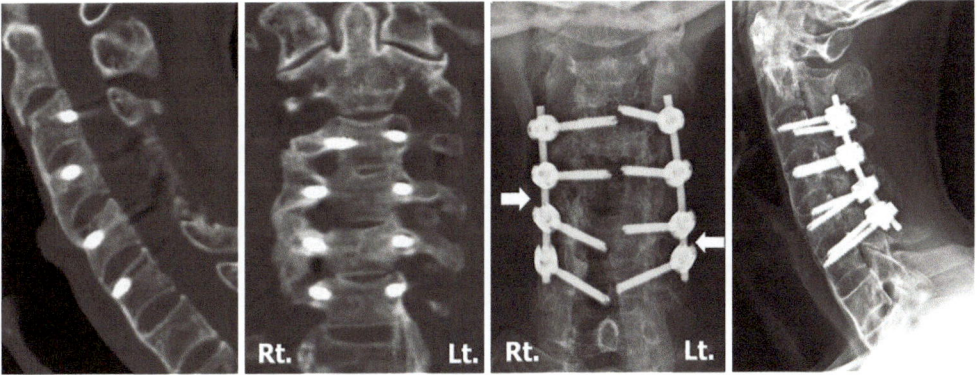

Fig. 4.29 Postoperative CT scan and MRI of unstable fracture in SLICS (6 points)

Tips and Pitfalls

The management guideline and controversy for the subaxial cervical spinal fracture-dislocation

Cervical facet dislocations occur as a result of flexion and distraction forces (with or without rotational forces) acting on the subaxial cervical spine. Substantial controversy remains regarding the order of priority between MRI and closed reduction, the necessity of closed reduction attempts prior surgical open reduction despite of the possibility of the closed reduction, and the choice of surgical approach among anterior, posterior, or both [9, 29–32]. According to the AANS/CNS guideline for subaxial cervical spinal facet dislocation, the general consensus was suggested for these situations [33, 34] (Fig. 4.30).

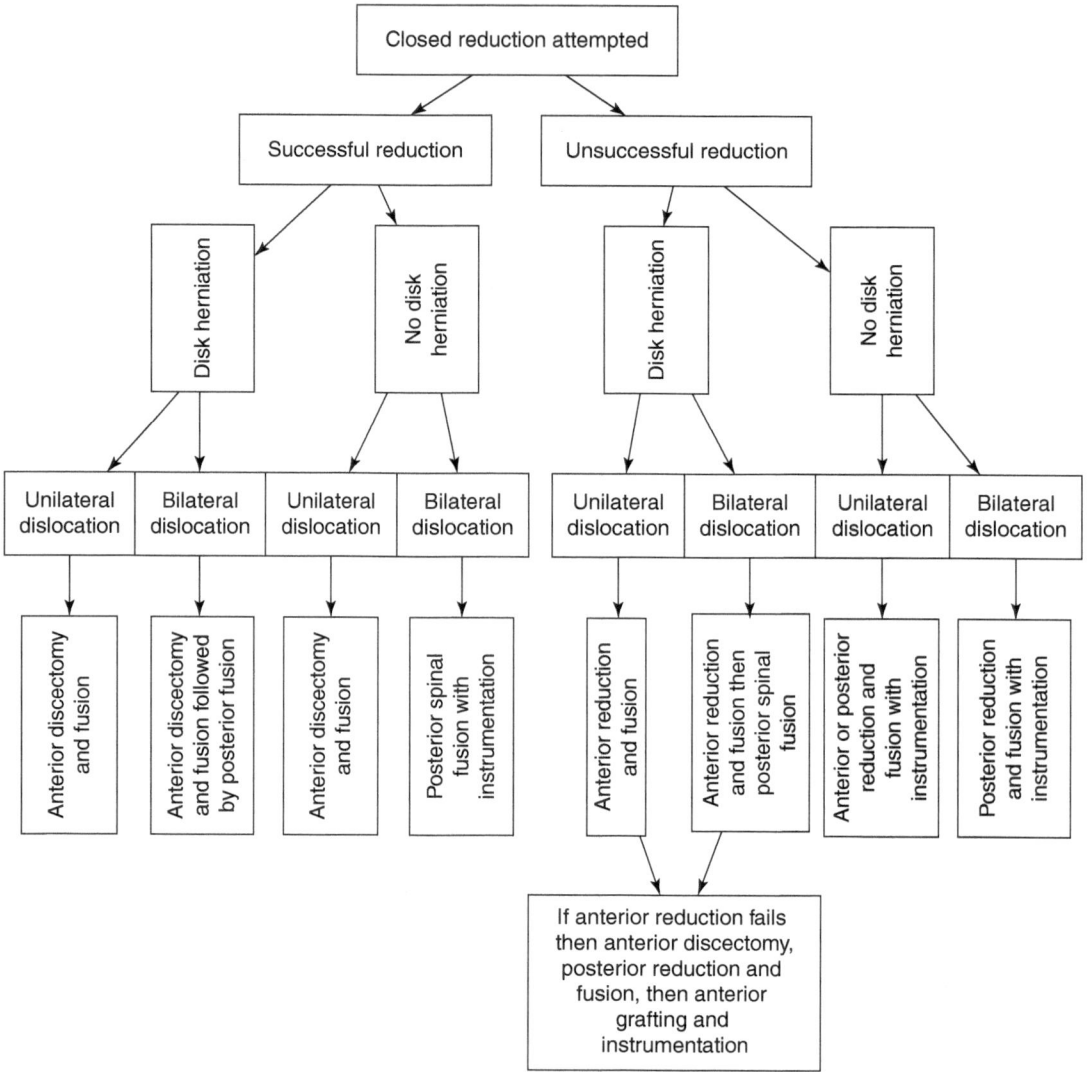

Fig. 4.30 Flow diagrm for the treatment of Cervical spinal facet dislocation [33, 34]

4.5.6 Cervical Spinal Cord Injury Without Bone and Disc Injury (Central Cord Syndrome)

Cervical spinal cord injury without bone and disc injury tends to be caused by a hyperextension force to the neck. Cervical spinal cord contusion even after minor hyperextension trauma could be developed especially when a patient had previously asymptomatic but degenerative changes such as osteophytes, disc bulging, hypertrophy or ossification of ligamentum flavum (OLF), or ossification of posterior longitudinal ligament (OPLL). Usually MRI shows high signal intense cord signal change and index-level cord compression even without bony fracture or dislocation (Fig. 4.31).

Fig. 4.31 MRI and CT scan of patient with central cord syndrome

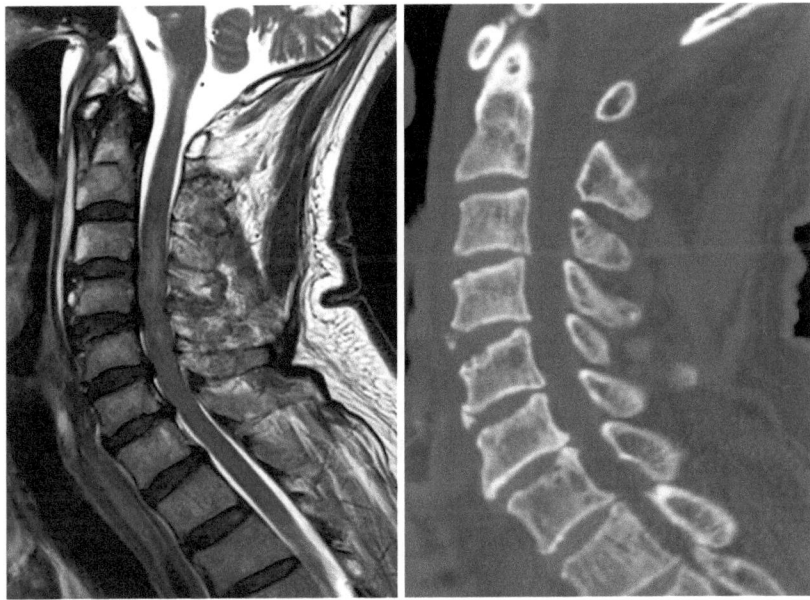

4.5.7 Thoracic and Lumbar Spine Injuries and Treatment Guideline According to TLICS System

This kind of patients usually shows worse upper extremity weakness than lower extremity because their central cord injury tends to be more severe. Although there have been controversies between the surgery and conservative treatment [35–38], recent several prospective studies suggested that only early surgery (i.e., less than critical time point like 24 hrs) could make better surgical outcome [7, 39–41].

The other management protocol for this traumatic patient should be followed spinal cord injury protocol described previously in this chapter.

4.5.8 Thoracolumbar Spine Injury and Treatment Guideline According to TLICS System

Like cervical spinal injury, there is thoracolumbar injury classification and severity score (TLICS) system for the assessment of thoracic and lumbar spinal injury [28] (Table 4.3).

Table 4.3 Thoracolumbar injury classification and severity score (TLICS)

Injury parameter	Points
Morphology	
No abnormality	0
Compression fracture	1
Burst fracture	2
Translation or rotation	3
Distraction (circumferential disruption of all spinal elements)	4
Discoligamentous complex	
Intact	0
Indeterminate (isolated interspinous widening or MRI signal change)	2
Disrupted (translation, interspinous widening, or disrupted PLC on MR)	3
Neurological status	
Intact	0
Nerve root compression	2
Complete spinal cord or conus medullaris injury	2
Incomplete spinal cord or conus medullaris injury	3
Cauda equina syndrome	3

ASIA American Spinal Injury Association International Standards for Neurological Classification of Spinal Cord Injury Impairment Scale grade, *MRI* magnetic resonance imaging, *PLC* posterior ligamentous complex

This is also described under the three core mechanisms and assigned 1–4 points reflecting severity. Patients with a score sum of 3 or less are considered acutely stable and therefore candidates for nonoperative management with brace immobilization and rapid ambulation.

Patients with a score sum of 5 or greater are considered acutely unstable and thus recommended for operative intervention for acute spinal stabilization, deformity correction, and neurological decompression if necessary. A patient with a score sum equal to 4 points can be considered for either operative or nonoperative treatment. However, we should keep in mind that there might be some exceptional cases.

According to above criteria, 19-year-old male patient with L1, L2, and L3 compression and burst fractures, but no neurological deficit and no ligament injury on MRI, indicated only 2 points

on TLCIS system was treated nonsurgically and kept TLSO brace for 2 months and showed no pain and normal global alignment but only L1 segmental kyphosis on whole spine lateral X-ray image after 2 years. After 3 years, patient showed mild back pain, but good global alignment on whole spine lateral X-ray and nearly normal daily life (Fig. 4.32).

The other 59/M patient showed L1 and T11 burst fractures and T7

The other 52-year-old male patient showed T12, T11, and T9 burst fractures and indeterminate ligament injury on MRI with normal neurological status (Fig. 4.33). This patient indicated 4 points on TLCIS system was treated nonsurgically and kept TLSO brace for 2 months. After 3 months, the CT scan showed bony healing in the body and facet joint. After 4 years, the patient showed no back pain and good global alignment on whole spine lateral X-ray.

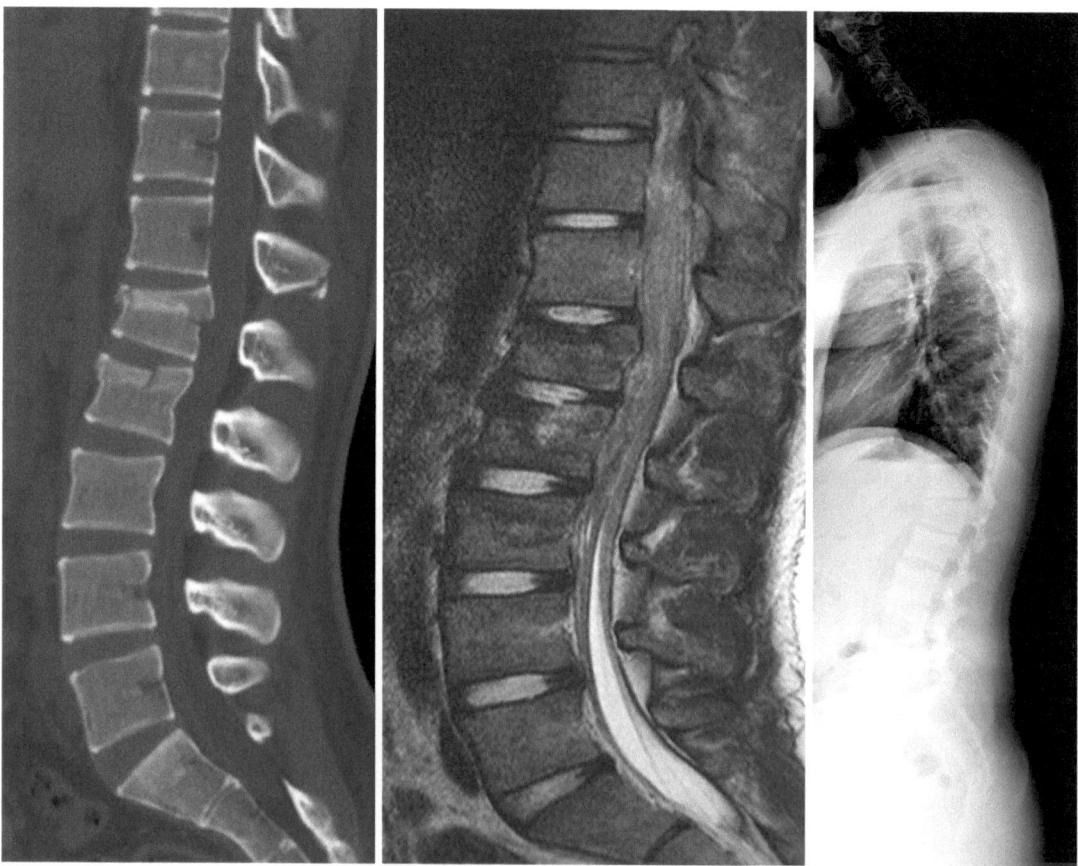

Fig. 4.32 CT scan and MRI amd X-ray of stable fracture in TLICS (2 points)

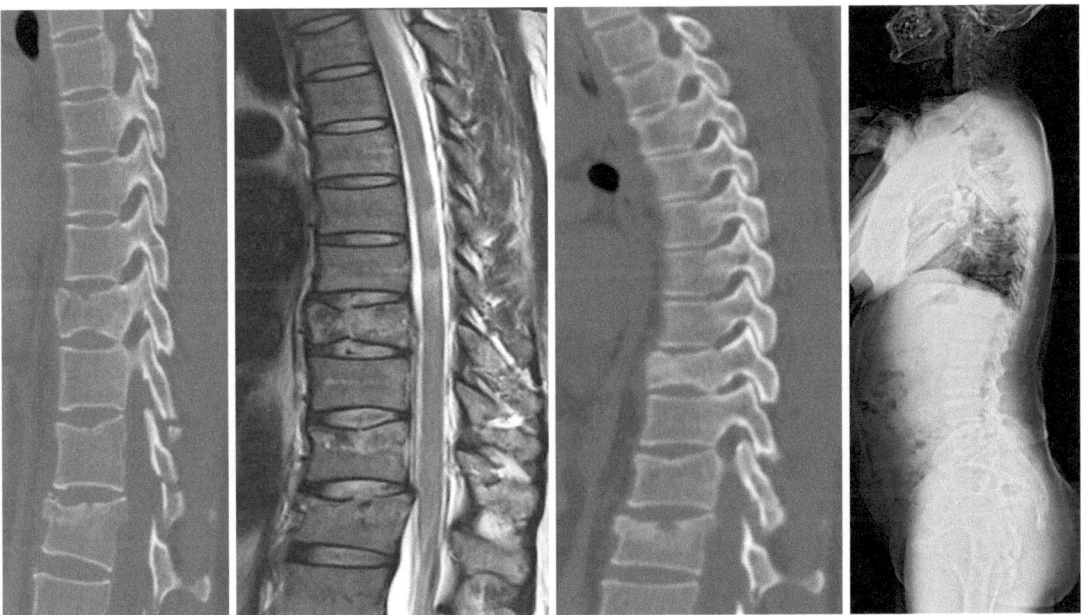

Fig. 4.33 CT scan and MRI amd X-ray of stable fracture in TLICS (4 points)

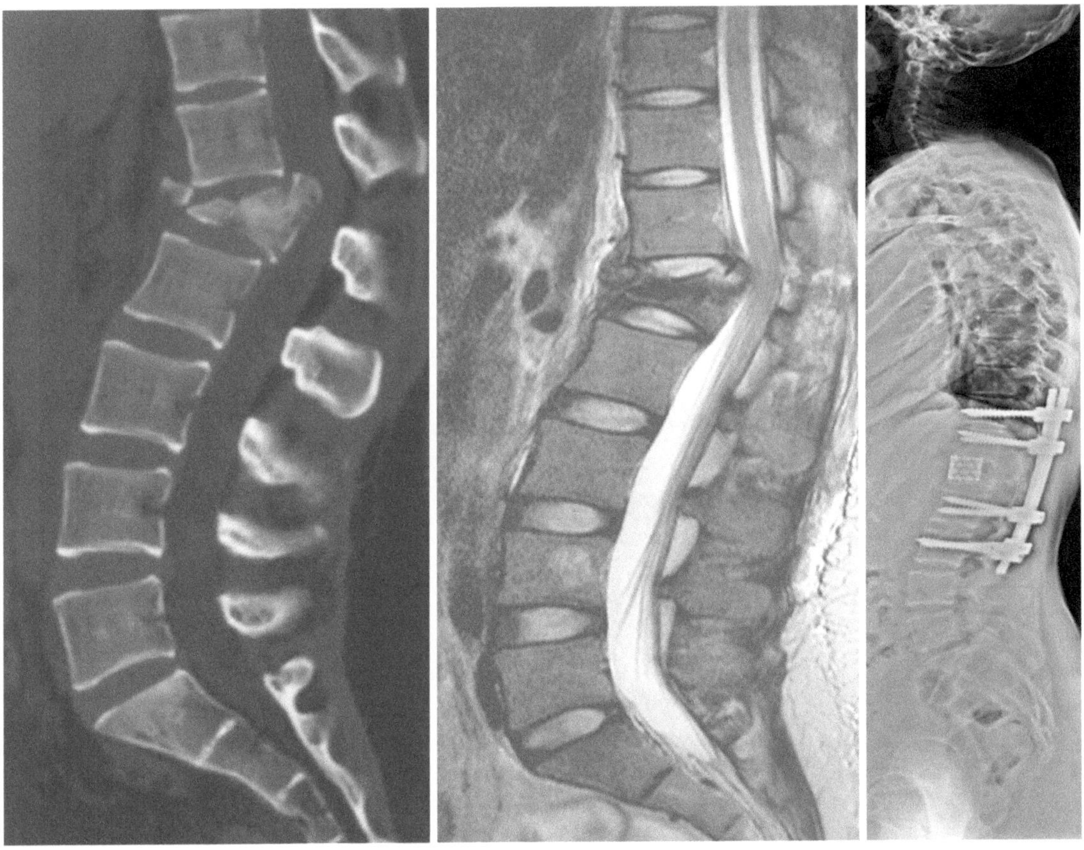

Fig. 4.34 CT scan and MRI amd postoperative X-ray of unstable fracture in TLICS (10 points)

However, a 30-year-old female patient showed ASIA B neurological status after trauma. A CT scan and MRI showed L1 burst fracture (circumferential disruption of all spinal elements) and disrupted posterior ligament (Fig. 4.34). On TLICS system, distraction (4 points), disrupted PLC 3 points), and incomplete cord or conus medullaris injury (3 points) led us to do a surgical treatment (total 10 points). Open reduction with kyphosis correction through removal of fractured upper body and stabilization was done. After 3 years, patient showed complete recovery (AISA E) with normal daily life, and whole spinal lateral image also showed good global balance.

The other a 40-year-old male patient visited our emergency center due to paralysis following a trauma (ASIA B). CT scan showed a L3 burst fracture and dislocated L2-3 facet joint. MRI showed severe canal compression and posterior ligament injury (Fig. 4.35). On TLICS system, distraction distracted burst fracture (4 points), disrupted PLC (3 points), and cauda equina syndrome (3 points) led us to do a surgical treatment (total 10 points). Open reduction, removal of comminuted fractured body, and stabilization were done. After 2 years, the patient improved into ASIA E with normal daily life and good alignment on whole spinal lateral image.

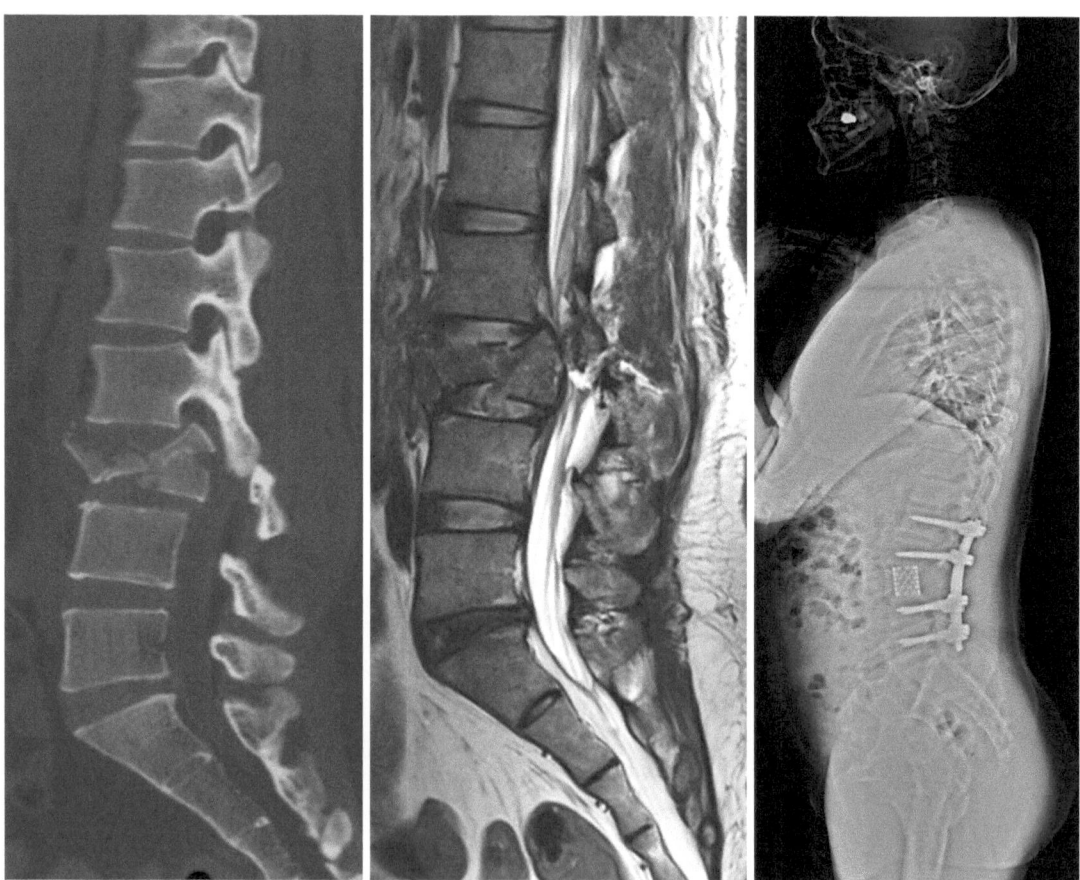

Fig. 4.35 CT scan and MRI amd postoperative X-ray of unstable fracture in TLICS (10 points)

Summary

1. The possibility of an unstable spine must be considered as well as an airway, breathing, and circulation when transferring the patient. This airway can be managed using the chin lift and jaw-thrust technique and the removal of obstructed material.

2. Specific image choices depend on patient condition and different protocol at each center. The CT scan and MRI with angiography can be possibly included in the traumatic SCI setting. Whole-body CT scan followed by special image can be one of best choice in the emergent traumatic setting.

3. Surgical treatment for the traumatic spine should be necessary when neural element compression and unstable spine are detected according to the published guidelines, such as TLICS and SLICS, etc.

References

1. Hoffman JR, Wolfson AB, Todd K, Mower WR. Selective cervical spine radiography in blunt trauma: methodology of the National Emergency X-Radiography Utilization Study (NEXUS). Ann Emerg Med. 1998;32(4):461–9.

2. Ryken TC, Hurlbert RJ, Hadley MN, Aarabi B, Dhall SS, Gelb DE, et al. The acute cardiopulmonary management of patients with cervical spinal cord injuries. Neurosurgery. 2013;72(Suppl 2):84–92.

3. Mukherjee S, Beck C, Yoganandan N, Rao RD. Incidence and mechanism of neurological deficit after thoracolumbar fractures sustained in motor vehicle collisions. J Neurosurg Spine. 2016:24(2):323–31.

4. Ahn H, Singh J, Nathens A, MacDonald RD, Travers A, Tallon J, et al. Pre-hospital care management of a potential spinal cord injured patient: a systematic review of the literature and evidence-based guidelines. J Neurotrauma. 2011;28(8):1341–61.

5. Huber-Wagner S, Lefering R, Kanz K-G, Biberthaler P, Stengel D. The importance of immediate total-body CT scanning. Lancet. 2017;389(10068):502–3.

6. American Spinal Injury Association. International standards for the neurological classification of spinal cord injury. Chicago: American Spinal Injury Association; 2002.

7. Park JH, Kim JH, Roh SW, Rhim SC, Jeon SR. Prognostic factor analysis after surgical decompression and stabilization for cervical spinal-cord injury. Br J Neurosurg. 2017;31(2):194–8.

8. Finfer S, Bellomo R, Boyce N, French J, Myburgh J, Norton R. A comparison of albumin and saline for fluid resuscitation in the intensive care unit. N Engl J Med. 2004;350(22):2247–56.

9. Park JH, Roh SW, Rhim SC. A single-stage posterior approach with open reduction and pedicle screw fixation in subaxial cervical facet dislocations. J Neurosurg Spine. 2015;23(1):35–41.

10. Coleman WP, Benzel D, Cahill DW, Ducker T, Geisler F, Green B, et al. A critical appraisal of the reporting of the National Acute Spinal Cord Injury Studies (II and III) of methylprednisolone in acute spinal cord injury. J Spinal Disord. 2000;13(3):185–99.

11. Hurlbert RJ, Hadley MN, Walters BC, Aarabi B, Dhall SS, Gelb DE, et al. Pharmacological therapy for acute spinal cord injury. Neurosurgery. 2013;72(Suppl 2):93–105.

12. Short DJ, El Masry WS, Jones PW. High dose methylprednisolone in the management of acute spinal cord injury – a systematic review from a clinical perspective. Spinal Cord. 2000;38(5):273–86.

13. Geisler FH, Coleman WP, Grieco G, Poonian D. Recruitment and early treatment in a multicenter study of acute spinal cord injury. Spine. 2001;26(24 Suppl):S58–67.

14. Fehlings MG, Sekhon LH, Tator C. The role and timing of decompression in acute spinal cord injury: what do we know? What should we do? Spine. 2001;26(24 Suppl):S101–10.

15. Pourtaheri S, Emami A, Sinha K, Faloon M, Hwang K, Shafa E, et al. The role of magnetic resonance imaging in acute cervical spine fractures. Spine J. 2014;14(11):2546–53.

16. Sarani B, Waring S, Sonnad S, Schwab CW. Magnetic resonance imaging is a useful adjunct in the evaluation of the cervical spine of injured patients. J Trauma. 2007;63(3):637–40.

17. Como JJ, Diaz JJ, Dunham CM, Chiu WC, Duane TM, Capella JM, et al. Practice management guidelines for identification of cervical spine injuries following trauma: update from the eastern association for the surgery of trauma practice management guidelines committee. J Trauma. 2009;67(3):651–9.

18. Berry GE, Adams S, Harris MB, Boles CA, McKernan MG, Collinson F, et al. Are plain radiographs of the

spine necessary during evaluation after blunt trauma? Accuracy of screening torso computed tomography in thoracic/lumbar spine fracture diagnosis. J Trauma. 2005;59(6):1410–3; discussion 3.

19. Antevil JL, Sise MJ, Sack DI, Kidder B, Hopper A, Brown CV. Spiral computed tomography for the initial evaluation of spine trauma: a new standard of care? J Trauma. 2006;61(2):382–7.

20. Sheridan R, Peralta R, Rhea J, Ptak T, Novelline R. Reformatted visceral protocol helical computed tomographic scanning allows conventional radiographs of the thoracic and lumbar spine to be eliminated in the evaluation of blunt trauma patients. J Trauma. 2003;55(4):665–9.

21. Pizones J, Sanchez-Mariscal F, Zuniga L, Alvarez P, Izquierdo E. Prospective analysis of magnetic resonance imaging accuracy in diagnosing traumatic injuries of the posterior ligamentous complex of the thoracolumbar spine. Spine. 2013;38(9):745–51.

22. Vaccaro AR, Hulbert RJ, Patel AA, Fisher C, Dvorak M, Lehman RA Jr, et al. The subaxial cervical spine injury classification system: a novel approach to recognize the importance of morphology, neurology, and integrity of the disco-ligamentous complex. Spine. 2007;32(21):2365–74.

23. Theodore N, Aarabi B, Dhall SS, Gelb DE, Hurlbert RJ, Rozzelle CJ, et al. The diagnosis and management of traumatic atlanto-occipital dislocation injuries. Neurosurgery. 2013;72(Suppl 2):114–26.

24. Theodore N, Aarabi B, Dhall SS, Gelb DE, Hurlbert RJ, Rozzelle CJ, et al. Transportation of patients with acute traumatic cervical spine injuries. Neurosurgery. 2013;72(Suppl 2):35–9.

25. Kakarla UK, Chang SW, Theodore N, Sonntag VK. Atlas fractures. Neurosurgery. 2010;66(3 Suppl):60–7.

26. Anderson LD, D' Alonzo RT. Fractures of the odontoid process of the axis 1974. J Bone Joint Surg Am Vol. 2004;86-a(9):2081.

27. Apfelbaum RI, Lonser RR, Veres R, Casey A. Direct anterior screw fixation for recent and remote odontoid fractures. J Neurosurg. 2000;93(2 Suppl):227–36.

28. Keynan O, Fisher CG, Vaccaro A, Fehlings MG, Oner FC, Dietz J, et al. Radiographic measurement parameters in thoracolumbar fractures: a systematic review and consensus statement of the spine trauma study group. Spine. 2006;31(5):E156–65.

29. Hart RA. Cervical facet dislocation: when is magnetic resonance imaging indicated? Spine. 2002;27(1):116–7.

30. Lee JY, Nassr A, Eck JC, Vaccaro AR. Controversies in the treatment of cervical spine dislocations. Spine J. 2009;9(5):418–23.

31. Wimberley DW, Vaccaro AR, Goyal N, Harrop JS, Anderson DG, Albert TJ, et al. Acute quadriplegia following closed traction reduction of a cervical facet dislocation in the setting of ossification of the posterior longitudinal ligament: case report. Spine. 2005;30(15):E433–8.

32. Gelb DE, Aarabi B, Dhall SS, Hurlbert RJ, Rozzelle CJ, Ryken TC, et al. Treatment of subaxial cervical spinal injuries. Neurosurgery. 2013;72(Suppl 2):187–94.

33. Gelb DE, Hadley MN, Aarabi B, Dhall SS, Hurlbert RJ, Rozzelle CJ, et al. Initial closed reduction of cervical spinal fracture-dislocation injuries. Neurosurgery. 2013;72(Suppl 2):73–83.

34. Nassr A, Lee JY, Dvorak MF, Harrop JS, Dailey AT, Shaffrey CI, et al. Variations in surgical treatment of cervical facet dislocations. Spine. 2008;33(7):E188–93.

35. Pollard ME, Apple DF. Factors associated with improved neurologic outcomes in patients with incomplete tetraplegia. Spine. 2003;28(1):33–9.

36. Fehlings MG, Perrin RG. The timing of surgical intervention in the treatment of spinal cord injury: a systematic review of recent clinical evidence. Spine. 2006;31(11 Suppl):S28–35; discussion S6.

37. Papadopoulos SM, Selden NR, Quint DJ, Patel N, Gillespie B, Grube S. Immediate spinal cord decompression for cervical spinal cord injury: feasibility and outcome. J Trauma. 2002;52(2):323–32.

38. Uribe J, Green BA, Vanni S, Moza K, Guest JD, Levi AD. Acute traumatic central cord syndrome-experience using surgical decompression with open-door expansile cervical laminoplasty. Surg Neurol. 2005;63(6):505–10; discussion 10.

39. Fehlings MG, Vaccaro A, Wilson JR, Singh A, WC D, Harrop JS, et al. Early versus delayed decompression for traumatic cervical spinal cord injury: results of the Surgical Timing in Acute Spinal Cord Injury Study (STASCIS). PLoS One. 2012;7(2):e32037.

40. Anderson KK, Tetreault L, Shamji MF, Singh A, Vukas RR, Harrop JS, et al. Optimal timing of surgical decompression for acute traumatic central cord syndrome: a systematic review of the literature. Neurosurgery. 2015;77(Suppl 4):S15–32.

41. Kepler CK, Kong C, Schroeder GD, Hjelm N, Sayadipour A, Vaccaro AR, et al. Early outcome and predictors of early outcome in patients treated surgically for central cord syndrome. J Neurosurg Spine. 2015;23(4):490–4.

Thoracic Injury

Dong Kwan Kim and Geun Dong Lee

5.1 Introduction

Thoracic trauma accounts for 20–25% of all trauma-related deaths [1, 2]. Prompt assessment and immediate treatment can reduce the mortality rate. Initial evaluation and treatment of the patient include the primary survey, resuscitation, a detailed secondary survey, and definitive treatments. Most treatments are available without surgery if implemented quickly. Therefore, the clinicians should be well informed of assessment and treatment in advance for prompt and accurate management.

5.2 Primary Survey: Life-Threatening Injuries

For injuries found during the primary survey, immediate treatment should be performed including airway and shock managements. If necessary, the placement of the large-bore needle or chest tube should be performed promptly.

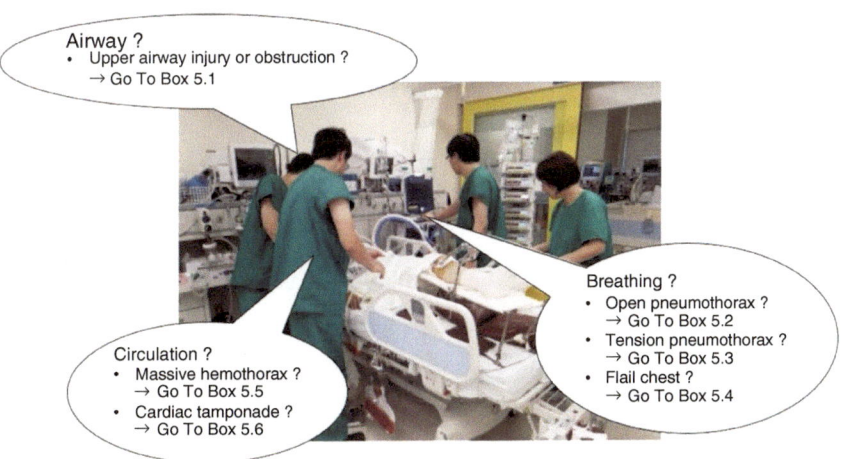

D. K. Kim (✉) · G. D. Lee
Department of Thoracic and Cardiovascular Surgery,
Asan Medical Center, University of Ulsan College of Medicine,
Seoul, South Korea
e-mail: dkkim@amc.seoul.kr

© Springer Nature Singapore Pte Ltd. 2019
S.-K. Hong et al. (eds.), *Primary Management of Polytrauma*,
https://doi.org/10.1007/978-981-10-5529-4_5

Key Points

1. The primary survey starts with the ABC (Airway, Breathing, Circulation).
2. Airway injury or obstruction: It is essential to check the open state of the airway. High level of suspicion is imperative for diagnosis.
3. Open pneumothorax: Sucking wounds should be covered with a clean plastic sheet, and only three sides of the sheet should be covered so that the other side can act like a one-way valve which requires for prevention of tension pneumothorax.
4. Tension pneumothorax: If clinical symptoms and physical examination are suspected, do not wait for an x-ray or other radiological examination. Emergency needle decompression should be considered.
5. Flail chest: If paradoxical movement is present, proper pain control and supportive ventilation should be done. If necessary, endotracheal intubation should be performed.
6. Massive hemothorax: Chest tube insertion should be performed, and the need for thoracotomy should be assessed and prepared. Patients with suspected cardiovascular injury or severe hypotension should consider emergency procedure with minimal investigation.
7. Cardiac tamponade: Diagnosis can be made with clinical symptoms and confirmed by ultrasound. Once confirmation is complete, proper fluid therapy, pericardiocentesis, and surgical treatment should be carried out.

Box 5.1 Upper Airway Injury and Obstruction

It is crucial to recognize upper airway injury during the primary survey. Though trauma in the larynx or trachea is rare and initially seen as insignificant, it can quickly deteriorate and be life-threatening with the mortality rate up to 40%.

1. Symptoms and signs:
   A. Presentation of respiratory distress, hemoptysis, subcutaneous emphysema
2. Diagnosis:
   A. Use the chest x-ray, chest computed tomography (CT) (Fig. 5.1)
3. A careful bronchoscopic examination including inspection of the tracheobronchial tree is required. This may involve the withdrawal of the endotracheal tube in an intubated patient to diagnose proximal tracheal tears.
4. Managements:
   A. Bypassing the lesion with endobronchial intubation is necessary.
   B. Primary surgical repair of the injured airway should be considered (Fig. 5.1).

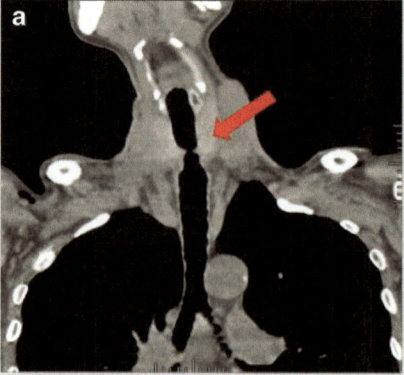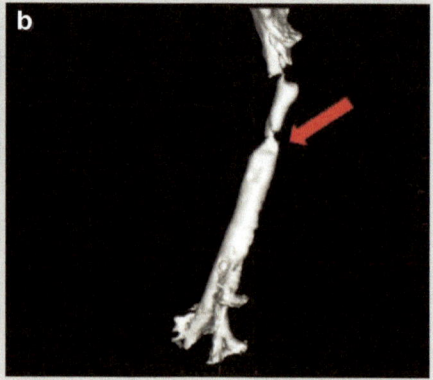

Fig. 5.1 Traumatic tracheal injury: (**a**) CT scan shows disruption of the cervical trachea (red arrows), (**b**) 3D reconstructed image of injured trachea

Airway Obstruction Due to the Posterior Dislocation of Clavicle (Fig. 5.2)

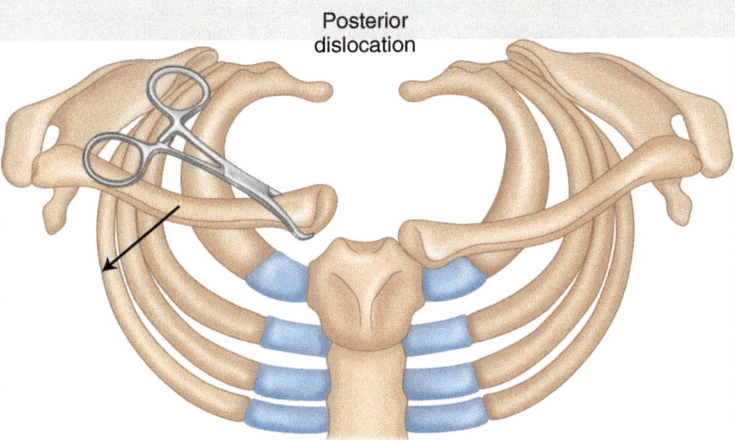

Fig. 5.2 Sternoclavicular joint injuries resulting posterior dislocation of the clavicle head can cause upper airway obstruction. Closed reduction entails shoulder extension, grasping the clavicle with a pointed instrument such as a towel clamp, and manual reduction. Reduction of the dislocated clavicle should not be delayed because of the correction of fractures. Once adjusted, it is rare to dislocate again

Box 5.2 Open Pneumothorax

Open pneumothorax can cause paradoxical respiration where the chest wall moves inward on inspiration and outward on expiration, the opposite of normal breathing. It is important to prevent respiratory insufficiency until the patient arrives at the hospital. And also, care must be taken to avoid infections by the inflow of external contaminants to the chest wall and thoracic cavity.

Skill I: Dressing for Open Pneumothorax

A temporary dressing should be applied to the wound at the scene of accident in an attempt to improve ventilation. Open sucking wounds should be covered with a clean square gauze or plastic sheet which is taped only on three sides ("three-way dressing") to avoid a tension pneumothorax. Packing or suturing the wound before inserting the thoracostomy tube also can cause tension pneumothorax. Usually, it is better to insert the chest tube through the normal skin away from the wound (Fig. 5.3).

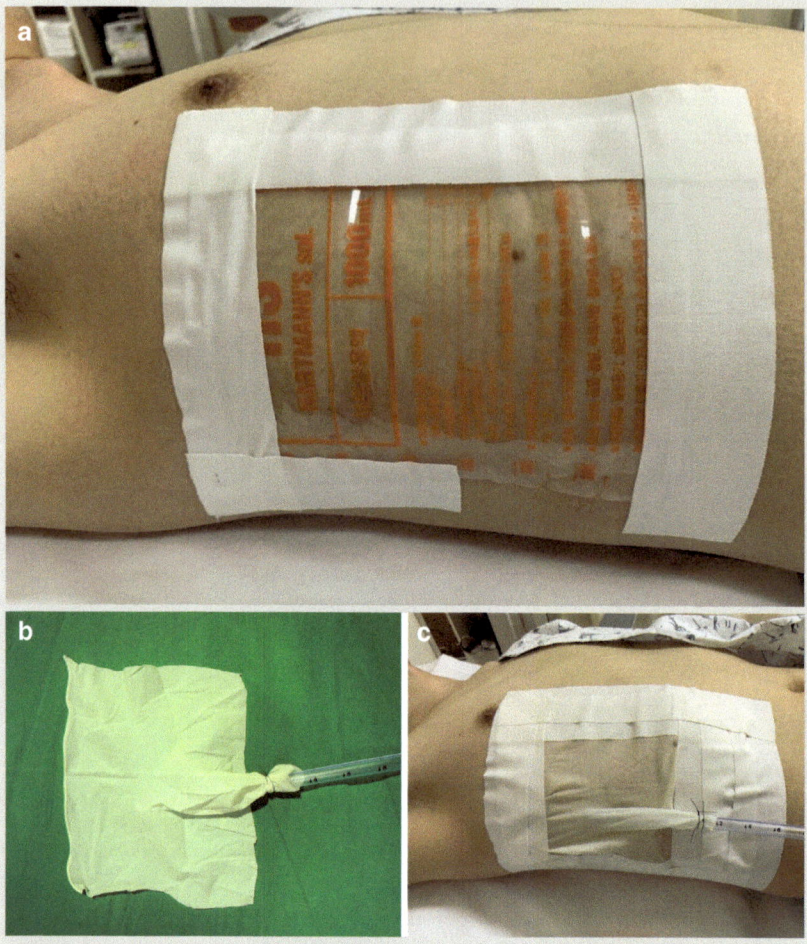

Fig. 5.3 Various dressing methods for open pneumothorax. (**a**) The "three-way dressing," placing a plastic sheet sealed on three sides, leaving the fourth one unsealed (at least a few inches) can create a one-way valve dressing. (**b**) Dressing method using a surgical glove, cut the surgical glove around the area containing the thumb to an appropriate size. Then, insert a chest tube through the finger tip of the glove. (**c**) Seal the open wound using the glove

---

Box 5.3 Tension Pneumothorax

Tension pneumothorax is a life-threatening condition requiring immediate treatment. Tension pneumothorax is caused by progressive building up of air within the pleural space, usually due to the laceration of the lung which allows air to escape into the pleural space without returning. Positive pressure ventilation may exacerbate this "one-way valve" effect. Progressive buildup pressure in the pleural space pushes the mediastinum to the opposite hemithorax and disrupts the veins from returning to the heart. This can destabilize the circulatory system and may result in traumatic arrest.

1. Symptoms and signs: the symptoms are usually quite severe.
    A. Severe dyspnea, tachypnea
    B. Hypotension, shock, neck vein distention
    C. Unilateral absence of breathing sound, hyperresonance on affected side
2. Diagnosis: chest x-ray (treatment should not be delayed for radiologic evaluation) (Fig. 5.4)

A. Deviation of the trachea away to the opposite site
B. Shift of the mediastinum
C. Depression of the hemidiaphragm

3. Managements:
   A. If tension pneumothorax is suspected, decompression of the intrathoracic pressure should be performed, immediately.
   B. Emergency needle decompression is first to be carried out to release trapped air in the pleural space, followed by the insertion of a chest tube.

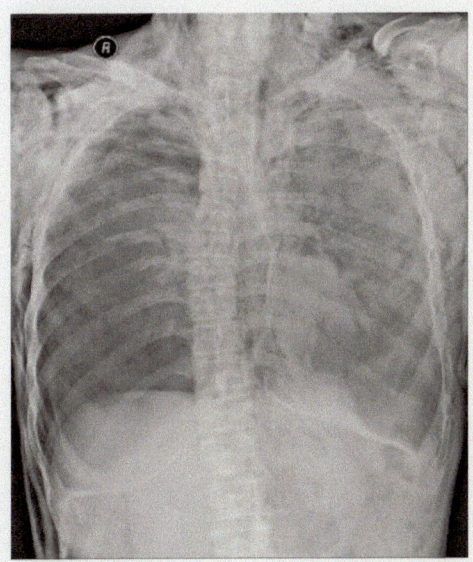

Fig. 5.4 Chest x-ray of tension pneumothorax: deviation of the trachea to the opposite side of the tension, shift of the mediastinum, depression of the hemidiaphragm

Skill II: Emergency Needle Decompression
Tension pneumothorax can be relieved by emergency needle decompression. Use a large diameter needle with sufficient length (16–18 gauge, greater than 4.5 cm in length). If air is not released immediately, needle should be repositioned. It should be taken into account that this method is not always successful (Fig. 5.5).

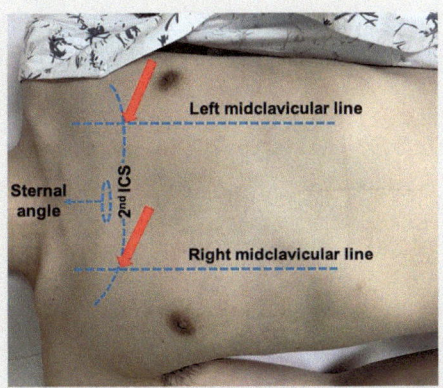

Fig. 5.5 Emergency needle decompression sites; most common location of the needle decompression is at the junction between the midclavicular line and the second intercostal space (red arrows) of the affected hemithorax

Skill III: Chest Tube Thoracostomy
Chest tube thoracostomy is a definite first-line treatment of a tension pneumothorax. Puncture of the pleura after blunt dissection decompresses the air and allows the chest tube to be placed into the pleural cavity to drain the air. The most common area for tube thoracotomy is 4–6th intercostal space, anterior to the midaxillary line. This area is referred to as the "triangle of safety," which borders the pectoralis major muscle anteriorly, latissimus dorsi muscle posteriorly, base of the axilla superiorly, and a horizontal line below the nipple inferiorly (Fig. 5.6).

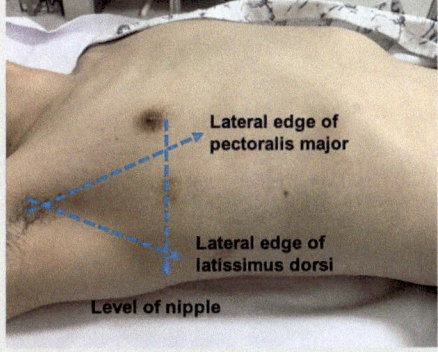

Fig. 5.6 "Safety triangle," preferred site for chest tube thoracostomy. This area is bounded by the pectoralis major muscle, latissimus dorsi, axilla, and the nipple [3]

Box 5.4 Flail Chest

Flail chest is defined radiographically as three or more consecutive rib fractures in two or more places, either unilateral or bilateral, thus causing thoracic cage instability. Patients with flail chest are distinct from those with multiple rib fractures as they are at a higher risk of respiratory compromise and often require early intervention [4, 5].

1. Symptoms and signs
   A. Asymmetrical movement of the chest wall or reverse motion of the chest wall is a distinctive sign of the flail chest. Reverse motion of chest wall is called paradoxical respiration, which is a type of breathing where the chest wall moves inward upon inspiration and outward upon expiration (Fig. 5.7).
   B. It is very important for examiners to keep the level of their eyes at the level of the patient's chest. The mechanical ventilator can make the diagnosis difficult for its positive pressure enables the chest moves simultaneously.

2. Managements
   A. Continuous close monitoring and serial arterial blood gas analysis (ABGA) are required, though initial ABGA is normal.
   B. For patients with normal oxygen saturation (SaO2) and ABGA, analgesia is indicated.
   C. Mechanical ventilation with endotracheal intubation is indicated for patients with respiratory failure with a respiratory rate of more than 40 breaths per minute or a partial pressure of oxygen (PO2) less than 60 mmHg despite applying of a face mask with 60% oxygen.
   D. Surgical fixation of fractured ribs can be useful in patients who are unable to wean the ventilator [2, 6–8].

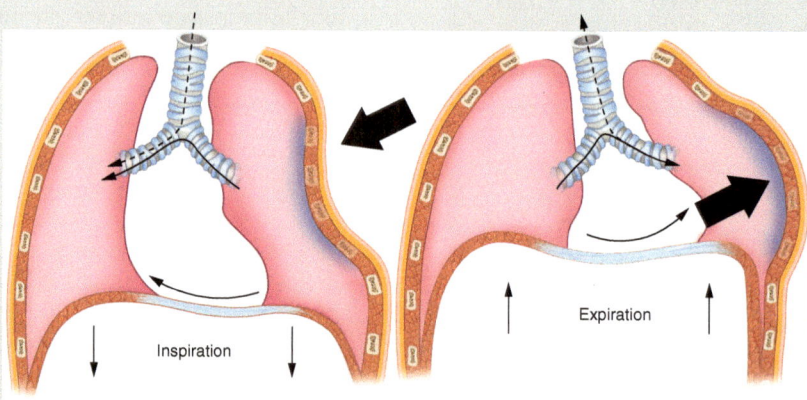

Fig. 5.7 Paradoxical movement in patient with flail chest. Reverse motion of chest wall is called paradoxical respiration, which is a type of breathing where the chest wall (red arrow) moves inward upon inspiration (**a**) and outward upon expiration (**b**)

Tips and Pitfalls

Rib Fixation Surgery

There has been growing evidence to suggest that open reduction and internal fixation of ribs benefit the patient. The surgical indications are limited to severely injured patients with flail chest (Fig. 5.8, Table 5.1).

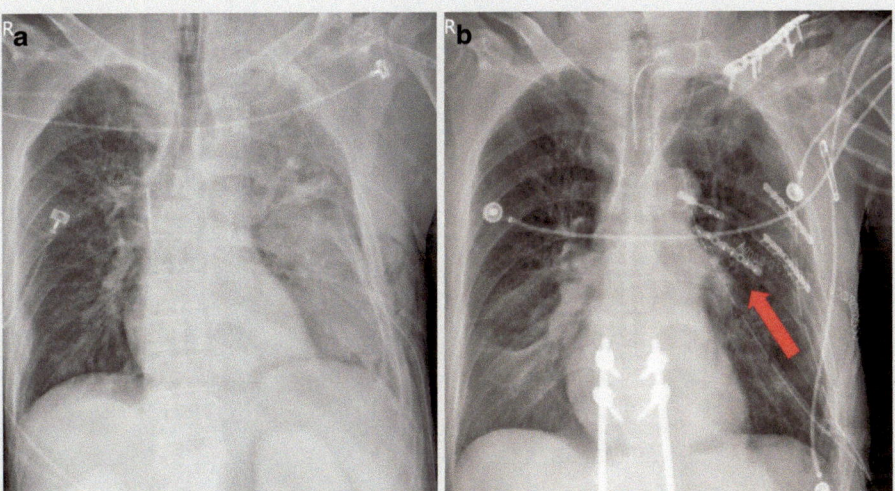

Fig. 5.8 Rib fixation surgery in patient who failed ventilator weaning due to flail chest: (**a**) preoperative chest x-ray, (**b**) chest x-ray after rib fixation surgery with titanium plates (red arrow). Surgery for clavicle fracture was performed simultaneously

Table 5.1 Indication of rib fixation surgery [8]

Recommended
≥5 rib flail chest requiring mechanical ventilation
Symptomatic nonunion
Severe displacement found during a thoracotomy for another reason
Relative indications
≥3 rib flail not requiring mechanical ventilation
≥3 ribs with severely displaced fractures (bi-cortical displacement)
≥3 ribs with mild to moderate displacement and 50% reduction of expected forced vital capacity percent despite optimal pain management
Contraindication
Contaminated field
Relative contraindications
Severe lung contusion requiring prolonged mechanical ventilation
High cervical spine injury requiring mechanical ventilation

Box 5.5 Massive Hemothorax

Massive hemothorax is defined as more than 1500 ml of bleeding from the chest or one-third of the pleural cavity filled with blood. Penetration of the chest cavity or blunt trauma can cause significant bleeding. Injuries of the great vessels such as the pulmonary artery, vein, and right atrium should be suspected first, and early surgical intervention should be considered.

1. Symptoms and signs
   A. Patients may have dyspnea, tachypnea, and hypovolemia. However, patients may often be asymptomatic in an early stage.
   B. Patients may present a shock with the absence of breath sounds and/or dullness to percussion on one side of the chest.

2. Diagnosis
   A. Radiographic image of a large hemothorax may be similar to that of pleural effusion. It is almost impossible to differentiate a hemothorax from other causes of pleural effusions (Fig. 5.9).
   B. Ultrasound has a very high sensitivity (92%), specificity (100%), positive predictive values (100%), and negative predictive values (98%) in detection of a hemothorax after trauma.
   C. CT is useful in determining the nature of the pleural fluid in the setting of trauma by assessing the attenuation value. Blood in the pleural space typically has an attenuation of 35–70 Hounsfield units (HU).

3. Managements
   A. Restoration of blood volume is a priority goal.
      1. Ensure large caliber IV lines, and crystalloid fluid should be infused rapidly.
      2. ABO compatible blood should be prepared and administered promptly.
   B. Decompression of the chest cavity
      1. Insert single large-bore chest tube (more than 28 French).
      2. Emergency thoracotomy or emergency surgery should be considered if 1500 mL of blood has evacuated initially or more than 200 mL/hour of bleeding persists for 2–4 hours.

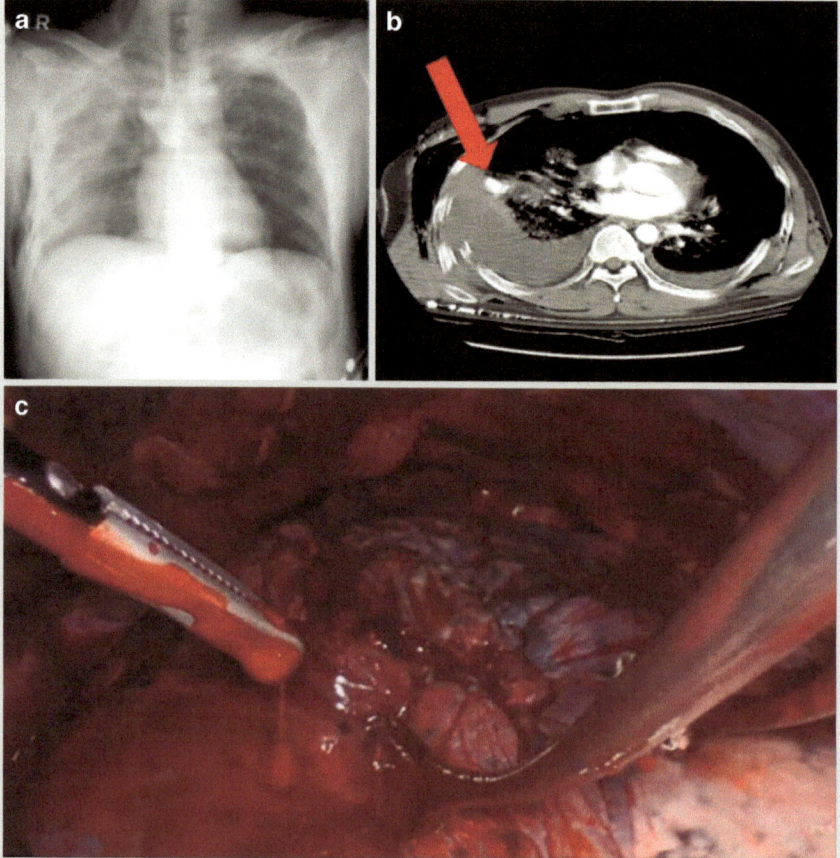

Fig. 5.9 Traumatic hemothorax: (**a**) Chest x-ray shows opacification of the right hemothorax. (**b**) Chest CT image reveals tear in the lung parenchyme, extravasation of contrast dye (red arrow), and a large hemothorax. (**c**) Intraoperative image of a massive hemothorax due to traumatic pulmonary laceration

Box 5.6 Cardiac Tamponade

Cardiac tamponade occurs when there is increased pressure and volume in the pericardium interrupting the blood flow which enters the ventricle, thus resulting in decreased cardiac output. It is a condition which can develop pulmonary edema, shock, and even death. Even a small amount of blood (60–100 ml) in the pericardium developed in a short time can cause symptoms of cardiac tamponade. Cardiac tamponade should be ruled out in patients with a stabbing wound in the chest or upper abdomen.

1. Symptoms and signs
   A. Symptoms include the rare Beck's triad (hypotension with a narrowed pulse pressure, jugular venous distention, muffled heart sounds). Muffled heart sounds are often difficult to detect in emergency situations. In addition, the jugular vein distension does not appear well in patients with hypovolemic shock. Therefore, if Beck's triad does not appear, it is not possible to exclude cardiac tamponade.
   B. Cardiac tamponade should be considered if the central venous pressure is increased to 15–20 cmH20 or more with persistent hypotension and tachycardia despite adequate fluid supply.
   C. Kussmaul's sign (a raise in central venous pressure during inspiration) is a true paradoxical venous pressure abnormality associated with tamponade.
2. Diagnosis
   A. If there is fluid in the pericardium and the right atrium and right ventricle is flattened during diastole
   B. Most chest x-rays showing normal findings
   C. Echocardiography
3. Managements: Evacuation of pericardial fluid is indicated for patients who do not respond to the usual management of resuscitation for hemorrhagic shock.
   A. Pericardiocentesis: Removing approximately 5–10 ml of blood from the pericardium may increase the output by 25–50%. Under the guidance with ultrasound, the Seldinger technique for insertion of flexible catheter is ideal. Pericardiocentesis may not be diagnostic or therapeutic when the blood in the pericardial sac has clotted. Complications may include cardiovascular damage or cardiac puncture or arrhythmia. Although cardiac tamponade is relieved by pericardiocentesis, surgery should be considered.
   B. Pericardiotomy via sternotomy or thoracotomy is indicated only when a qualified surgeon is available.
   C. All patients with an acute tamponade and a positive pericardiocentesis will require surgery to examine the heart and repair the injury (Fig. 5.10).

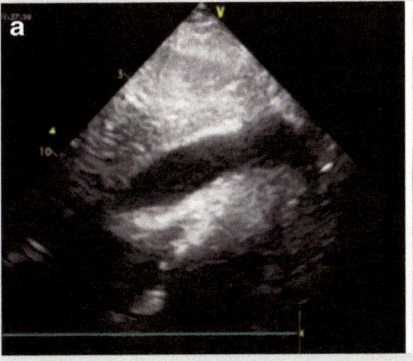
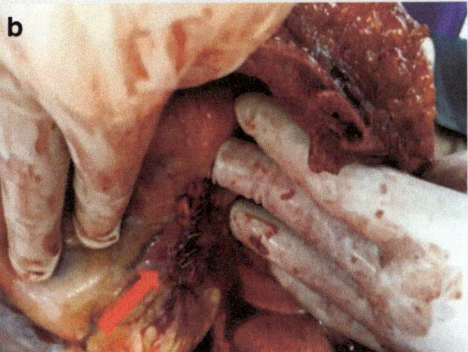
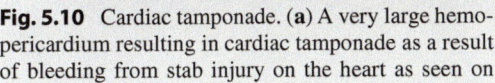

Fig. 5.10 Cardiac tamponade. (**a**) A very large hemopericardium resulting in cardiac tamponade as a result of bleeding from stab injury on the heart as seen on ultrasound (FAST, subxiphoid view). (**b**) Stab wound (red arrow) of the heart results in bleeding into pericardial sac

Box 5.7 Indications for Emergency Department Thoracotomy

Emergency thoracotomy clearly plays a role in the cases of penetrating thoracic trauma, particularly for trauma patients with cardiac tamponade from penetrating chest injuries [9] although the indications for emergency thoracotomy have been widely debated [10]. A qualified surgeon must be present to determine the need and potential for success of a resuscitative thoracotomy [11] (Table 5.2).

Table 5.2 Indications and contraindications for emergency department thoracotomy [12]

Accepted indications
Unresponsive hypotension (systolic blood pressure < 60 mmHg)
Rapid exsanguination from indwelling chest tube (>1500 ml)
Traumatic arrest with previously witnessed cardiac activity after penetrating thoracic injuries
Persistent hypotension (systolic blood pressure < 60 mmHg) with diagnostic cardiac tamponade, air embolism
Relative indications
Traumatic arrest with previously witnessed cardiac activity after blunt trauma
Traumatic arrest without previously witnessed cardiac activity after penetrating thoracic injuries
Prehospital cardiopulmonary resuscitation less than 10 min in intubated patients, 5 min in non-intubated patients
Contraindication
Blunt thoracic injuries with no previously witnessed cardiac activity
Multiple blunt trauma
Severe head injury

Skill IV: Bilateral Anterior Thoracotomy (Clamshell Incision) for Emergency Thoracotomy

Emergency thoracotomy is a procedure that provides rapid access to the intrathoracic structures for thoracic trauma patients. In severe cases of thoracic trauma, specific injuries, even if suspected, is difficult to detect. In this case, the surgical approach should be accessible to all thoracic structures for rapid assessment and management (Fig. 5.11). Therefore, the clamshell approach in the supine position could be a good option in those hemodynamically unstable patients particularly when lateral position is intolerable [13].

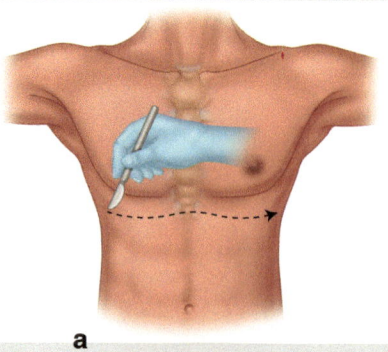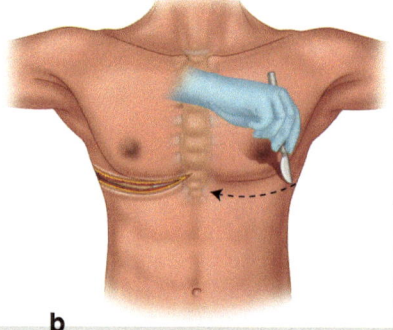
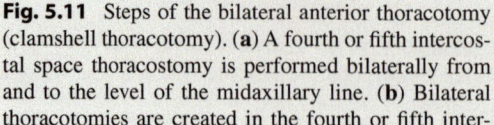

Fig. 5.11 Steps of the bilateral anterior thoracotomy (clamshell thoracotomy). (**a**) A fourth or fifth intercostal space thoracostomy is performed bilaterally from and to the level of the midaxillary line. (**b**) Bilateral thoracotomies are created in the fourth or fifth intercostal spaces by starting from the thoracostomy and extending incisions to the sternum. (**c**) The sternum is cut with heavy plaster or "paramedic" scissors. (**d**) A retractor is placed with the bar on the right side. (**e**) Open chest with rib spreader in situ [13, 14]

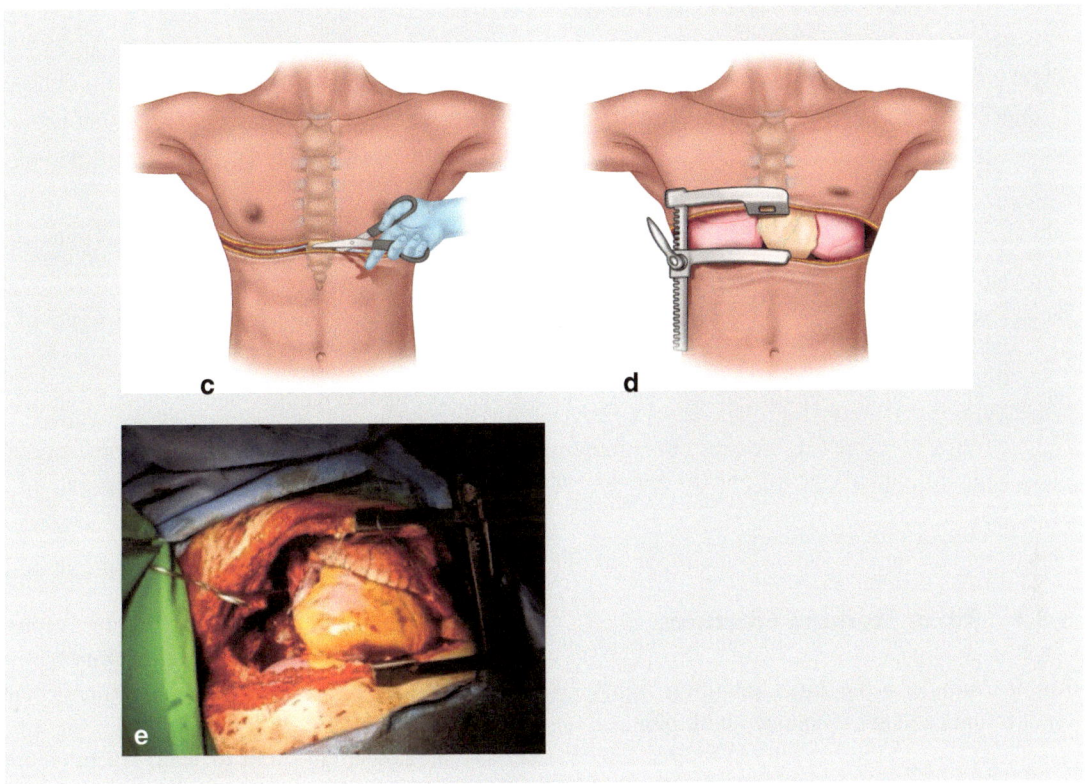

5.3   Secondary Survey: Potentially Life-Threatening Injuries

Secondary assessments include more detailed physical and radiological tests, cardiac monitors, and oxygen saturation tests. This condition can be life-threatening if not found immediately after the damage.

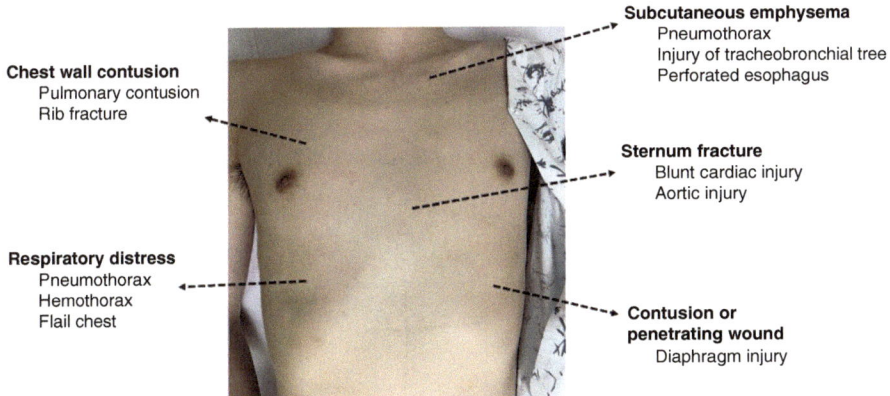

Key Points

During the secondary survey, the following injuries should be identified and treated:

1. Rib fracture or sternal fracture: The extent and location of the rib fracture can be used to assess the degree of damage to the internal organs.
2. Pneumothorax or hemothorax: Diagnose with a chest x-ray and CT; chest tube insertion is necessary in most cases.
3. Pulmonary contusion: Diagnose using a chest x-ray and CT, proper fluid therapy and ventilatory control are needed, and if necessary, endotracheal intubation should be performed.
4. Blunt cardiac injury: Common complications are arrhythmia. Treat with other associated injuries.
5. Aortic disruption: Chest x-ray shows mediastinal widening and chest CT is useful for diagnosis.
6. Rupture of the diaphragm: It is easy to miss if clinicians do not doubt. Most require surgical treatment.
7. Blunt rupture of esophagus: Mortality can be reduced by performing surgery quickly.

5.3.1 Rib or Sternum Fractures

Rib fractures are the most common injury of chest trauma and are associated with pain.

1. Symptoms and signs include localized pain, tenderness on palpation, and crepitation.
2. Diagnosis
   A. Chest x-ray (including rib series) required. However, fracture at the costochondral junction may not be seen on chest x-rays.
   1. Upper rib (first to third) fractures illustrate the magnitude of the injury.
   2. Middle rib (4th to 9th) fractures occur in majority of blunt trauma.
   3. Lower rib (10th to 12th) fractures can cause intra-abdominal injuries as well as hepatosplenic injuries.
   B. CT scan can be utilized as an adjunct.
   C. Bone scan can be an effective method in detecting missed fractures among patients with trauma induced.

3. Managements.
   A. Most of the uncomplicated rib fractures do not require surgical treatment; however, it is important to identify the associated injuries.
   B. Early and aggressive pain control is important.

5.3.2 Pneumothorax

Pneumothorax can be treated differently depending on its volume and cause. In patients with traumatic pneumothorax, the closed thoracostomy should be performed before general anesthesia or positive pressure ventilation or transfer to other hospitals. Otherwise, it may evolve into tension pneumothorax due to the positive pressure ventilation, which may pose as a life threat.

1. Symptoms and signs
   A. Patients are often asymptomatic.
   B. Dyspnea and tachypnea are the main symptoms.
2. Diagnosis
   A. An upright expiratory chest x-ray aids in the diagnosis.
   B. Chest CT is often performed to identify other lesions in the thorax.
3. Managements: Drainage actually depends on physiologic status of patient.

A. Oxygen administration is required first.

B. Stable pneumothorax less than 25% can be managed without drainage. Serial x-ray after 6–8 hours for reassessment is recommended. Air slowly resorbs from the pleural space at a rate of approximately 1.5%/day. This rate will increase with use of supplemental oxygen.

C. Significant pneumothorax greater than 25% usually requires chest tube drainage. If the patient is undergoing mechanical ventilation or undergoing air transport prior to transfer to another facility, pneumothorax should be treated with thoracostomy tubes.

Tips and Pitfalls (Fig. 5.12)

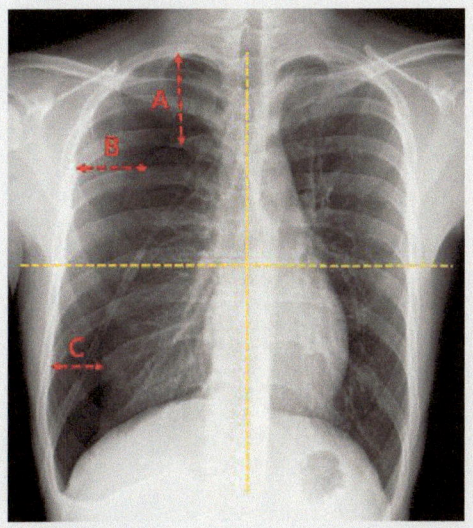

Fig. 5.12 Pneumothorax volume calculation. Diagram showing location of interpleural distance measurements on the chest x-ray (A, interpleural distance (cm) between apex and apex of the lung; B, interpleural distance (cm) at midpoint of the upper half; C, interpleural distance (cm) at midpoint of the lower half). Calculated percentage pneumothorax = 4.2 + (4.7 × (A + B + C) % [15]

5.3.3   Hemothorax

1. Causes include laceration of the lung, intercostal vessel or internal mammary artery, or thoracic spine fracture.

2. Diagnosis
   A. Diagnosis can be achieved using a chest x-ray.
   B. Ultrasonography confirms fluid retention in the pleural cavity, which is helpful for the diagnosis of hemothorax [16].
   C. A chest CT is often performed to identify other lesions in the thorax.

3. Managements
   A. Asymptomatic patients with a normal chest radiograph can be safely observed [17]. A serial chest x-ray at 6–8 hours seems to be a reasonable time period to see signs and symptoms of a delayed hemothorax or pneumothorax.
   B. If the hemothorax is visible on the x-ray, it is ideal to insert a large chest tube (28–32 Fr.).
   C. The indications for surgical exploration are as follows:
      1. Initial chest tube drainage more than 1500 ml of blood.
      2. Drainage of more than 200 ml/hour for 2–4 consecutive hours after chest tube placement [18].

Tips and Pitfalls
If the patient has more than 200–300 ml of blood, an x-ray in a standing position can be utilized to diagnose the condition. However, in the supine position, even if the blood is greater than 1000 ml, the diagnosis occasionally cannot be made.

5.3.4   Pulmonary Contusion

Blunt thoracic trauma manifests in various ways, depending on the structures injured and type of injury, commonly manifested as parenchymal contusion [19]. A pulmonary contusion refers to an interstitial and/or alveolar lung injury without any frank laceration. Although pulmonary contusions are generally associated with concomitant thoracic cage damage, it can be isolated without evident rib fracture [18].

1. Symptoms and signs
   A. The usual clinical manifestations include hemoptysis, cough, dyspnea, chest pain, fever, and leukocytosis.

2. Diagnosis
   A. Chest x-ray is the first evaluation method.
   B. A CT scans are superior for detecting pulmonary contusion.

3. Managements
   A. Oxygen administration is required first.
   B. If respiratory failure is present, mechanical ventilation is required. Patients with significant hypoxia ($PaO_2 < 65$ mmHg, $SaO_2 < 90\%$) should be intubated and ventilated within 1 hour after the injury [18].

Tips and Pitfalls
Traumatic Pulmonary Pseudocyst
The parenchyma gets lacerated in a bursting manner resulting in a cavity formation. Traumatic pulmonary pseudocysts may appear immediately or within a few hours after injury, and their sizes range from 2 to 14 cm in diameter. Traumatic pulmonary pseudocysts are usually benign lesions which mostly needs conservative management unless complications arise. Traumatic pseudocysts usually resolve within 4 months (Fig. 5.13).

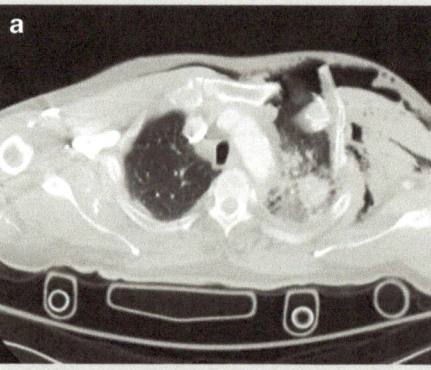
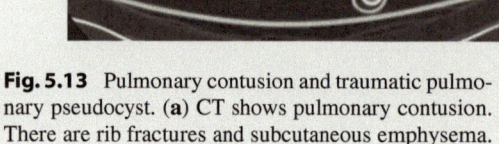
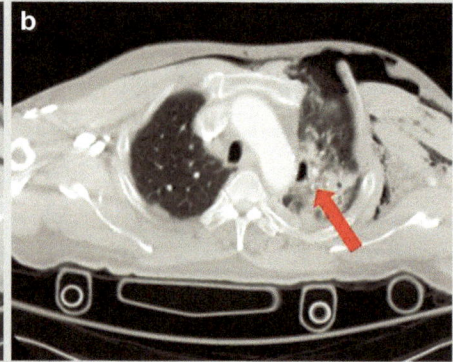

Fig. 5.13 Pulmonary contusion and traumatic pulmonary pseudocyst. (**a**) CT shows pulmonary contusion. There are rib fractures and subcutaneous emphysema. (**b**) CT demonstrates cystic structure (red arrow) in the left upper lobe surrounded by pulmonary contusion

5.3.5 Tracheobronchial Tree Injury

More than 80% of tracheobronchial ruptures occur within 2.5 cm of the carina. In only 30% of cases is a definitive diagnosis made within 24 hours of injury. For proper diagnosis, high level of suspicion is imperative.

1. Symptoms and signs
   A. Persistent pneumothorax with massive air leakage or incomplete expansion of the lung after placement of chest tube.

2. Diagnosis
   A. Chest x-ray and chest CT can demonstrate pneumothorax, pneumomediastinum, or subcutaneous emphysema.
   B. A careful bronchoscopic examination is required.

3. Managements
   A. Airway patency should be the first step. If patients are in acute stage with severe air leakage with respiratory difficulties and unstable condition, patients should be intubated. Temporary intuba-

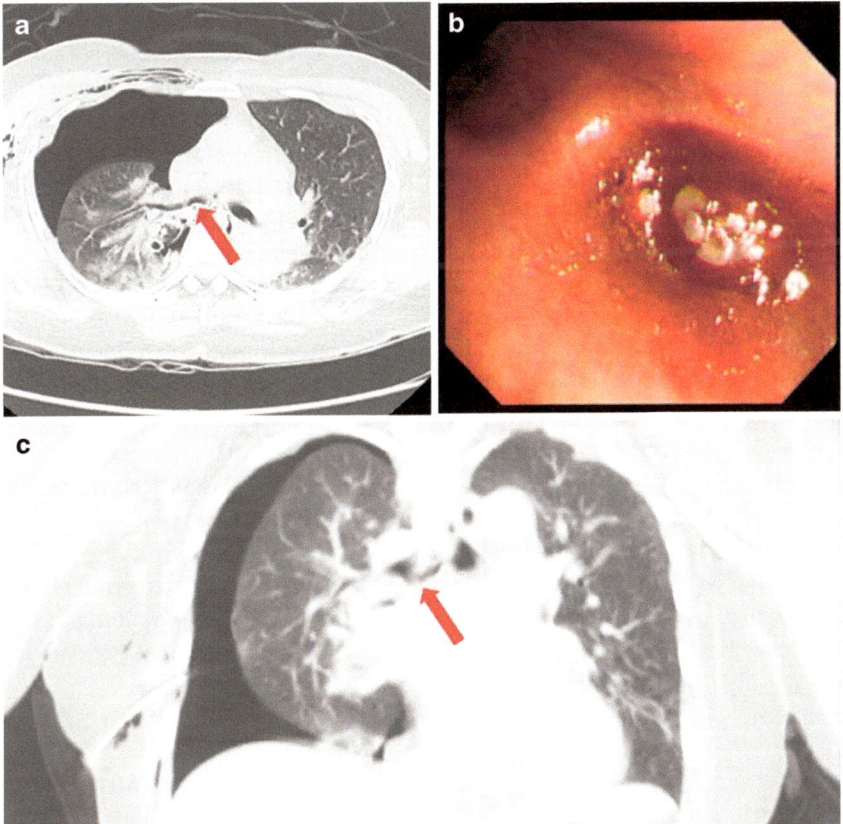

Fig. 5.14 Traumatic bronchial injury. (**a**) Axial CT image of the chest in lung window settings shows an injury at the right main bronchus (red arrow), right pneumothorax with underlying collapse of the right lung, and subcutaneous emphysema over right side. (**b**) The bronchoscopic image indicates that the right main bronchus is full of hematoma. (**c**) Coronal reconstructed image

tion of the opposite main stem bronchus may be required to provide adequate oxygenation.

B. In principle, rupture of the trachea and bronchus should be operated as soon as possible. Early repair on healthy tissue with quick improvement of the dysfunction of ventilation can provide better clinical outcome.

C. In stable patients, surgery may be delayed until acute inflammation and edema resolve (Fig. 5.14).

5.3.6 Blunt Cardiac Injury

It may vary from asymptomatic or symptomatic cardiac contusion to full cardiac rupture. Direct blunt trauma over the precordium or rapid deceleration accidents can cause blunt cardiac injury in the anterior aspect of the right ventricle, interventricular septum, and left ventricle.

1. Symptoms and signs
   A. Patients are often asymptomatic. However, blunt cardiac trauma may be associated with cardiac failure, cardiac arrhythmia, and hypotension.
2. Diagnosis: For proper diagnosis, a high level of suspicion is imperative.
   A. A FAST exam can diagnose tamponade due to cardiac rupture.
   B. New-onset tachyarrhythmias, especially sinus tachycardia, are the most common findings on an ECG. This initial ECG is the best indicator of blunt cardiac injury [20].

C. Initial cardiac enzyme measurement on admission and following measurement is required 6–8 hours later. Troponin I have been shown to have the highest specificity. An elevation of troponin signifies the presence of blunt myocardial injury [21].

D. Normal ECG and cardiac enzyme on admission reliably exclude any significant cardiac contusion.

3. Managements

A. If a patient shows no symptoms or evidence of cardiac enzyme abnormality with normal readings on the ECG, the patient can be discharged and monitored through outpatient clinic.

B. If a patient shows an abnormality in the ECG with no clinical symptoms, the patient should be monitored for 24 hours.

C. Patients with abnormal ECG and elevated cardiac enzymes should be hospitalized due to the high likelihood of subsequent cardiac complications.

5.3.7 Traumatic Aortic Injury

The thoracic great vessels consist of the aorta and its major intrathoracic branches. The site of injury is usually to the aortic isthmus (medial descending aorta at the ligamentum arteriosum), where shear forces caused by rapid deceleration result in a tear at this point of fixation of the vasculature. A high index of suspicion in a patient who has suffered a high-speed collision is critical as approximately half of the patients with contained aortic rupture have no external signs of trauma [22].

1. Symptoms and signs include chest and back pain, hoarseness (compression of the recurrent laryngeal nerve), and hypertension in the arms with hypotension in the legs.

2. Diagnosis

A. Chest x-ray shows mediastinal widening (usually more than 8 cm at the upper mediastinum). However, sometimes the chest x-ray may be normal.

B. Contrast-enhanced CT scan has been shown to be an accurate screening method for patients with suspected aortic injury.

C. Transesophageal echocardiogram (TEE) can be performed for patients in intensive care unit who cannot be moved for CT scan or aortography.

3. Managements

A. Maintain the systolic blood pressure at 90–100 mmHg to minimize the risk of free rupture. The aortic repair can be delayed for a few days given the blood pressure is controlled.

B. Thoracic endovascular aortic repair (TEVAR) is an acceptable approach for the treatment of traumatic aortic injury [23].

C. For injuries involving aortic arch which cannot be treated with TEVAR, open surgical repair is required. A qualified surgeon should treat patients with traumatic aortic injury.

5.3.8 Diaphragm Injury

In blunt trauma the diaphragmatic rupture is usually secondary to severe abdominal trauma resulting in abrupt increase in intra-abdominal pressure. Fractured ribs can also cause a diaphragmatic tear. Deceleration injuries may result in avulsion of the diaphragm from its peripheral attachments. Most (approximately 70%) of the injuries involve the left diaphragm [24, 25]. Rupture of the right diaphragm requires a greater intense force and is almost always associated with other intra-abdominal injuries.

1. Symptoms and signs

A. Patients are often asymptomatic, especially in small penetrating injuries.

B. Blood loss, cardiopulmonary distress due to massive diaphragmatic hernia, and abdominal visceral obstruction can occur.

C. A diaphragmatic hernia may occur within minutes, hours, weeks, or years after the injury. The stomach, colon, and omentum

Tips and Pitfalls

Thoracic endovascular aortic repair (TEVAR) for the management of traumatic aortic dissection (Fig. 5.15)

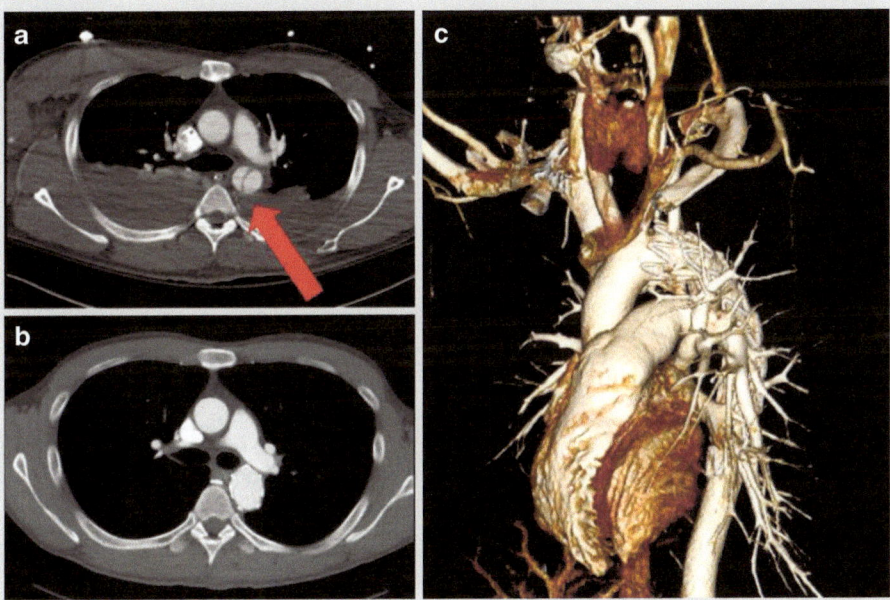

Fig. 5.15 (**a**) Preinterventional chest CT in young male patient injured in pedestrian traffic accident. A typical traumatic dissection flap (red arrow) is observed in the aortic isthmus region. This patient was treated with emergency TEVAR. (**b**) An 8-month fol- low-up CT shows a complete expansion of the stent graft inside the aorta. (**c**) Multi-detector CT scan, with 3D volume rendering reconstruction, shows complete exclusion of the lesion of proximal descending tho- racic aorta with adequate remodeling of the aorta

are the most commonly herniated visceral organ.

2. Diagnosis: Early diagnosis and treatment are very important because complicated diaphrag- matic hernias are associated with high mor- bidity and mortality. High index of suspicion is the most important determinant for early diagnosis. Every penetrating wound over the lower chest should be considered as involving the diaphragm injury.

   A. Chest x-ray may show an elevated hemi- diaphragm, air fluid levels, or an air- containing viscus in the chest. However, in approximately half the cases of diaphrag- matic injuries, the chest x-ray usually shows a nonspecific hemopneumothorax. If the stomach is suspected to be in the chest, a chest x-ray after the insertion of the nasogastric tube is beneficial.

   B. CT scan can be helpful in diagnosing dia- phragmatic hernias; however they do not detect small uncomplicated diaphragmatic perforations.

   C. Laparoscopy and/or thoracoscopy is uti- lized for asymptomatic patients with pen- etrating injuries below the nipple line and above the costal margin for the diagnosis of diaphragmatic injury. Prior to laparos- copy, an observation period of 6–8 hours is recommended to exclude any intra- abdominal injuries.

3. Managements

   A. If a diaphragmatic hernia is suspected, do not insert a chest tube preoperatively.

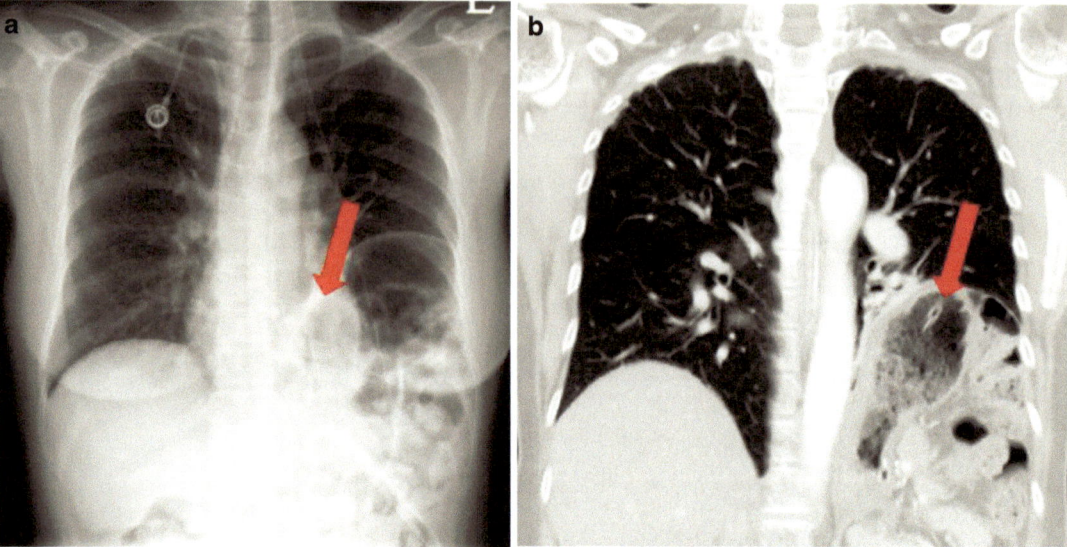

Fig. 5.16 Diaphragm rupture: (**a**) Chest x-ray shows a stomach projects in the lower left hemithorax. The position of nasogastric tube (red arrow) indicates the stomach is located in the left thoracic cavity. (**b**) CT scan shows left diaphragmatic rupture with herniation of the stomach into the left thoracic cavity

B. Diaphragmatic ruptures should be repaired surgically as soon as possible. Surgical repair with laparoscopy or with open laparotomy is necessary.

C. Small perforations in the posterior right diaphragm do not require repair because the liver protects it from herniation. However, anterior injuries should be repaired as herniation can occur.

D. Thoracoscopy is rarely used during the acute stages. It might be the approach of choice in the presence of associated significant residual hemothorax requiring evacuation (Fig. 5.16).

5.3.9 Esophageal Injury

Trauma to the esophagus is rare due to the location of the thoracic esophagus in the posterior mediastinum [26]. Traumatic esophageal injury is mainly caused by penetrating injury with approximately 1% caused by blunt trauma. Cervical esophageal injury is the most common and is often associated with tracheal injury. Damage caused by blunt trauma occurs when the contents of the stomach are ejected into the esophagus causing damage to the lower esophagus.

1. Symptoms and signs: It is necessary to suspect an esophageal injury given the patient has the following unique symptoms:
   A. Neck pain, dysphagia, or hematemesis
   B. Left pneumothorax without rib fracture or hemothorax
   C. Foreign body in the chest tube
2. Diagnosis
   A. Chest x-ray may show mediastinal emphysema.
   B. CT scan can be helpful, but unable to detect small esophageal perforations.
   C. If the patient is stable, esophagography using a water-soluble contrast medium (Gastrografin) is performed. Negative study should be followed with barium.
   D. Esophagoscopy is useful in patients unable to swallow. Esophagoscopy has been reported to have higher sensitivity than contrast studies [27].
3. Managements: Greater than 90% of patients require surgical treatment (Fig. 5.17).

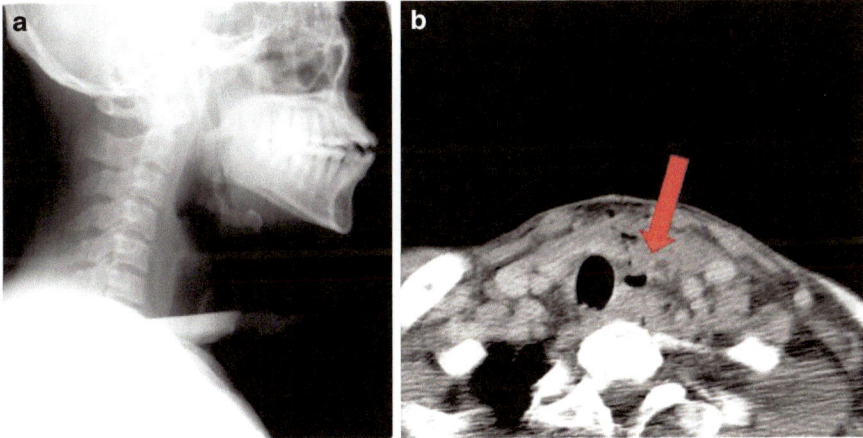

Fig. 5.17 Traumatic cervical esophageal perforation. (**a**) Stab injury on x-ray. (**b**) CT scan shows the esophageal perforation with subcutaneous emphysema (red arrow) in the soft tissues of the neck

5.4   Summary

5.4.1   Primary Survey

The first line of assessment of chest trauma begins from the ABC (Airway, Breathing, Circulation). The aim of the primary survey is to identify the life-threatening injuries requiring immediate treatment.

- Airway injury or obstruction
- Open pneumothorax
- Tension pneumothorax
- Flail chest
- Massive hemothorax
- Cardiac tamponade

5.4.2   Secondary Survey

Secondary survey entails a more precise physical examination, radiologic evaluation, electrocardiogram monitoring, and oxygen saturation. It could be fatal if treatment is delayed. Therefore, an accurate diagnosis is essential.

- Rib or sternal fractures
- Pneumothorax or hemothorax
- Pulmonary contusion
- Blunt cardiac injury

- Traumatic aortic injury
- Diaphragmatic injury
- Esophageal injury

Acknowledgments We would like to thank Dr. Dae Sung Ma and Hong Jun Bae for their photographic materials and Byung Kwon Chong, Yong Ho Jeong, Yooyoung Chong, Jae Kwang Yun, and Wayne Ser for the English proofreading.

References

1. LoCicero J 3rd, Mattox KL. Epidemiology of chest trauma. Surg Clin North Am. 1989;69(1):15–9.
2. Richardson JD, Franklin GA, Heffley S, Seligson D. Operative fixation of chest wall fractures: an underused procedure? Am Surg. 2007;73(6):591–6; discussion 6–7.
3. Dev SP, Nascimiento B Jr, Simone C, Chien V. Videos in clinical medicine. Chest-tube insertion. N Engl J Med. 2007;357(15):e15.
4. Freedland M, Wilson RF, Bender JS, Levison MA. The management of flail chest injury: factors affecting outcome. J Trauma. 1990;30(12):1460–8.
5. Velmahos GC, Vassiliu P, Chan LS, Murray JA, Berne TV, Demetriades D. Influence of flail chest on outcome among patients with severe thoracic cage trauma. Int Surg. 2002;87(4):240–4.
6. Balci AE, Eren S, Cakir O, Eren MN. Open fixation in flail chest: review of 64 patients. Asian Cardiovasc Thorac Ann. 2004;12(1):11–5.
7. Bemelman M, de Kruijf MW, van Baal M, Leenen L. Rib fractures: to fix or not to fix? An evidence-

based algorithm. Korean J Thorac Cardiovasc Surg. 2017;50(4):229–34.

8. de Moya M, Nirula R, Biffl W. Rib fixation: who, what, when? Trauma Surg Acute Care Open. 2017;2(1):e000059.

9. Lewis G, Knottenbelt JD. Should emergency room thoracotomy be reserved for cases of cardiac tamponade? Injury. 1991;22(1):5–6.

10. Mejia JC, Stewart RM, Cohn SM. Emergency department thoracotomy. Semin Thorac Cardiovasc Surg. 2008;20(1):13–8.

11. Alexander RH, Proctor HJ, American College of Surgeons. Committee on Trauma. Advanced trauma life support program for physicians : ATLS. 5th ed. Chicago: American College of Surgeons; 1993.

12. Working Group AHSoOACoSCoT. Practice management guidelines for emergency department thoracotomy. Working Group, Ad Hoc Subcommittee on Outcomes, American College of Surgeons-Committee on Trauma. J Am Coll Surg. 2001;193(3):303–9.

13. Simms ER, Flaris AN, Franchino X, Thomas MS, Caillot JL, Voiglio EJ. Bilateral anterior thoracotomy (clamshell incision) is the ideal emergency thoracotomy incision: an anatomic study. World J Surg. 2013;37(6):1277–85.

14. Wise D, Davies G, Coats T, Lockey D, Hyde J, Good A. Emergency thoracotomy: "how to do it". Emerg Med J. 2005;22(1):22–4.

15. Collins CD, Lopez A, Mathie A, Wood V, Jackson JE, Roddie ME. Quantification of pneumothorax size on chest radiographs using interpleural distances: regression analysis based on volume measurements from helical CT. AJR Am J Roentgenol. 1995;165(5):1127–30.

16. Sisley AC, Rozycki GS, Ballard RB, Namias N, Salomone JP, Feliciano DV. Rapid detection of traumatic effusion using surgeon-performed ultrasonography. J Trauma. 1998;44(2):291–6; discussion 6–7.

17. Brown PF 3rd, Larsen CP, Symbas PN. Management of the asymptomatic patient with a stab wound to the chest. South Med J. 1991;84(5):591–3.

18. Sellke FW, Del Nido PJ, Swanson SJ. Sabiston & Spencer surgery of the chest. 9th ed. Philadelphia: Elsevier; 2016. 2 volumes (xxix, 2410, 48 pages) p.

19. Bastos R, Calhoon JH, Baisden CE. Flail chest and pulmonary contusion. Semin Thorac Cardiovasc Surg. 2008;20(1):39–45.

20. Foil MB, Mackersie RC, Furst SR, Davis JW, Swanson MS, Hoyt DB, et al. The asymptomatic patient with suspected myocardial contusion. Am J Surg. 1990;160(6):638–42; discussion 42–3.

21. Sybrandy KC, Cramer MJ, Burgersdijk C. Diagnosing cardiac contusion: old wisdom and new insights. Heart. 2003;89(5):485–9.

22. Mattox KL. Approaches to trauma involving the major vessels of the thorax. Surg Clin North Am. 1989;69(1):77–91.

23. Rousseau H, Elaassar O, Marcheix B, Cron C, Chabbert V, Combelles S, et al. The role of stent-grafts in the management of aortic trauma. Cardiovasc Intervent Radiol. 2012;35(1):2–14.

24. Shah R, Sabanathan S, Mearns AJ, Choudhury AK. Traumatic rupture of diaphragm. Ann Thorac Surg. 1995;60(5):1444–9.

25. Al-Refaie RE, Awad E, Mokbel EM. Blunt traumatic diaphragmatic rupture: a retrospective observational study of 46 patients. Interact Cardiovasc Thorac Surg. 2009;9(1):45–9.

26. Bryant AS, Cerfolio RJ. Esophageal trauma. Thorac Surg Clin. 2007;17(1):63–72.

27. Bastos RB, Graeber GM. Esophageal injuries. Chest Surg Clin N Am. 1997;7(2):357–71.

Abdominal Injury

Suk-Kyung Hong

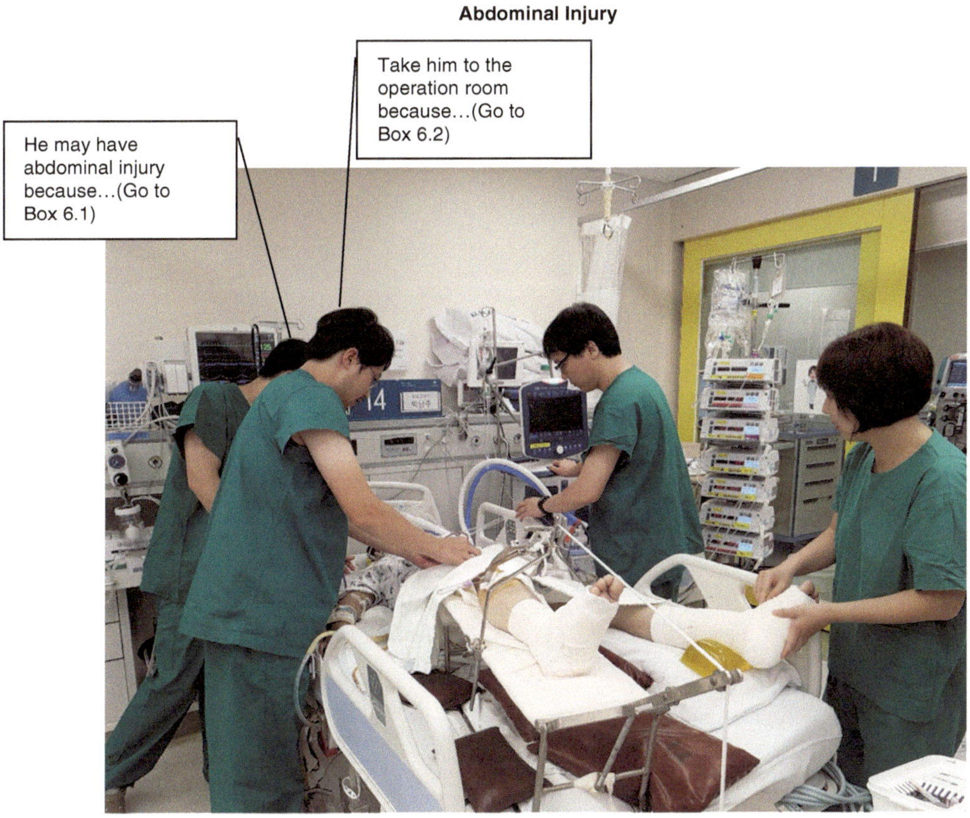

Fig. 6.1 Multidisciplinary approach to abdominal injury patient

S.-K. Hong (✉)
Division of Acute Care Surgery, Department of
Surgery, Asan Medical Center, University of Ulsan
College of Medicine, Seoul, South Korea
e-mail: skhong94@amc.seoul.kr

© Springer Nature Singapore Pte Ltd. 2019
S.-K. Hong et al. (eds.), *Primary Management of Polytrauma*,
https://doi.org/10.1007/978-981-10-5529-4_6

Box 6.1

Abdominal injury is suspected, when patients show the findings from ① to ④:

① Abdominal pain.
② Abdominal bruise, seat belt sign.

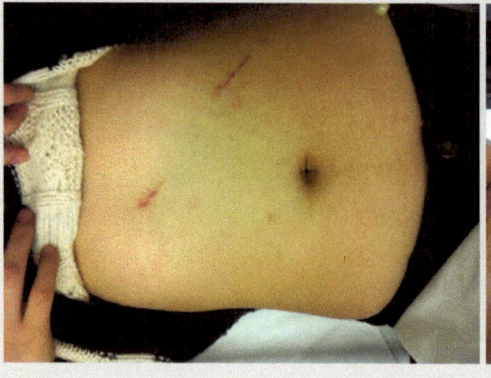 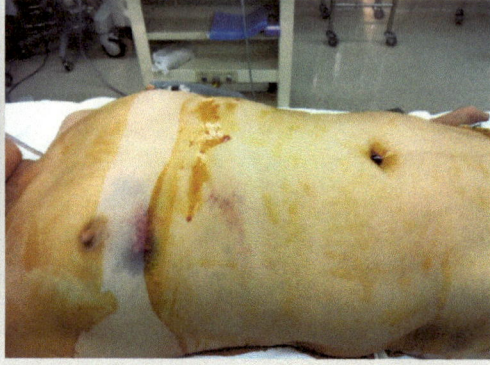

③ If unconscious, patient is under shock.
④ If unconscious, abdomen is distended.

Box 6.2

Take the patient to operation room, when:

① Hypotensive blunt trauma with a positive FAST or clinical evidence of intraabdominal bleeding
② Hypotensive penetrating abdominal trauma
③ Free air or retroperitoneal air
④ Peritonitis

⑤ Diaphragmatic hernia
⑥ Evisceration

The abdomen can be injured in many types of trauma; injury may be confined to the abdomen or be accompanied by severe, multisystem trauma. The nature and severity of abdominal injuries vary widely depending on the mechanism and forces involved, thus generalizations about mortality and need for operation tend to be misleading (Fig. 6.1).

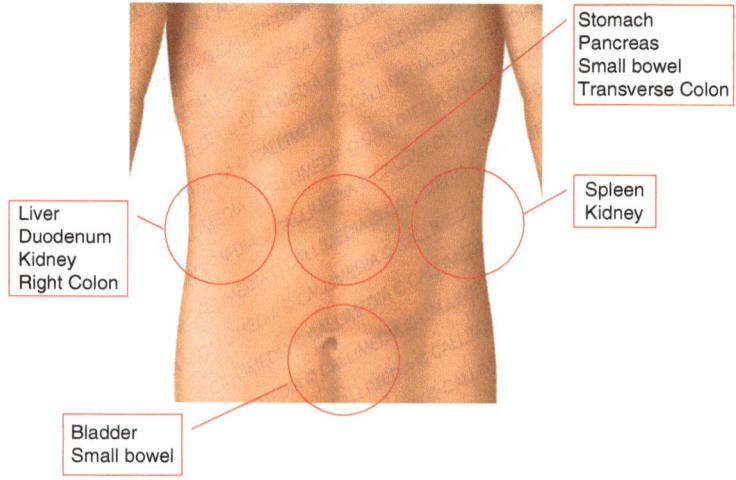

Stomach
Pancreas
Small bowel
Transverse Colon

Spleen
Kidney

Liver
Duodenum
Kidney
Right Colon

Bladder
Small bowel

6.1 Mechanism of Injury

Blunt trauma may involve a direct blow (e.g., kick), impact with an object (e.g., fall on bicycle handlebars), or sudden deceleration (e.g., fall from a height, vehicle crash). The spleen is the organ damaged most commonly, followed by the liver and hollow viscus (typically the small intestine) [1].

Penetrating injuries may or may not penetrate peritoneum and if they do, may not cause organ injury. Stab wounds are less likely than gunshot wounds to damage intra-abdominal structures; in both, any structure can be affected. Penetrating wounds to the lower chest may cross the diaphragm and damage abdominal structures.

6.2 Diagnosis

6.2.1 Clinical Evaluation

Blunt abdominal trauma can be produced not only by direct contusion to the abdomen but also by deceleration injury or falls. Serious, devastating intra-abdominal injuries may be present despite the absence of external signs of trauma. Therefore, a thorough physical examination, the judicious use of diagnostic modalities, and careful follow-up should be followed [2].

A complete history of the mechanism of injury can help identify the potential for intra-abdominal injuries. Information may be provided by the patients, other passengers, the police, or emergency medicine personnel. Injury can be characterized as blunt or penetrating. The most common mechanism of blunt trauma includes vehicular crashes, pedestrian crashes, falls, occupational injuries, and recreational injuries. In patients with penetrating injury, time of injury, type of weapon, distance of weapon, the location of the impact, the mass, and the velocity of weapon can be included. In a motor vehicle crash, speed of crash, type of collision (ex frontal impact, lateral impact, side swipe, rear impact, or rollover), types of restraints used, deployment of air bags, and location of the victim in the vehicle are included.

Physical examination in patients with injury alone has a sensitivity of only 35%, positive predictive value of 30–50%, and a negative predictive value of about 60%. As many as 40% of patients with hemoperitoneum show no findings on initial physical examination. While patients with gastric injuries show significant peritoneal sign due to the leakage of the low pH content of the stomach, peritoneal sign with penetrating trauma to the small intestine may be minimal.

Tips and Pitfalls
For cal examination must be repeated serially by the same experienced trauma surgeons and considered with diagnostic imaging.

The physical examination in patients under unconsciousness, especially alcohol or drug intoxication, spinal cord injury, and pregnancy.

No laboratory studies including hematocrit, WBC, and amylase are useful in initial diagnosis of abdominal injury.

FAST (focused assessment by sonography for trauma) is a useful tool if the patient's hemodynamics is unstable to transport to the CT scanner. FAST is specific for blood in the peritoneum, but it is operator-dependent. FAST includes the following view: pericardial view, the spaces between the liver and kidney (Morison's pouch) and between the spleen and kidney (splenorenal recess), and suprapubic space [3, 4].

Tips and Pitfalls
A positive FAST with unstable hemodynamics is an indication for laparotomy.

However, a negative FAST does not exclude intra-abdominal bleeding. If the patients are under shock, repeated FAST or other investigations need to be considered.

CT scan is highly sensitive and very reliable diagnostic modality diagnostic modality in hemodynamically stable blunt trauma patients [5, 6]

6.3 Management

6.3.1 General Principle

Patients are given intravenous fluid resuscitation as needed, typically with isotonic balanced solution. However, patients who appear to be in hemorrhagic shock should receive damage control resuscitation until hemorrhage can be controlled. Damage control resuscitation uses blood products in an approximately 1:1:1 ratio of plasma to platelets to red blood cells to minimize the use of crystalloid solutions. Some hemodynamically unstable patients are necessary for immediate exploratory laparotomy [7, 8]. For the majority of patients who do not require immediate surgery but who have intra-abdominal injuries identified during imaging, management options include observation, angiographic embolization, and less frequently operative intervention. Prophylactic antibiotics are not indicated when patients are managed without surgery. However, antibiotics are often given before surgical exploration when patients develop an indication for surgery.

At first, the most important thing is to identify whether ongoing bleeding or peritonitis is present.

6.3.1.1 Ongoing Bleeding
- Worsening hemodynamic status
- Significant ongoing transfusion needs (e.g., more than four units over a 1-h period)
- A significant decrease in Hct (e.g., by >10–12%)

6.3.2 Damage Control Surgery

Damage control surgery is one of the major advances in surgical technique in the past 20 years. The principles of damage control have been slow to be accepted by surgeons around the world [9].

Staged Laparotomy

| er | Or | iCU | | Or | iCU |

TIME ⟶

The central concept of damage control surgery is that patients can die from a triad of *coagulopathy*, *hypothermia*, and *metabolic acidosis* in patients with exsanguinating intra-abdomninal bleeding.

Damage control emerged as a way of halting this rapid physiologic deterioration by quickly managing bleeding, providing aggressive resuscitation, and leaving more definitive reconstruction for a time when stability has been established. Damage control surgery is the most technically demanding and challenging surgery a trauma surgeon can perform. There is no margin for error and no place for careless surgery.

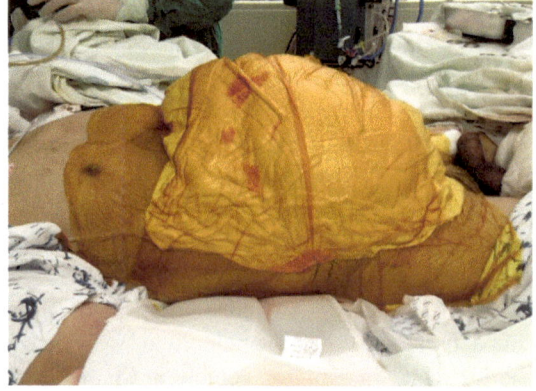

6.3.3 Specific Injuries

6.3.3.1 Splenic Injury (Fig. 6.2)

The organ spleen is the most commonly injured abdominal. Contrast-enhanced abdominal CT is the most valuable diagnostic modality for identifying and characterizing splenic injuries [10].

Angiography with embolization represents the most recent advance in the evaluation and management of spleen injuries [11]. Operative management of splenic injuries may be required in the setting of instability at the time of admission or after failed nonoperative management. When careful selection of patients is applied, many patients with blunt splenic trauma can be managed without splenectomy. It is critical that only patients who are stable and have no evidence of ongoing blood loss be considered for nonoperative management. It should not be overlooked that the definitive management for splenic bleeding remains splenectomy.

Postsplenectomy vaccines must be provided to ensure protection from encapsulated bacteria, including *Streptococcus pneumoniae*, *Neisseria meningitidis*, and *Haemophilus influenzae* [12].

6.3.3.2 Hepatic Injury (Fig. 6.3)

Hepatic injuries are extremely common after blunt and penetrating trauma.

Hepatic injuries can be diagnosed for free fluid on FAST examination in hemodynamically unstable patient. Free fluid on FAST especially around Morisson's pouch suggests bleeding from injured intra-abdominal organs. However, abdominal CT remains gold standards in diagnosing intra-abdominal injuries providing excellent anatomic details that allows highly accurate characterization of injuries.

The free fluid on FAST examination may require immediate interventions. In appropriately selected patients, angioembolization has improved the rate of successful nonoperative management with a reduction in conversion to surgical treatment. Nonoperative management of liver injuries has been shown to demonstrate excellent results [13]. Even though there have been great advances in the nonoperative management of hepatic injuries, it should not be overlooked that operative management is mandatory in hemodynamically unstable patients require operative management of bleeding.

The natural history of hepatic pseudoaneurysms is not entirely elucidated, but it is believed that may be associated with an increased risk of delayed bleeding, especially when they are associated with hepatic arterial branches.

6.3.3.3 Pancreatic Injury (Fig. 6.4)

Pancreatic injuries remain uncommon and no single institution has extensive experience. However, delays in diagnosis and management contribute to significant mortality rates [14, 15]. If diagnose is delayed, pancreatic enzymes are causing massive systemic inflammation and subsequent poor out-

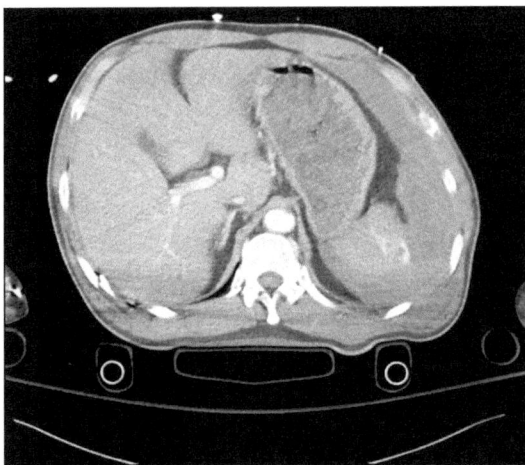

Fig. 6.2 Splenic injury

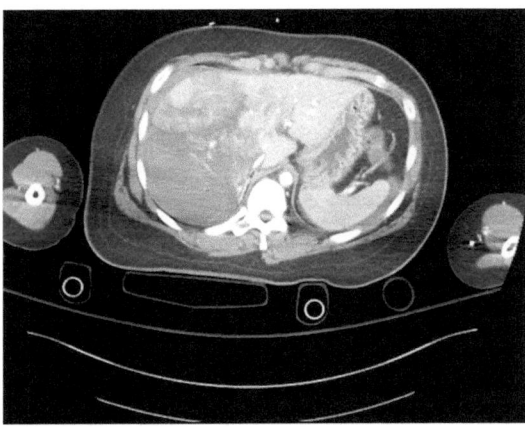

Fig. 6.3 Hepatic injury

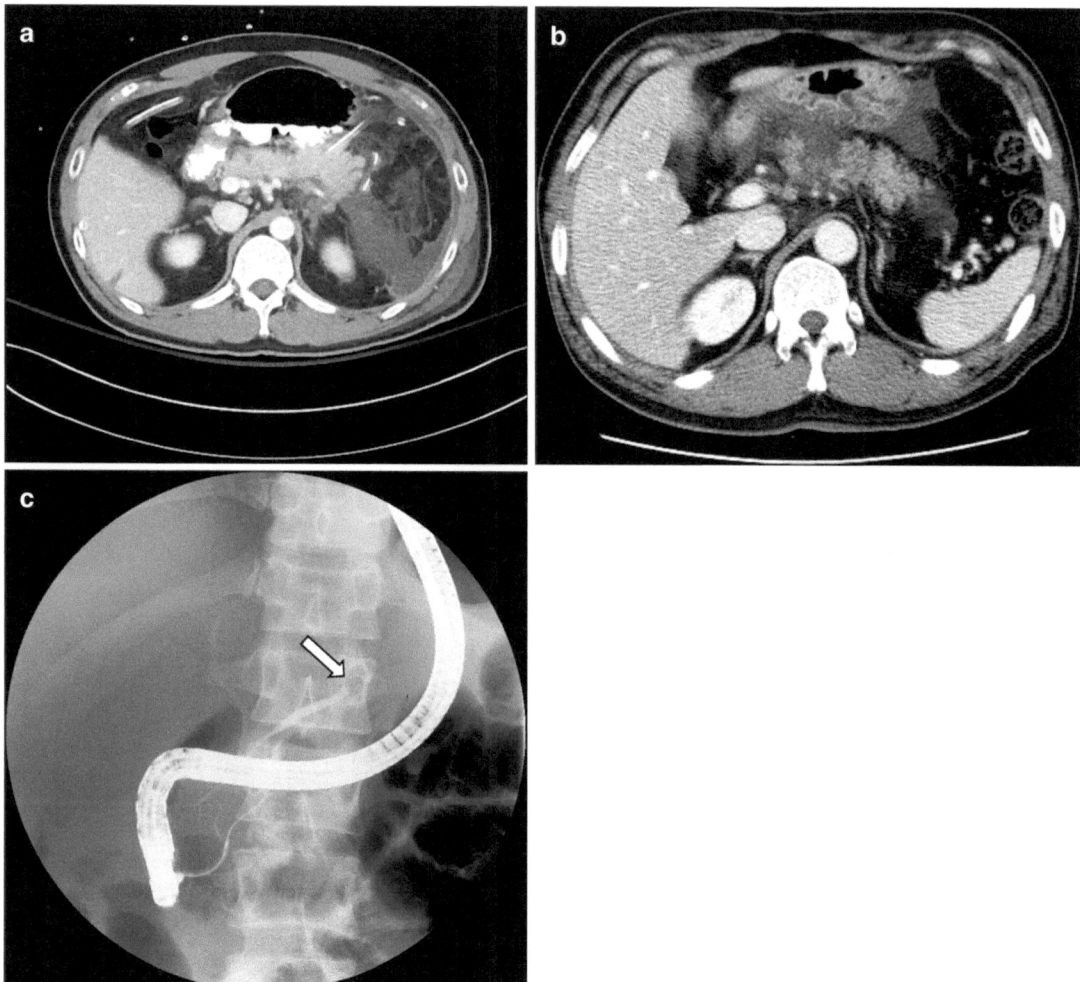

Fig. 6.4 Pancreatic injury. (**a**) Grade III, CT scan, (**b**) Grade IV, CT scan, (**c**) Pancreas duct injury (arrow), ERCP

comes. Pancreas tissue injury can result from direct laceration or through the transmission of blunt force energy to the retroperitoneum. A common mechanism of blunt pancreatic injury involves the crushing of the body of the pancreas, such as a steering wheel or seat belt, and the vertebral column.

The retroperitoneal location of the pancreas makes physical examination findings less helpful for diagnosis. Injury to the pancreas is significantly challenging. The level of serum amylase is relatively sensitive but is lacking in specificity and therefore is of limited value. Abdominal CT is more helpful to diagnose the pancreas and associated injuries. Repeated CT imagings may suggest a pancreatic

injury that requires time to develop radiographically evident pancreatic inflammation. Imaging of the pancreatic ducts with ERCP or magnetic resonance cholangiopancreatography may be helpful, especially for those patients who have a suggestion of pancreatic injuries. Pancreatic injuries of any significance require surgical management [16].

6.3.3.4 Kidney Injury (Fig. 6.5)
The presence of gross hematuria is the most valuable screen for injuries to the genitourinary organs. IV contrast–enhanced CT frequently identifies injuries to the genitourinary organs [17]. Abdominal CT reveals injuries to the kidneys or

adjacent adrenal glands and can demonstrate findings suggestive of urine extravasation. Presence of injury to the bladder can be evaluated by obtaining a CT cystogram [18]. Blood at the urethral meatus or a displaced prostate on rectal examination are suggestive of a urethral injury and requires additional evaluation. Urethral injuries can be confirmed by the retrograde urethrog-

raphy, especially before placement of a urinary catheter. Penetrating genitourinary injuries may be first identified at the time of laparotomy or diagnosed with imaging studies. Penetrating injuries to the back benefit from CT, which can characterize the injury track and delineate adjacent organs.

6.3.3.5 Diaphragm Injury (Fig. 6.6)

Diaphragmatic injury after penetrating injury (10~15%) is more common than blunt injury (1~7%). Left side is more common than right side. The higher energy impact is necessary to make right-sided rupture. Diaphragmatic injury is often asymptomatic, or dominant symptom is from associated injury. Therefore, diaphragmatic injury should be suspected with any wound of the thoracoabdominal regions [19].

Hollow viscus above diaphragm, abnormal position of nasogastric tube, elevation or blurring of the hemidiaphragm, and ipsilateral pleural effusion represent possible diaphragmatic injury. Confirmative CT scan is necessary.

Once diagnosis is made, operative repair should be accomplished. The principles of repairing acute diaphragmatic hernias are complete reduction of

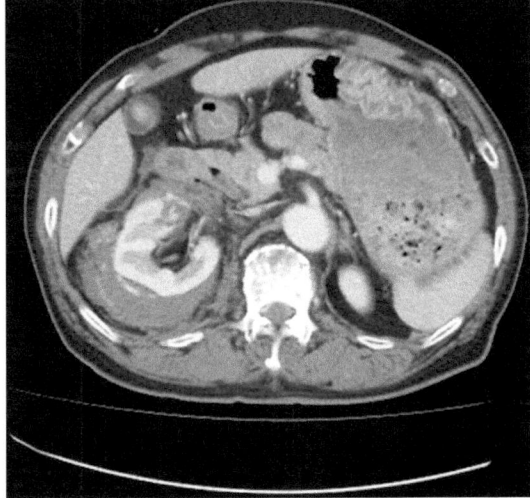

Fig. 6.5 Kidney injury

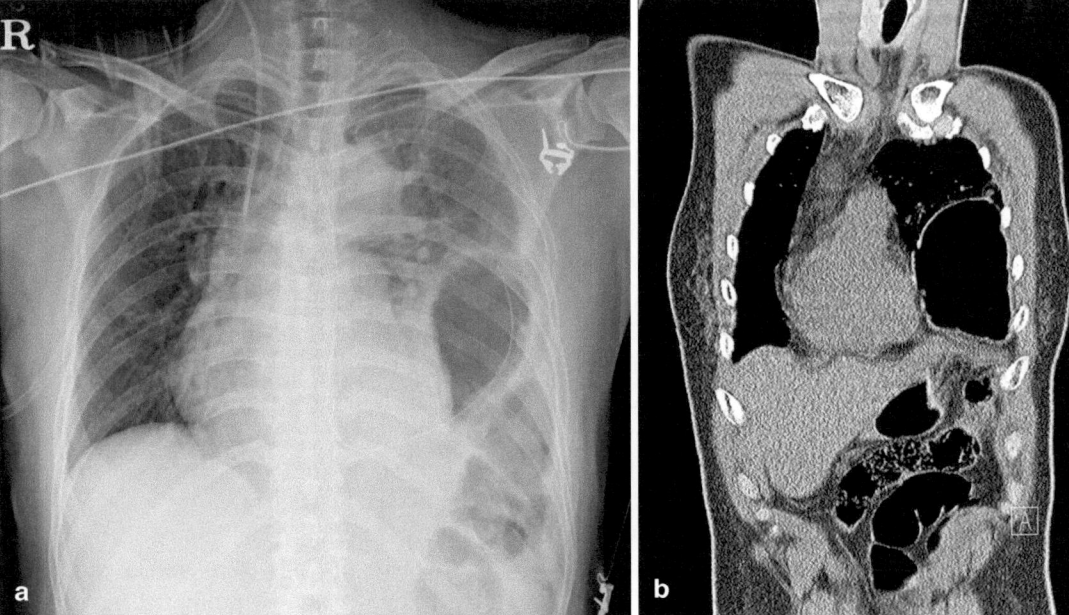

Fig. 6.6 Diaphragm injury (**a**) Chest radiograph, (**b**) CT scan

the herniated organs back into the abdominal cavity and closure the defect to prevent recurrence.

6.3.3.6 Gastric Injury

Penetrating gastric injuries can result in full-thickness perforations with likely spillage of gastric contents into the abdomen. Blunt gastric rupture is caused by an acute increase in intraluminal pressure from external forces that result in bursting of the gastric wall. Because of the high-energy nature of this mechanism, associated injury to the liver, spleen, pancreas, and small bowel is common, and mortality is frequently attributed to these associated injuries.

By physical examination, the presence of peritonitis and the location of penetrating wounds may be suggestive of gastric injury. Some gastric injuries are evident on abdominal CT, but the overall sensitivity for hollow visceral injury is limited. Operative management is mandatory including full-thickness repair, Billroth I or II gastroenterostomy, and Roux-en-Y esophagojejunostomy depending on the extent of the resection.

6.3.3.7 Duodenal Injury

Duodenal injuries are uncommon after blunt and penetrating trauma but can pose a diagnostic and therapeutic challenge. Penetrating duodenal injuries are often first diagnosed at laparotomy. Blunt duodenal injuries can be more challenging to identify and therefore require a high index of suspicion to avoid missed injuries. Physical examination findings can be lacking because of the retroperitoneal location of the duodenum. Even full-thickness duodenal perforations may not demonstrate peritoneal signs unless the perforation involves an intraperitoneal segment [20, 21].

Abdominal CT may demonstrate a thickened duodenal wall, air or fluid outside the bowel lumen, or extravasation of contrast material if an oral contrast agent was administered. Upper gastrointestinal contrast studies, diagnostic peritoneal lavage, and laboratory studies such as serum amylase level determination may provide additional information but have a limited role in the evaluation of duodenal injuries.

The approach to management of duodenal injuries depends on the location of the injury and the amount of tissue destruction. Hematomas of the duodenal wall will often resolve without intervention and are an issue only if they cause a gastric outlet obstruction. Most duodenal wall perforations should be repaired primarily by a single- or double-layer approach after debridement of devitalized tissue. Complete mobilization of the duodenum with a wide Kocher maneuver may be required to provide necessary exposure and to ensure a tension-free repair.

6.3.3.8 Small Bowel Injuries

The small intestine is one of the more frequently injured organs after penetrating abdominal trauma. Blunt injuries of the small bowel are relatively less common. At the tissue level, injury can be secondary to crushing, rupture, and shearing mechanisms. Direct tissue injury can occur when the small bowel is crushed between the steering wheel or seat belt and a rigid structure, such as the vertebral column. Deceleration mechanisms can result in a shearing effect throughout a segment of small bowel. Finally, injuries to the small bowel mesentery can result in devascularization and subsequent intestinal necrosis without direct tissue injury [22].

Patients may have peritonitis on examination at the time of presentation, or their abdominal examination findings may worsen in the hours after presentation. Abdominal CT imaging has significant limitations, and a high index of suspicion must exist to avoid a missed injury.

6.3.3.9 Colon Injuries

Colon and rectal injuries occur most commonly after penetrating abdominal trauma and rarely after blunt mechanisms. Colonic tissue loss from penetrating injuries can range in severity, depending on the level of energy associated with the mechanism. From an examination standpoint, the retroperitoneal location of the right and left colon can obscure findings and injury identification. Colon injuries may first be identified at the time of laparotomy that was prompted by hemodynamic instability or a suggestive penetrating mechanism. The evaluation of the colon is similar to that of the small bowel. Abdominal CT is limited in capability, although it may demonstrate colonic wall thickening with surrounding stranding or fluid. Furthermore, imaging may identify the track of a penetrating mechanism, allowing the surgeon to assess proximity to the colon. Finally, care must be taken to adequately assess the segments of the colon that are retroperitoneal in location.

References

1. Dischinger PC, Cushing BM, Kerns TJ. Injury patterns associated with direction of impact: drivers admitted to trauma centers. J Trauma. 1993;35:454–9.
2. Liu M, Lee C, Veng F. Prospective comparison of diagnostic peritoneal lavage, computed tomographic scanning, and ultrasonography for the diagnosis of blunt abdominal trauma. J Trauma. 1993;35:267–70.
3. Boyle RB, Rozycki GS, Mewman PG, Cubillos JE, Ingram WL, Feliciano DV. An algorithm to reduce the incidence of false-negative FAST examinations inpatients at high risk for occult injury. J Am Coll Surg. 1999;189(2):145–50.
4. Nordenholz KE, Rubin MA, Gularte GG, liang HK. Ultrasound in the evaluation and management of blunt abdominal trauma. Ann Emerg Med. 1997;29(3):357–66.
5. Meyer DM, Thal ER, Weigelt JA. The role of abdominal CT in the evaluation of stab wounds to the back. J Trauma. 1989;29:1226–30.
6. Phillips T, Scalfani SJA, Goldstein A, Scalea T, Panetta T, Shaftan G. Use of the contrast-enhanced CT enema in the management of penetrating trauma to the frank and back. J Trauma. 1986;26:593–601.
7. Fabian TC, Croce MA. Abdominal trauma, including indications for laparotomy. In: Mattox, Feliciano DV, Moore EE, editors. Trauma. East Norwalk: Appleton & Lango; 2000. p. 583–602.
8. Zan LF, Ivatury RR, Smith RS. Diagnostic and therapeutic laparoscopy for penetrating abdominal trauma: a multicenter experience. J Trauma. 1997;42(5):825–9.
9. Rotondo MF, Schwab CW, McGonigai MD, Phillips GR, Fruchterman TM, Kauder DR, et al. Damage control: an approach for improved survival in exsanguinating penetrating abdominal Injury. J Trauma. 1993;35(3):375–82.
10. Peitzman AB, Heil B, Rivera L, Federle MB, Harbrecht BG, Clancy KD, et al. Blunt splenic injury in adults: multi-institutional study of the Easte Association for the surgery of trauma. J Trauma. 2000;49(2):177–87.
11. Demetriades D, Hadjizacharia P, Constantinou C, Brown C, Inaba K, Thee P, et al. Selective non-operative management of penetrating abdominal solid organ injuries. Ann surg. 2006;244:620–8.
12. Lynch AM, Kapila R. Overwhelming postsplencetomy infection. Infect Dis Clin North Am. 1996;10:693–707.
13. Malhorta AK, Fabian TC, Croce MA, Gavin TJ, Kudsk KA, Minard G, et al. Blunt hepatic injury: a paradigm shift from operative to nonoperative management in the 1990s. Ann Surg. 2000;231:804–13.
14. Vasquez JC, Coimbra R, Hoyt DB, Fortlage D. Management of penetrating pancreas trauma: an 11-year experience of a level-1 trauma center. Injury. 2001;32:753–9.
15. Takishima T, Hirata M, Kataoka Y, Asari Y, Ohwada T, Kakita A. Pancreaticographic classification of pancreatic ductal injuries caused by blunt injury to the pancreas. J Trauma. 2000;48:745–52.
16. Bhasin DK, Rana SS, Rawal P. Endoscopic retrograde pancreaticography in pancreas trauma.: need to break the mental barrier. J Gastroenterol Hepatol. 2009;24:720–8.
17. Lynch TH, Martinez-pineiro L, Plas E, Serafetinidis E, Turkery L, Hohenfellner M. European Association of Urology. EAU guidelines on urologic trauma. Eur Urol. 2005;47:1.
18. Kuan JK, Wright JL, Nathens AB, Rivara FP, Wessells H, American Association for the Surgery of Trauma. American association for the surgery of trauma organ injury scale for kidney injuries predicts nephrectomy, dialysis and death in patients with blunt injury and nephrectomy for penetrating injuries. J Trauma. 2006;50:351.
19. Meyers BF, McCabe CJ. Traumatic diaphragmatic hernia. Ann Surg. 1993;218:782–90.
20. Shorr RM, Greaney GC, Donovan AJ. Injuries of the duodenum. Am J Surg. 1987;154:93–8.
21. Ivatury RR, Nallatham M, Gaudino J, Rohman M, Tahl WM. Penetrating duodenal injuries:analysis of 100 consecutive cases. Ann Surg. 1985;202:153–8.
22. Malharta AK, Fabian TC, Katsis SB, Gavant ML, Croce MA. Blunt bowel and mesenteric injuries: the role of screening computed tomography. J Trauma. 2000;48(6):991–8.

Ji Wan Kim

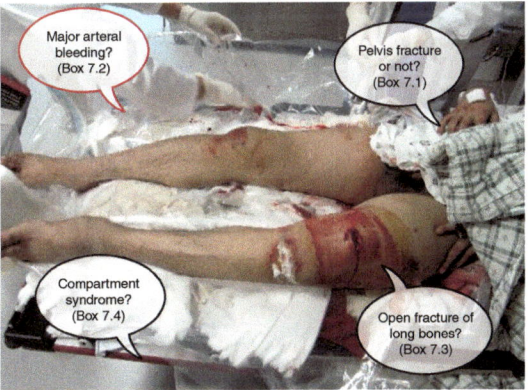

Fig. 7.1 Approach to patients with musculoskeletal injury

Box 7.1 Pelvic Ring Injury
When a polytrauma patient shows the following features, they should be evaluated for pelvic fracture (Fig. 7.1):

1. Pain in pelvis
2. Tenderness
3. External wound
4. If the patient is hemodynamically unstable or unconscious

5. If there is a high energy injury.

For diagnosis we can check pelvic X-ray, and pelvic computed tomography (CT) scans. Hemodynamic instability with pelvic ring injury was defined as a persistent systolic blood pressure <90 mmHg after receiving 2 L of intravenous crystallid and a negative FAST scan [3].

Sources of hemorrhage in pelvic fracture:

1. Pelvic artery injury
2. Fracture site hemorrhage
3. Pelvic venous plexus injury.

85% of hemorrhages were due to venous injury and fracture sites [4].

- Treatment of hemorrhage

There are various methods for hemostasis, which are performed according to the patient's condition and the availability of medical resources and medical staff. In general, methods such as a pelvic binder (sling), external fixation, internal fixation, direct surgical vascular ligation, and pelvic packing are used.

J. W. Kim (✉)
Department of Orthopedic Surgery, Asan Medical Center, University of Ulsan College of Medicine, Seoul, South Korea

© Springer Nature Singapore Pte Ltd. 2019
S.-K. Hong et al. (eds.), *Primary Management of Polytrauma*,
https://doi.org/10.1007/978-981-10-5529-4_7

Tips and Pitfalls on the Diagnosis of Pelvic Ring Injury

- A pelvic stability test is performed by exerting gentle rotational force on each iliac crest only once, and abnormal lower extremity positioning is a clue indicating pelvic ring injury.
- Scrotal, labial, or perineal hematoma and swelling; flank hematoma; perineal laceration; and degloving injury (Morel-Lavallee lesion) indicate a high possibility of pelvic ring injury.

Predictors of mortality in hemodynamically unstable pelvic ring injury are [5]:

- Old age
- Injury severity
- Head injury.
- Amount of blood transfusion, which can be reduced by early bleeding control.

Skill I. Pelvic Binder

The pelvic binder is located at the level of the greater trochanter, not the iliac crest (Figs. 7.2 and 7.3).

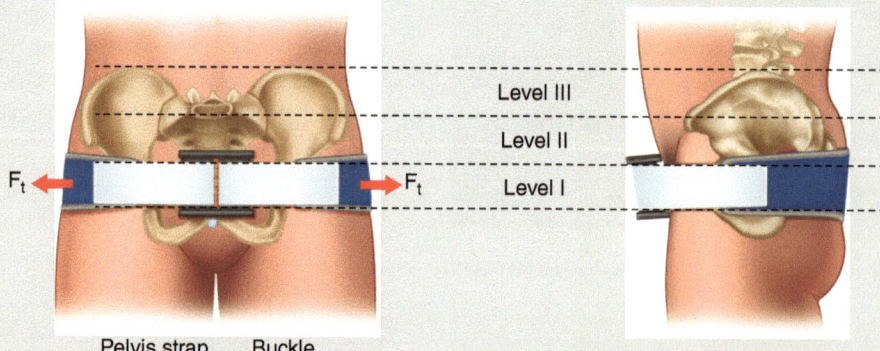

Fig. 7.2 Appropriate position of pelvic binder

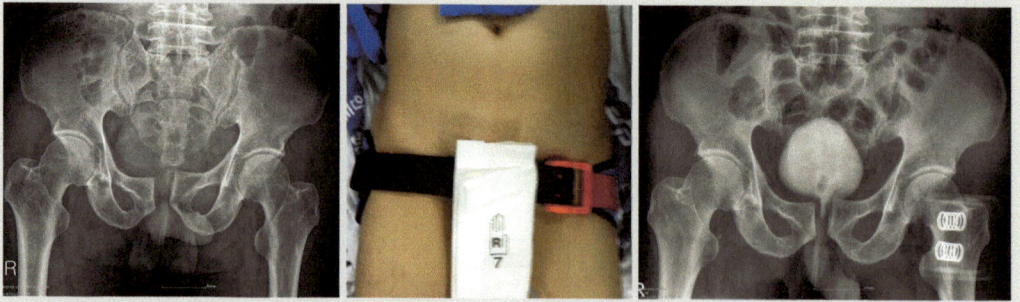

Fig. 7.3 Example of application of pelvic binder

Skill II. C-Clamp (Fig. 7.4)
Application of C-clamp

1. Draw a line from the anterior superior iliac spine to the posterior superior iliac spine.
2. Palpate the greater femoral trochanter and draw a line along the axis of the femoral shaft perpendicular to the first line (A).
3. A small skin incision for the entry point is made at the junction of the two lines.
4. Let a pin glide into the depression between the oblique orientation of the iliac wing and the vertical part of the posterior iliac wing until the center of the cavity is reached (B).
5. If available, an image intensifier should be used in the lateral projection to confirm that the entry point overlies the center of the S1 body.

6. The pelvis should be realigned as well as possible before the C-clamp is applied.
7. The side struts with attached nails are advanced through the incisions to the bone until the tips have a firm hold in the lateral cortex at the correct entry point (C).

- (Reference: AO surgery reference, External fixation: Emergency stabilization with a C-clamp [39].)
- The surgeon must be aware of the inherent risks and potential technical complications of using the C-clamp, owing to the learning curve and required experience for safe application.
- The following factors are contraindications: (1) iliac wing fracture at C-clamp insertion site, (2) comminuted fracture of either innominate bone.

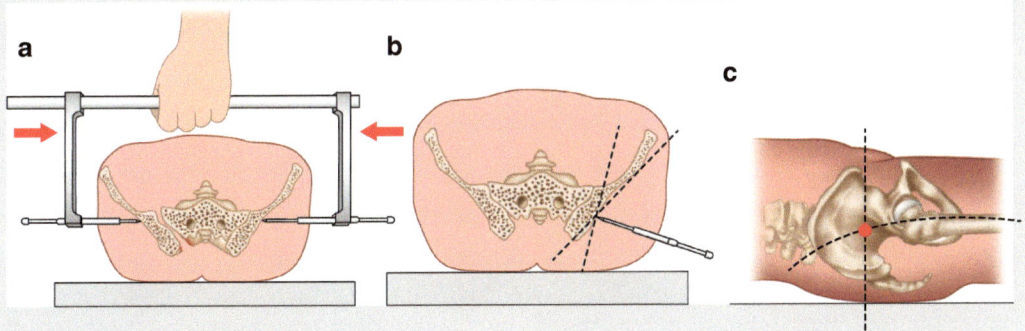

Fig. 7.4 Appropriate position of C-clamp

Case Scenario (Fig. 7.5)

A 25-year-old male. Admission after motor-cycle accident.

Initial blood pressure (BP) 40/22 mmHg, heart rate (HR) 130 beats per min, body temperature (BT) 35.0 °C.

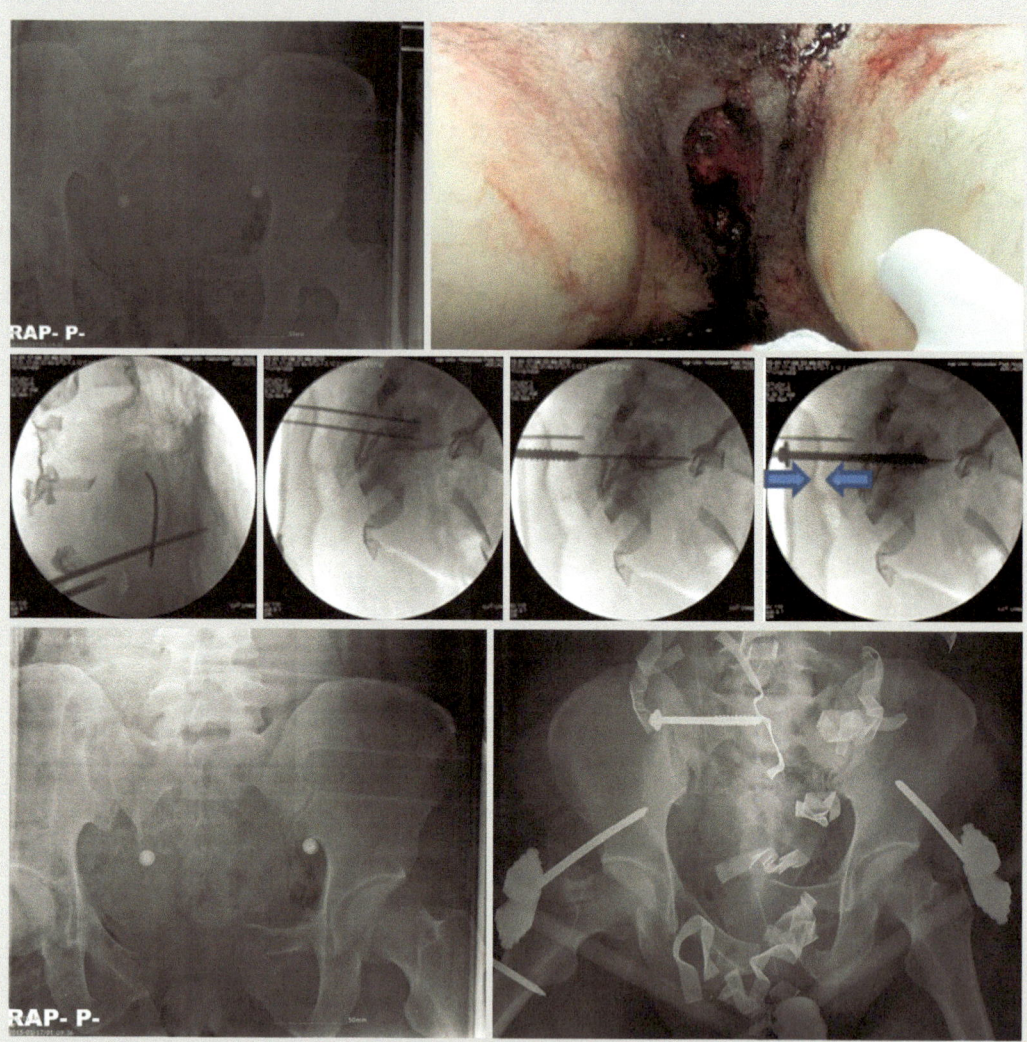

Fig. 7.5 After initial resuscitation, the hemodynamic status of the patient was still unstable and he was transferred to the operation theater. External fixation was applied to the anterior ring, but the posterior ring was still widened and unstable. The posterior ring was fixed with an iliosacral screw. After the posterior fixation, the patient's vital signs responded to resuscitation

Box 7.2 Major Arterial Bleeding

Trauma in an extremity can cause major arterial bleeding, which can be massive and result in possible life- or limb-threatening injury. This injury usually presents as a penetrating wound, or fractures disrupting an artery, or often as a combined open fracture. Sometimes arterial occlusion results from the trauma, and it is a potential limb-threatening injury. For example, popliteal artery injury occurs in 7–15% of knee dislocations and is rare in tibial plateau fracture.

We should suspect arterial compromise if the patient shows the following findings:

① Cold, pale, or pulseless distal extremity
② Rapidly expanding hematoma.

Careful examination and inspection of the limb, including pulse, capillary refill, and skin color is the most important aspect of diagnosis.

For diagnosis we can check the ankle brachial index (ABI), angiography, and CT angiography.

Treatment

1. Direct pressure.
2. Temporary pneumatic tourniquet
3. Immediate consultation
4. Correct coagulopathy and commence hemostatic resuscitation as required.

• Physicians should remember that the number one priority in arterial injury is 'life first'. Despite current improvements in reconstructive surgery, reconstruction is to be considered when the patient's life is not in jeopardy (Fig. 7.6).
• When arterial repair or bypass is carried out, fasciotomy should be performed to avoid compartment syndrome.

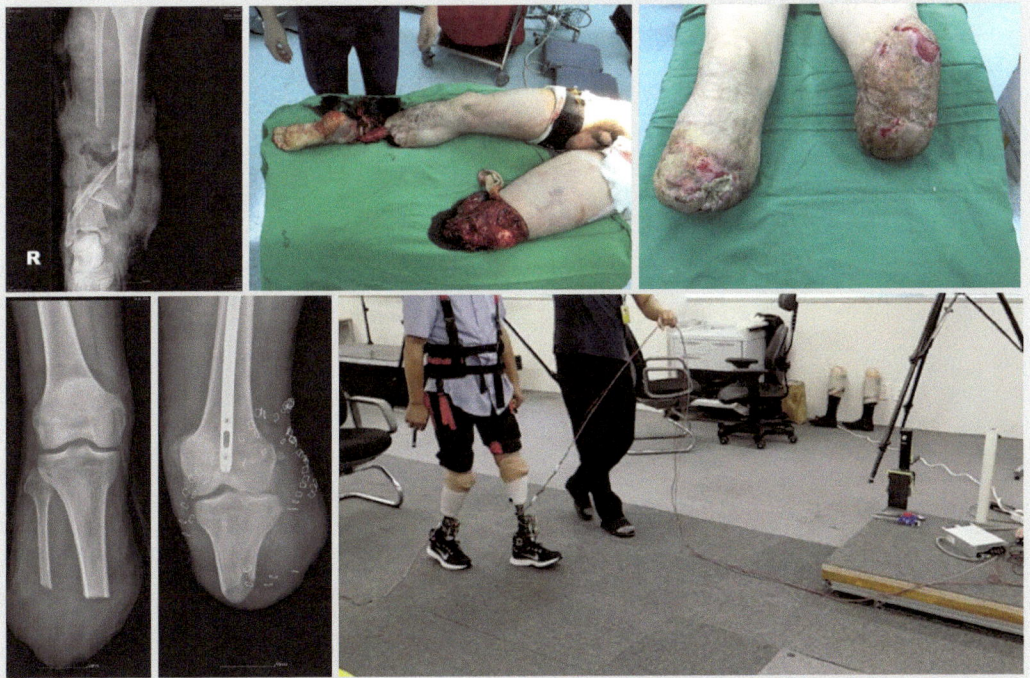

Fig. 7.6 Case. A 57-year-old male vehicle driver. Bilateral major arterial injury resulted in hypovolemic shock, which caused me to decide on amputation rather than reconstruction

Tips and Pitfalls of the major arterial injury

The ankle brachial index (ABI) is a reliable test. The ABI is the ratio of the blood pressure at the ankle to the blood pressure in the upper arm (brachium). Compared with the blood pressure in the arm, a lower blood pressure in the leg sug- gests blocked arteries due to peripheral artery disease, including arterial rupture or occlusion; an ABI of 0.90 or greater has a 100% negative predictive value, and a value of less than 0.90 indicates the need for further arterial screening with angiography or CT angiography.

Box 7.3 Open Fracture

There is a higher risk of infection or nonunion in open fractures than in closed fractures; there- fore, proper wound treatment and prevention of infection are important in open fractures.

The site of the injury should be fully exposed, enabling the confirmation of damage to all nerves and blood vessels. Open fractures can also cause compartment syndrome and should be evaluated with this in mind. Because of the potential of displaced fractures to com- press the nerves and blood vessels, approxi- mate alignment recovery with careful traction is needed. Care should be taken to ensure that contaminants do not enter the fracture site while performing a thorough evaluation of an open wound. The size of the wound, the pres- ence of deep injury, and the degree of contam- ination should be determined.

Treatment

The time of debridement is important, and it has been recommended to perform it within 6 h after the injury. However, surgery may be delayed in patients with multiple trauma who have a poor general condition. Studies have shown that there is no statistically significant difference in the risk of infection between patients treated within 6 h and patients in whom treatment is delayed for more than 6 h. Therefore, thorough debride- ment within at least 24 h, as soon as possible, is effective in preventing infection.

Tips and Pitfalls of Performing Cultures in the Emergency Room (ER)

- Cultures in the ER are controversial.
- Early culture tests are not effective and they are not related to the actual infection; therefore wound culture is not performed in the ER.
- Although it is difficult to identify organ- isms after debridement, culture from debrided tissues in the operation room is recommended, because these cultures are known to be related to the infectious organism.

Tips and Pitfalls of Initial Treatment in the ER

- After the initial evaluation of nerves and open wounds, the sterile dressing used is covered with gauze soaked with normal saline solu- tion—rather than povidone-iodine solution— and a splint is applied to the limb.
- In the initial evaluation of an open wound, only easily removed foreign materials should be removed.
- Wound irrigation in the ER may be useful in severely contaminated wounds, but debridement of contaminated tissue should be done in the operating room as early as possible, within 24 h.
- Repeated evaluation of open wounds in the ER should be avoided because of the risk of secondary bacterial infections; therefore taking a photo of the wound may be useful.

Box 7.4 Compartment Syndrome

In compartment syndrome, elevation of interstitial pressure in the closed compartment causes tissue necrosis and results in functional loss of the limb. In severe cases, renal failure and death may result. Therefore, early diagnosis and treatment of compartment syndrome is important, and it is an orthopedic emergency [19–22].

Diagnosis

1. Clinical diagnosis
   - Early diagnosis is of paramount importance. Five 'P' signs: pain, pallor, pulseless, paresthesia, and paralysis, have been emphasized, but a palpable distal pulse is often present in a compartment syndrome.
   - The most important and early signs are 'pain out of proportion to injury' and 'pain greater than expected/increased by passive stretching of involved muscle'.
2. Measurement of compartment pressure
   In the case of an unconscious or anesthetized patient, compartment pressure should be measured (Fig. 7.7). Measurement of compartment pressure must be made in all compartments and within 5 cm of the fracture.

- Diagnostic criteria
  - Absolute pressure >30–50 mmHg
  - The most commonly used criteria are: ΔP (differential pressure)
  - (diastolic BP – compartment pressure) <30 mmHg
  - These values need to be considered in conjunction with clinical suspicions.

Treatment

- Surgical emergency with an immediate fasciotomy
- Single versus dual incision.

Wound management after fasciotomy

1. Early definitive skin graft
2. Vacuum-assisted wound care and shoelace technique closure (Fig. 7.8).
   - After finishing the fasciotomy, vacuum-assisted wound care is applied; this may reduce postoperative edema.
   - Nylon tape or elastic bands are used incrementally for wound closure, thus decreasing the need for a skin graft.

Skill III. Measurement of Compartment Pressure (Fig. 7.7)

Measurement of compartment pressure must be made in all compartments and within 5 cm of the fracture.

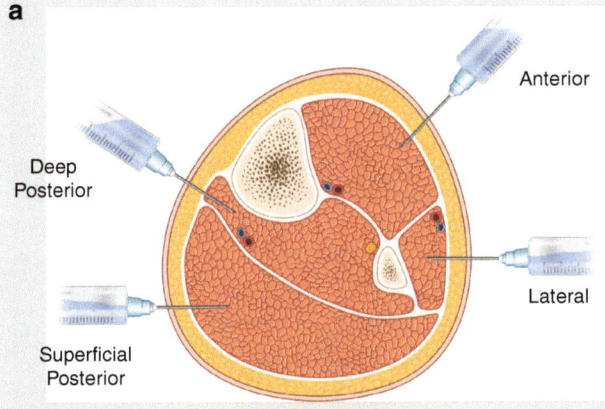
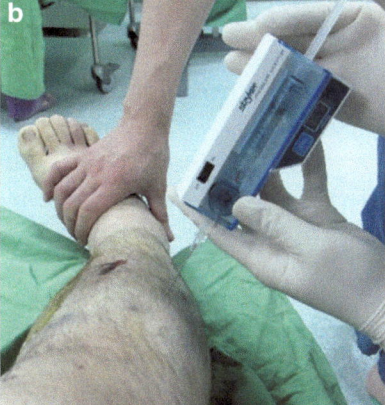

Fig. 7.7   Mesurement of compartment pressure (**a**) The four compartments of the lower leg. (**b**) Intracompartment measuring device

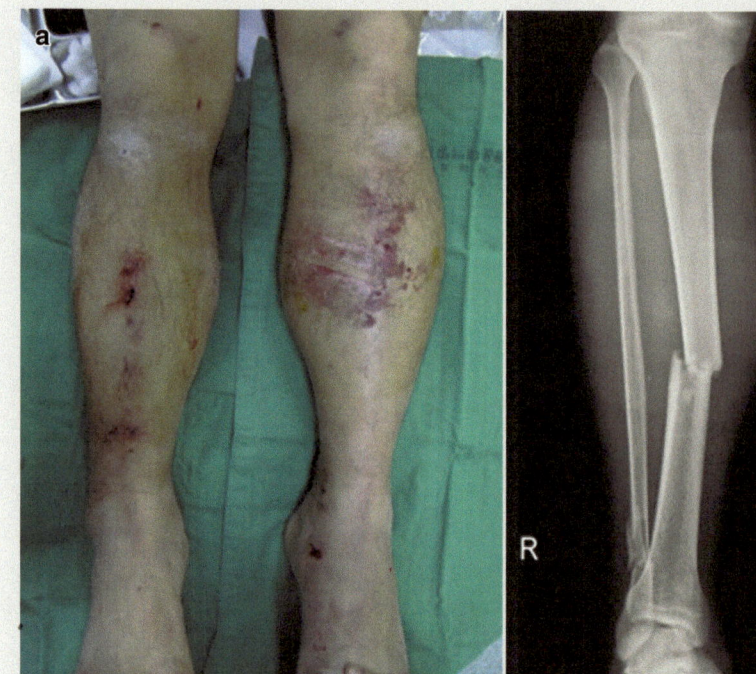

Fig. 7.8 Case (A) A 41-year-old male had both a tib-ial shaft fracture and severe swelling in the left leg, with pain. Emergency fasciotomy was performed with a double incision on the lateral side (B) and medial side (C). Photo at 4 days after injury shows that the shoelace technique and negative-pressure wound dressing was applied on the lateral (D) and medial (E) sides. Progressive wound closure was performed with the shoelace technique and negative-pressure wound dressing on the lateral side (F) and the medial side (G). At 16 days after the injury, complete wound closure was possible without skin graft (H, I)

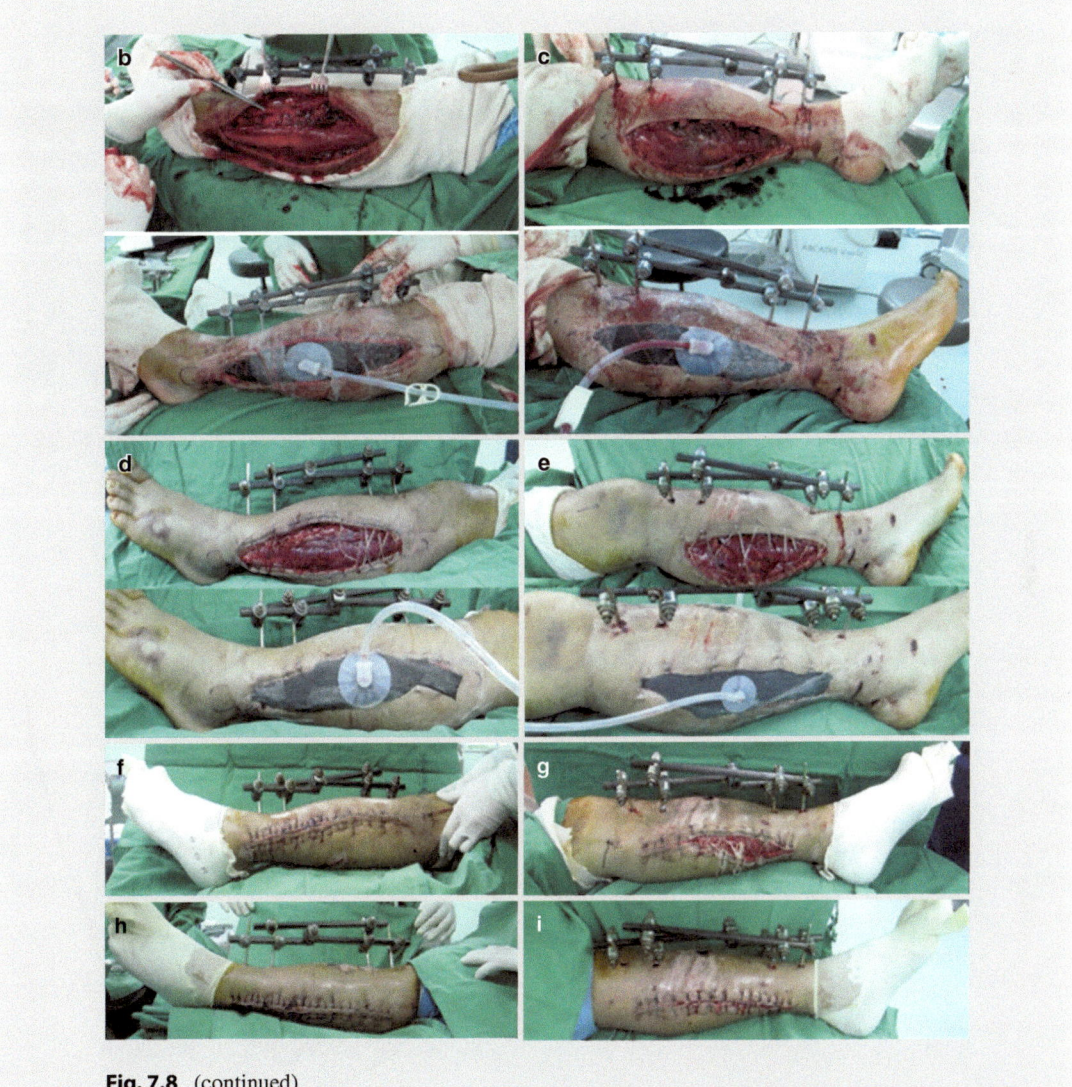

Fig. 7.8 (continued)

Skill IV. Single-Incision Fasciotomy (Fig. 7.9)

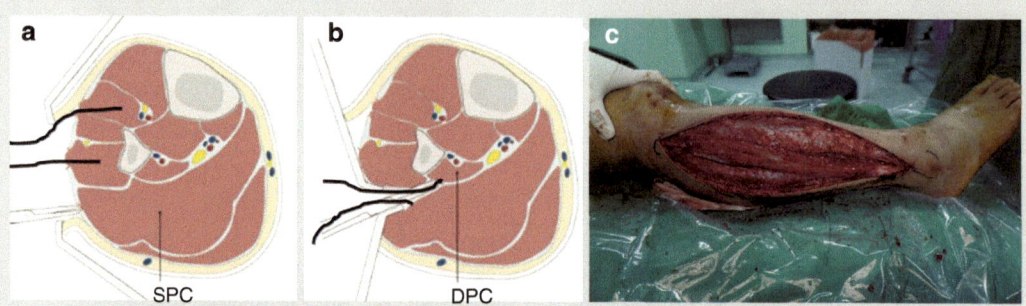

Fig. 7.9 (**a**) Release of anterior and lateral compartment of the lower leg. (**b**) Release of the posterior and deep posterior compartment after retraction of the lateral compartment anteriorly. (**c**) Single-incision fasciotomy. *SPC* superfical posterior compartment, *DPC* deep posterior compartment

Skill V. Double-Incision Fasciotomy (Fig. 7.10) [24]

1. Medial incision
    1. Incise skin along the medial tibia (1 cm posteriorly).
    2. Release superficial and deep posterior compartment.
2. Lateral incision
    1. Incise skin from the fibula head to the lateral malleolar tip 2 cm anterior to the fibula.
    2. Release anterior and lateral compartment.

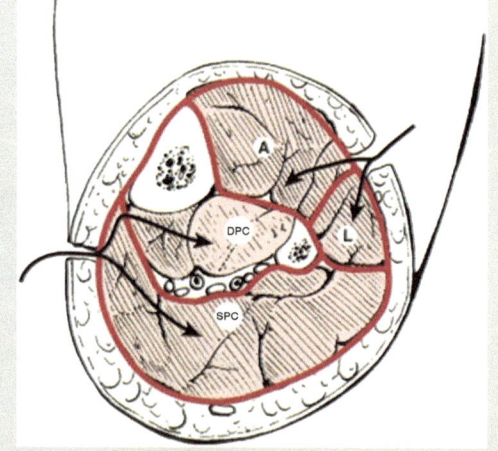

Fig. 7.10 Measurement of compartment pressure must be made in all compartments and within 5 cm of fracture. *SPC* superfical posterior compartment, *DPC* deep posterior compartment

Box 7.5 Timing of Surgery: Damage Control Operation (DCO) Versus Early Total Care (ETO)

Once the initial assessment and intervention is complete, patients should be placed into one of the four categories below in order to guide the subsequent approach to their care.

Classification systems for clinical patient assessment

	Parameter	Stable (grade I)	Borderline (grade II)	Unstable (grade III)	In extremis (grade IV)
Shock	Blood pressure (mmHg)	100 or more	80–100	60–90	<50–60
	Blood units (2 h)	0–2	2–8	5–15	>15
	Lactate levels	Normal range	Around 2.5	>2.5	Severe acidosis
	Base deficit (µmmol/L)	Normal range	No data	No data	>6–8
	ATLS classification	I	II–III	III–IV	IV
Coagulation	Platelet count (	>110	90–110	<70–90	<70
	Factors II and V (%)	90–100	70–80	50–70	<50
	Fibrinogen (g/dL)	1	Around 1	<1	DIC
	D-dimer	Normal range	Abnormal	Abnormal	DIC
Temperature		<33 °C	33–35 °C	30–32 °C	30 °C or less
Soft tissue injuries	Lung function; PaO$_2$/FiO$_2$	350–400	300–350	200–300	<200
	Chest trauma scores; AIS	AIS 1 or 2	AIS 2 or more	AIS 2 or more	AIS 3 or more
	Chest trauma score; TTS	0	I–II	II–III	IV
	Abdominal trauma (Moore)	< or = II	< or = III	III	III or > III
	Pelvic trauma (AO classification)	A type	B or C	C	C (crush, rollover abdomen)
	Extremities	AIS I–II	AIS II–III	AIS III–IV	Crush, rollover extremities

ATLS Advanced Trauma Life Support, *PAO2* Partial Pressure of Oxygen, *AIS* Abbreviated Injury Scale, *TTS* Thoracic Trauma Severity score, *DIC* Disseminated intravascular coagulation

Early total care (ETO)

- Definitive orthopedic surgery performed as soon as possible [24]
- Simultaneous operations: brain/head, abdomen/thorax, extremities [25]
- Early intramedullary nail for femur fracture (<24 h) reduced hospital stay, adult respiratory distress syndrome (ARDS), and mortality [39]

Damage control operation (DCO)

- To avoid worsening of the patient's condition by the "*second hit*" of a major orthopedic surgery [26].

- To delay definite fracture repair until a time when the *overall condition of the patient is optimized* (Fig. 7.11).
- To use *external fixation* as the means of provisional fixation [27].

Common indications for DCO

1. Femoral shaft fracture in multiple trauma [29]
2. Pelvic ring injury with substantial hemorrhage [30]
3. Polytrauma in geriatric patients [31].

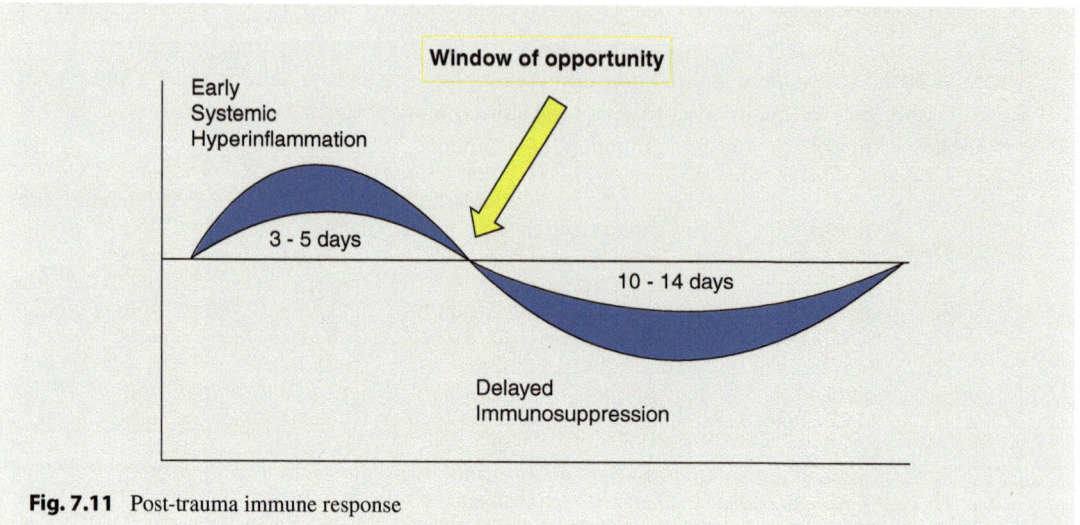

Fig. 7.11 Post-trauma immune response

Tips and Pitfalls: Clinical Parameters of ETO and DCO [28]
- Clinical parameters of ETO
  - Stable hemodynamics
  - No hypoxemia
  - Lactate level <2 mmol/L
  - No coagulopathy
  - Normothermia
  - Urine output >1 mL/kg/h
- Clinical parameters of DCO
  - Polytrauma with injury seventy score of >20 points and additional thoracic trauma (Abbreviated injury scale score of >2 points)
  - Polytrauma with abdominal and pelvic injuries and hemorrhagic shock (systolic blood pressure of <90 mmHg)
  - Injury severity score of ≥40 points without additional thoracic injury
  - Initial pulmonary artery pressure of >24 mmHg
  - Increased pulmonary artery pressure of >6 mmHg during intramedullary nailing
  - Difficult resuscitation
  - Platelet count <90,000/μL (<90 × 10⁹/L)
  - Hypothermia (e.g., temperature of <35 °C)
  - Transfusion of >10 units of blood
  - Bilateral lung contusion on initial chest radiograph
  - Multiple long-bone fractures and truncal injury
  - Prolonged duration of anticipated surgery (>90 min)

7.1 Hemodynamically Unstable Pelvic Ring Injury

High-energy injury can lead to pelvic ring injury with massive bleeding of pelvic soft tissues and fracture surfaces. In hemodynamically unstable pelvic ring injury, the mortality rate was 40% and cause of death was bleeding in early death, and sepsis and multi-organ failure in late death [1, 2, 40].

Although no definitive association exists between fracture pattern and bleeding, some fracture patterns, such as open book injury, are *associated* with a greater transfusion rate [23]—according to some studies [6]—and fracture classification is helpful to understand the injury mechanism and treatment plan. The use of pelvic X-ray in the emergency department is recommended in hemodynamically and mechanically unstable patients with pelvic trauma.

7.1.1   Radiographic Assessment

7.1.1.1 Pelvic X-Ray
Pelvic X-ray helps to identify pelvic ring injuries, but its execution must not delay proceeding with life-saving maneuvers. Pelvic X-ray clearly defines the injury pattern, which is helpful for the early planning of the subsequent diagnostic-therapeutic approach. A pelvic anteroposterior (AP) view is part of the initial advanced trauma life support (ATLS) evaluation, and an inlet/outlet view is the basic X-ray to evaluate the pelvis.

7.1.1.2 Computed Tomography (CT)
CT is the gold standard with sensitivity and specificity for bone fractures, and is routinely performed. Pelvic CT provides better characterization of the posterior ring and pelvic hematoma size than pelvic X-ray, and it also detects soft tissue injury and free peritoneal fluid, which can indicate life-threatening hemorrhage.

7.1.2   Fracture Classification

The AO/OTA classification (Fig. 7.12), one of various fracture classifications, is widely used because the stability of the pelvis can be determined. Type A is a stable type of fracture that does not involve the posterior ring of the pelvis, type B is a rotational unstable fracture, and type C is complete disruption of the posterior ring, resulting in vertical instability.

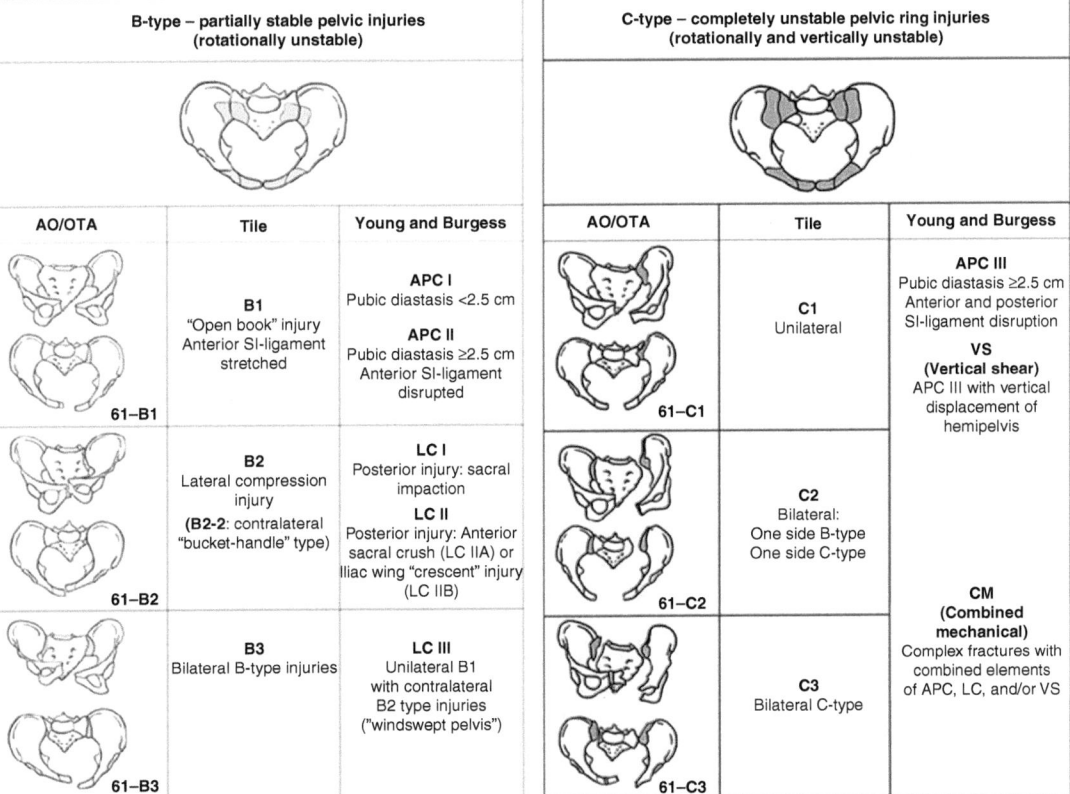

Fig. 7.12 Classification of pelvic ring injury. Type A, which does not involve the posterior arch (pelvic ring), is not shown

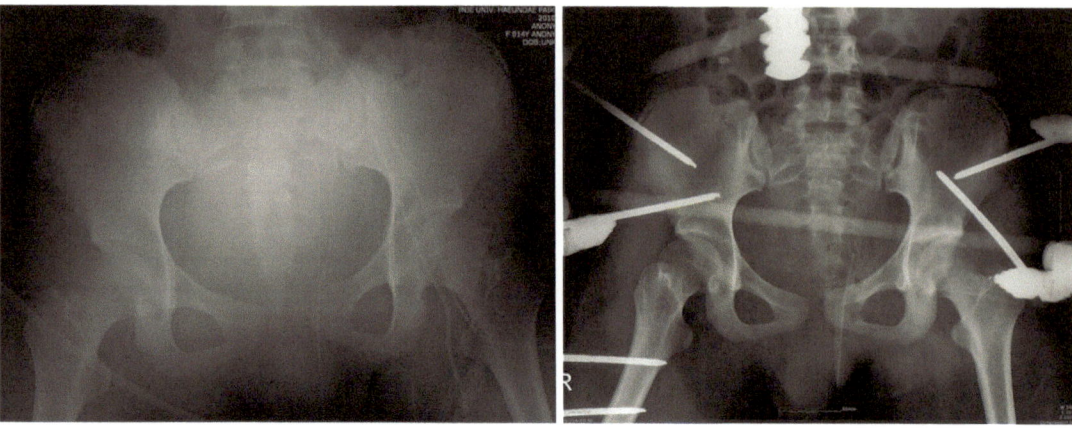

Fig. 7.13 External fixation in a hemodynamically unstable pelvic ring injury in a 14-year-old female who fell from a height

Although fracture pattern on pelvic X-ray does not single-handedly predict mortality or hemorrhage, in the open book fracture type, type B1 fracture and type C fracture are accompanied by massive bleeding and immediate treatment is needed. Diastasis of 3 cm of the symphysis pubis increases the pelvic volume by 1.5 L [7].

7.1.3 Management of Bleeding in Hemodynamically Unstable Pelvic Ring Injury

7.1.3.1 Pelvic Sheet or Binder
- Pelvic sheets or pelvic binders can be used easily in an emergency or in the emergency room.
- Be careful in a lateral compression type of pelvic fracture, as the use of a binder or sheet can make the fracture worse.
- Pelvic binders/sheets are helpful in reducing the enlarged pelvic volume in the open book fracture type, but there is controversy over whether the tamponade is effective, due to the damage of the posterior ring [7, 36].

7.1.3.2 External Fixation
- External fixations are effective methods of hemostasis through the reduction and provisional stabilization of the fracture; the tamponade effect that reduces the volume of the retroperitoneal space; and the hemostasis of the venous plexus, due to the formation of a retroperitoneal hematoma [8, 9].

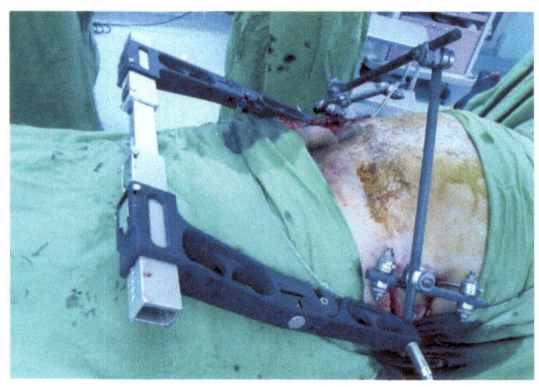

Fig. 7.14 C-clamp and external fixator

- Supra-acetabular pin placement has a very high pull-out resistance due to the solid supra-acetabular surgical corridor (Fig. 7.13).

7.1.3.3 C-clamp [10, 11, 37]
- Anterior ring fixation can be accomplished with external fixation, but posterior ring fixation can be achieved with a C-clamp.
- The C-clamp is indicated in posterior instability presenting with significant hemorrhage.
- Vertically unstable pelvic ring disruptions, such as vertical shear (VS) injuries, are best stabilized with a posterior C-clamp (Fig. 7.14).

7.1.3.4 Internal Fixation; Iliosacral Screw Fixation
In hemodynamically unstable patients, it is preferable to reduce the operation time as much as

possible using an external bone fixation device. However, iliosacral screw or internal fixation with plate are sometimes useful to manage bleeding, which is not usually indicated in the damage control operation, but it can be an option when performed by experts [12].

7.1.3.5 Angiographic Embolization

Angiographic embolization (AE) is the most common method used for arterial bleeding and external fixator placement is the most common method for venous bleeding. AE is the preferred treatment in some institutions and is a mainstay therapy in North America. AE reduces mortality in hemodynamically unstable pelvic ring injury, and it is recommended especially in patients who are aged 60 years or older [16]. However, arterial bleeding from a pelvic fracture occurs in 6–10% of patients [17], and the complication rate has been reported as 2–3%, including necrosis of soft tissues or internal organs [18]. Nonselective embolization of the internal iliac artery, especially bilateral embolization, has been suggested to have higher complication rates [35]. AE requires an interventional radiologist to be present at all times, which could delay action time at night or weekends [13, 14].

7.1.3.6 Preperitoneal Packing (PPP)

The notion of a mainly venous retroperitoneal bleeding source in pelvic fractures provides the main rationale for pelvic packing for acute surgical hemorrhage control. PPP combined with external fixation (EF) has been advocated to rapidly arrest hemorrhage, facilitate other emergent operative procedures, and provide the efficient use of AE. The use of PPP aims to compress the branches of the internal iliac vessels and venous plexus located lateral to the sacrum. Three sponges are placed sequentially in the space between the peritoneum and pelvic ring below the pelvic brim. The first sponge is placed posteriorly and below the sacroiliac joint. The second sponge is placed anterior to the previous sponge in the middle of the pelvic brim. The third sponge is placed in the retropubic space, deep and lateral to the bladder. Pelvic pack removal is performed at 24–48 h once physiological restoration is complete, and repacking of the pelvis should be avoided due to the risk of infection.

In hemodynamically and mechanically unstable pelvic fractures, PPP should be performed along with EF. Preperitoneal pelvic packing/external fixation with secondary AE provides optimal care for life-threatening hemorrhage from unstable pelvic fractures [15, 38].

7.2 Open Fractures

The wound of an open fracture site at the time of injury may cause infection, and infection of the fracture has a significant impact on fracture healing and prognosis. Therefore open fractures should be treated as emergency surgery to prevent infection and to heal injured soft tissue. Intravenous antibiotics should be instituted immediately, and initial debridement should take place as soon as the patient is hemodynamically stable. Wounds that are not evaluated within 24 h are likely to require more extensive and aggressive debridement.

7.2.1 Classification of Open Fractures

The most widely used classification is that of Gustilo and Anderson. This classification aims to predict the treatment outcome and prognosis based on the fracture and the degree of skin and soft tissue injury.

Type	
I	Clean wound, <1 cm Minimal soft tissue injury and comminution
II	Moderately contaminated wound, >1 cm Moderate soft tissue injury and comminution
III	Highly contaminated wound, >10 cm Severe soft tissue injury and comminution Adequate soft tissue coverage Requires flap for soft tissue coverage With a major vascular injury that requires repair for limb salvage. 　IIIA Adequate soft tissue coverage. 　IIIB Significant soft tissue loss with exposed bone that requires soft tissue transfer to achieve coverage. 　IIIC Associated vascular injury that requires repair for limb preservation.

7.2.2 Surgical Treatment

General anesthesia is recommended, because regional anesthesia may interfere with the diagnosis of compartment syndrome if this condition is suspected. Usually, a tourniquet is fitted but not inflated unless the bleeding is severe, because it is difficult to confirm muscle fatigue, and the tourniquet may disturb the blood circulation of the muscles and exacerbate the ischemic tissue damage.

7.2.2.1 Debridement [33]

The goal of debridement is to remove necrotic tissue and foreign bodies, reduce bacterial contamination, and promote healing without infection. Debridement is performed sequentially from the skin in the order of subcutaneous tissue and deep tissue. The contaminated skin or necrotic margins should be thoroughly removed, and in the subcutaneous tissue and fascia, which has poor blood supply, the contaminated part should be thoroughly removed. Muscle viability is determined by four criteria: color of muscle, consistency of muscle, capacity to bleed, and contractility of muscle. Of these criteria, contractility and consistency are clinically reliable indicators. Bone fragments that lack periosteum or soft tissue attachments should be excised, with the exception of major articular fragments of salvaged joints.

7.2.2.2 Irrigation

The advantage of irrigation is that it reduces the number of bacteria, removes the remaining contaminants, and removes the hematoma to make the wounds visible. Washing with a sufficient amount of normal saline will vary depending on the size of the wounds and the degree of contamination. Usually, 3 L is recommended for type I, 6 L for type II, and 9 L for type III open fractures. Wounds should be irrigated with warm, sterile fluids, either through low-pressure flow through sterile tubing, such as cystoscopy tubing, or through low-pressure pulse irrigation systems or arthroscopy pumps. While soaps and antibiotic solutions may lower initial bacterial counts, normal saline under low-pressure flow or bulb suction irrigation demonstrates decreased rebound bacterial counts, with less damage to native tissues, and it is currently the recommended method of irrigation. The use of antibiotics or disinfectants in addition to saline is controversial, but is not recommended because such addition reduces osteoblastic function and increases wound damage.

7.2.2.3 Wound Repair and Management

Early wound closure is ideal in open fractures, but early closures that are improperly or hastily sutured can increase the risk of infection, especially anaerobic infection. Methods of wound closure are classified into primary closure, delayed primary closure, and secondary closure; the method depends on the wound conditions. Primary closure is performed shortly after irrigation and debridement, and can be performed on type 1 and mild type 2 open fractures. The required condition for primary closure is that the wound must be clean, free from contamination, with all necrotic tissue and foreign bodies having been removed, the wound must have normal blood circulation and nerve function, and the patient should be in good general condition. It should also be possible to suture the skin without excessive stress and to avoid dead spaces inside the suture. Delayed primary suture is performed after 4–6 days. Sutures of the wound are performed with or without simple additional irrigation and debridement.

If there is a skin defect, vacuum-foam dressing is widely used to cover the wound and then converted to a skin graft or flap graft. In the treatment of soft tissue defects of type III open fractures, the use of vacuum-foam dressing can reduce the frequency of subsequent flap procedures or reduce the size of the implant. However, the incidence of infection and nonunion is not significantly different from that of conventional soft tissue treatment. Therefore, early bony fixation and flap can be considered as the ideal treatment method for soft tissue defects of open fractures.

7.2.2.4 Stabilization of Fracture

In open fractures, immobilization and stabilization of the fracture are very important for soft tissue and bone healing. The goal of early fixation in open fractures is to acquire early mobilization of the patient to prevent complications of bed rest, and for there to be less discomfort to the patient even though debridement may be performed several times through a stable fixation. The fixation should also be rigid enough to allow early joint motion.

Type I open fractures are treated in a manner similar to that used for closed fractures and the results are similar to those of closed fractures. The selection of the fixation in type II and III open fractures with severe open wounds is greatly influenced by the soft tissue. Internal fixation should be considered if the soft tissue can cover the implant, and it is advisable to approach through the wound as far as possible and avoid any further incisions. All surgical access and placement of external fixators should be located where they do not interfere with additional procedures. It may be better to fix with a temporary external fixator until the soft tissue condition improves. External fixation is most commonly used for fractures of the tibia type IIIB or IIIc, pelvic fractures, or severe soft tissue injuries. The EF in most cases is used as temporary fixation, and conversion to intramedullary nailing is recommended within two weeks if possible if there is no evidence of pin site infection.

7.3 Management of Multiply Injured Patient: Damage Control Operation Versus Early Total Care

7.3.1 Systemic Inflammatory Response and 'Second Hit'

The systemic response to severe injury involves interactions across the haemostatic, inflammatory, endocrine and neurological systems, aggravating initial damage caused by hypoperfusion (shock) and reperfusion. The systemic response has two components: the inflammatory response and counter-regulatory anti-inflammatory response. These two processes work in balance with each other to control the inflammatory response so that the patient's final outcome will be normalcy. If this balance is disturbed from severe injury, then significant complications can develop, such as the systemic inflammatory response syndrome (SIRS) or/and multiple organ failure. This response starts within thirty minutes of a major injury, and is an inflammatory response to blood loss and tissue damage rather than infection.

The injury represents a first hit, turning on the appropriate inflammatory response. Major surgical interventions has become a critical and debatable issue in regard to their potential to deliver a potent secondary immune stimulus ("second hit") within the host's innate immune response to the initial injury. Second hits such as infections, ischemia/reperfusion or early operations can further augment the pro-inflammatory immune response and have been correlated with the high morbidity and mortality including adult respiratory distress syndrome (ARDS) and multiple organ failure in the latter times after trauma (Fig. 7.15). The concept of damage control surgery developed in order to prevent secondary hits due to magnitude of surgery and involves doing the minimal in the shortest possible time followed by stabilization (Fig. 7.16).

7.3.2 Timing of Definite Fracture Fixation After DCO [33]

(i) *No major surgery between days 1–4 after trauma*
(ii) Optimal timing: *days 5–10 after trauma*
(iii) *No major surgery between days 10 and 21 after trauma.*

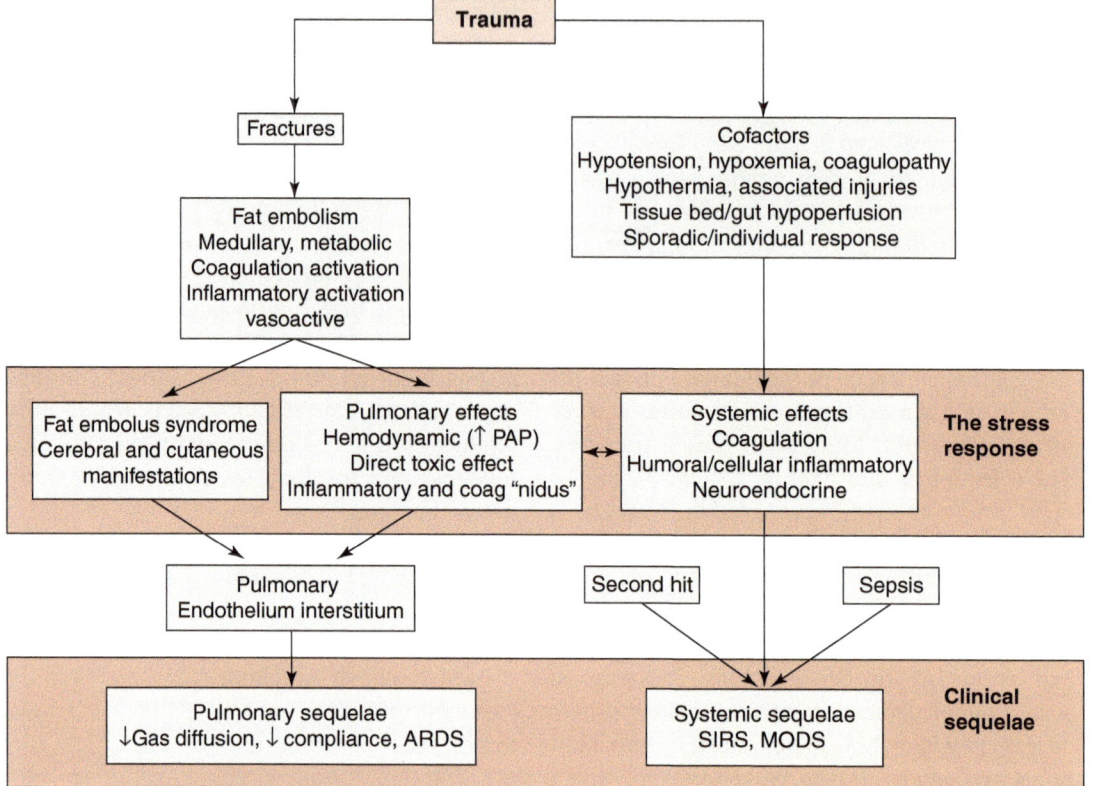

Fig. 7.15 Systemic inflammatory response

7.3.3 Criteria for Endpoints of DCO [32]

No increasing infiltrate on chest radiograph
Balanced or negative fluid balance
PaO_2/FiO_2 of >250
Pulmonary artery pressure of <24 mmHg
Platelet count >95,000/μl
Maximal inspiratory airway pressure of <35 mmHg
White blood cell count of <12,000/μl
Intracranial pressure of <15 cm H_2O

- Traumatic intracranial hemorrhage (ICH), pan-facial bone fracture, Multiple rib fracture with hemothorax

- Pelvic ring injury—open book type, open fracture. Distal femur, both, open fracture. Humerus right, fracture. Talar neck left, fracture. 3,4,5 metatarsal right (MT)., fracture. 2,3,4 MT left.

- Hemodynamically unstable, injury severity score (ISS) = 50

A damage control operation (DCO) was performed.

Ten days after the trauma, meeting the criteria of endpoint DCO, definitive fracture fixation was performed.

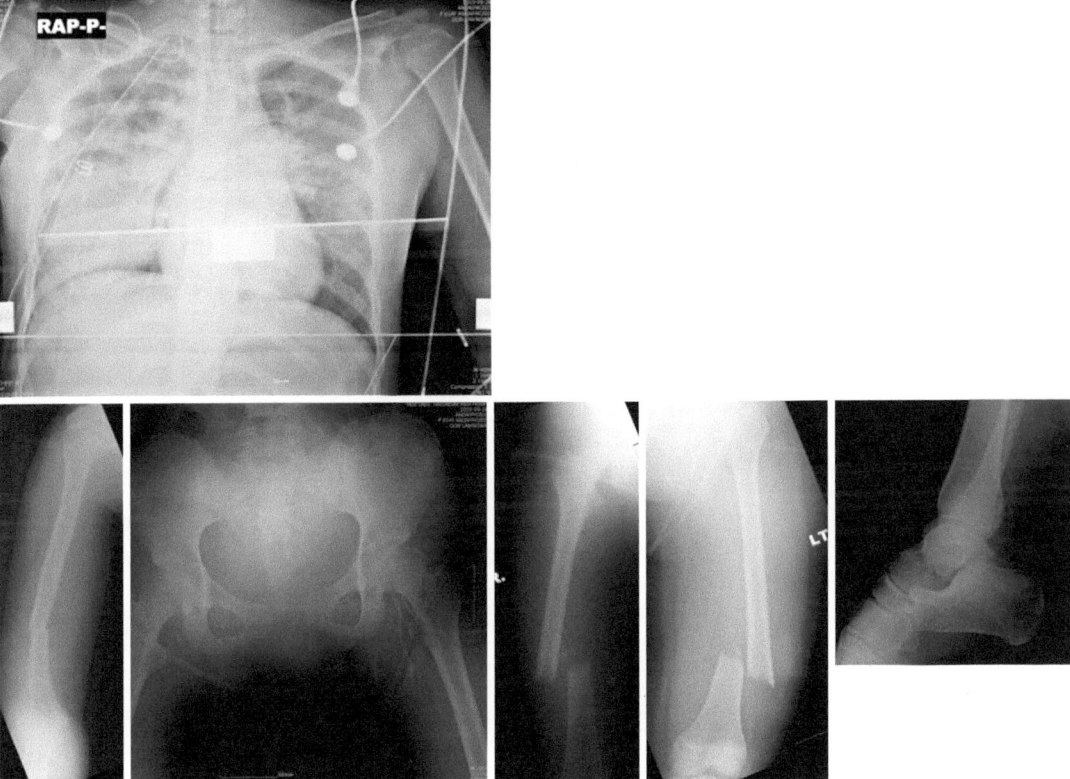

Fig. 7.16 Case. A 14-year-old female who fell from the 11th level of a building. A damage control operation (DCO) was performed. Ten days after the trauma, meeting the criteria of endpoint DCO, definitive fracture fixation was performed

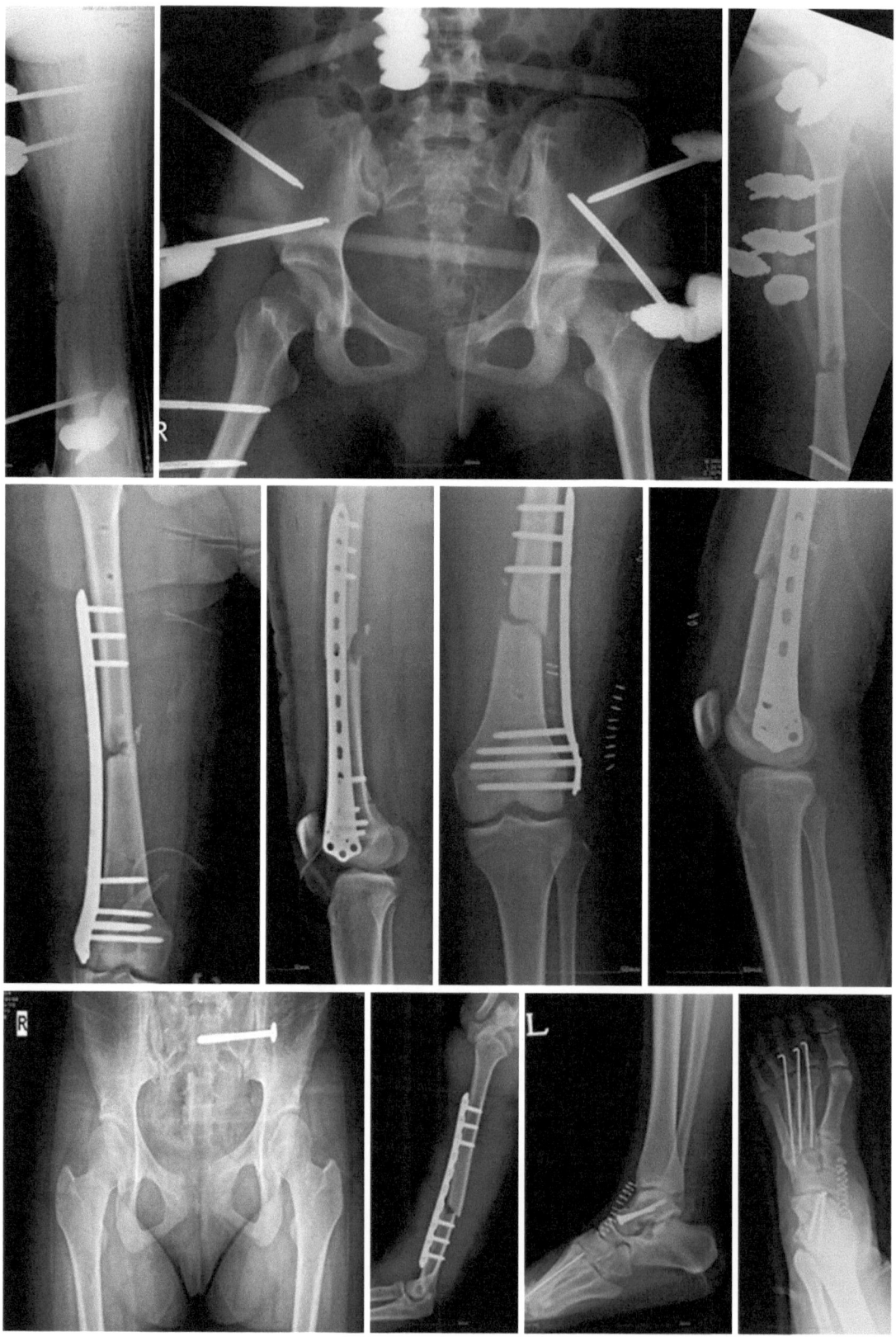

Fig. 7.16 (continued)

References

1. Miller PR, Moore PS, Mansell E, Meredith JW, Chang MC. External fixation or arteriogram in bleeding pelvic fracture: initial therapy guided by markers of arterial hemorrhage. J Trauma. 2003;54:437–43.

2. Eastridge BJ, Starr A, Minei JP, O'Keefe GE. The importance of fracture pattern in guiding therapeutic decision-making in patients with hemorrhagic shock and pelvic ring disruptions. J Trauma. 2002;53:446–51.

3. Tai D, Li W, Lee K, Cheng M, Lee K, Tang L, Lai A, Ho H, Cheung M. Retroperitoneal pelvic packing in the management of hemodynamically unstable pelvic fractures: a level I trauma center experience. J Trauma. 2011;71(4):1–8.

4. Brown JJ, Greene FL, McMillin RD. Vascular injuries associated with pelvic fractures. Am Surg. 1984;50:150–4.

5. Ali J, Ahmadi KA, Williams JI. Predictors of laparotomy and mortality in polytrauma patients with pelvic fractures. Can J Surg. 2009;52(4):271–6.

6. Burgess AR, Eastridge BJ, Young JW, et al. Pelvic ring disruptions: effective classification system and treatment protocols. J Trauma. 1990;30:848–56. https://doi.org/10.1097/00005373-199007000-00015.

7. Cryer HM, Miller FB, et al. Pelvic fracture classification: correlation with hemorrhage. J Trauma. 1988;28:973–80.

8. Ghanayem AJ, Wilber JH, Lieberman JM, Motta AO. The effect of laparotomy and external fixator stabilization on pelvic volume in an unstable pelvic injury. J Trauma. 1995;38:396–400.

9. Riemer BL, Butterfield SL, Diamond DL, Young JC, Raves JJ, Cottington E, Kislan K. Acute mortality associated with injuries to the pelvic ring: the role of early patient mobilization and external fixation. J Trauma. 1993;35:671–5; discussion 676–677.

10. Pohlemann T, Krettek C, Hoffmann R, Culemann U, Gansslen A. Biomechanical comparison of various emergency stabilization measures of the pelvic ring (in German). Unfallchirurg. 1994;97:503–10.

11. Ganz R, Krushell RJ, Jakob RP, Kuffer J. The antishock pelvic clamp. Clin Orthop Relat Res. 1991;267:71–8.

12. Routt ML Jr, Simonian PT, Mills WJ. Iliosacral screw fixation: early complications of the percutaneous technique. J Orthop Trauma. 1997;11:584–9.

13. Osborn PM, Smith WR, Moore EE, Cothren CC, Morgan SJ, Williams AE, et al. Direct retroperitoneal pelvic packing versus pelvic angiography: a comparison of two management protocols for haemodynamically unstable pelvic fractures. Injury. 2009;40:54–60.

14. Fangio P, Asehnoune K, Edouard A, Smail N, Benhamou D. Early embolization and vasopressor administration for management of life-threatening hemorrhage from pelvic fracture. J Trauma. 2005;58:978–84.

15. Burlew CC, Moore EE, Stahel PF, Geddes AE, Wagenaar AE, Pieracci FM, Fox CJ, Campion EM, Johnson JL, Mauffrey C. Preperitoneal pelvic packing reduces mortality in patients with life-threatening hemorrhage due to unstable pelvic fractures. J Trauma Acute Care Surg. 82(2):233–42.

16. Kimbrell BJ, Velmahos GC, Chan LS, et al. Angiographic embolization for pelvic fractures in older patients. Arch Surg. 2004;139:728–32; discussion 732–723.

17. Balogh Z, King KL, Mackay P, et al. The epidemiology of pelvic ring fractures: a population-based study. J Trauma. 2007;63:1066–73; discussion 1072–1063.

18. Namasivayam S, Kalra MK, Torres WE, et al. Adverse reactions to intravenous iodinated contrast media: an update. Curr Probl Diagn Radiol. 2006;35:164–9.

19. Oh CW, Lee H. Acute compartment syndrome after trauma. J Korean Fract Soc. 2010;23:399–403.

20. Elliott KG, Johnstone AJ. Review article: diagnosing acute compartment syndrome. J Bone Joint Surg Br. 2003;85:625–32.

21. Fulkerson E, Razi A, Tejwani N. Review: acute compartment syndrome of the foot. Foot Ankle Int. 2003;24:180–7.

22. Frink M, Hildebrand F, Krettek C, Brand J, Hankemeier S. Compartment syndrome of the lower leg and foot. Clin Orthop Relat Res. 2010;468:940–50.

23. Moore FA, Moore EE. Evolving concepts in the pathogenesis of postinjury multiple organ failure. Surg Clin North Am. 1995;75:257–77.

24. Riska EB, Von Bonsdorff H, Hakkinen S. Primary operative fixation of long bone fractures in patients with multiple injuries. J Trauma. 1977;17(2):111–21.

25. Seibel R, LaDuca J, Hassett JM. Blunt multiple trauma (ISS 36), femur traction, and the pulmonary failure-septic state. Ann Surg. 1985;202(3):283–95.

26. Pape HC, Stalp M, Griensven MV, Weinberg A, Dahlweit M, Tscherne H. Optimal timing for secondary surgery in polytrauma patients: an evaluation of 4314 serious-injury cases. Chirurg. 1999;70(11):1287–93.

27. Carson JH. Damage control orthopedics-when and why. The Journal of Lancaster General Hospital. 2007;2(3):103–5.

28. Pape HC, Giannoudis PV, Krettek C, Trentz O. Timing of fixation of major fractures in blunt polytrauma: role of conventional indicators in clinical decision making. J Orthop Trauma. 2005;19:551–62.

29. Canada LK, Taghizadeh S, Murali J, et al. Retrograde intramedullary nailing in treatment of bilateral femur fractures. J Orthop Trauma. 2008;22(8):530–4.

30. Giannoudis PV, Pape HC, et al. Damage control orthopaedics in unstable pelvic ring injuries. Injury. 2004;35(7):671–7.

31. Tornetta P 3rd, Mostafavi H, Riina J, Turen C, Reimer B, Levine R, Behrens F, Geller J, Ritter C, Homel P. Morbidity and mortality in elderly trauma patients. J Trauma. 1999;46(4):702–6.

32. Tscherne H, Regel G, Pape HC, Pohlemann T, Krettek C. Internal fixation of multiple fractures in patients with polytrauma. Clin Orthop Relat Res. 1998;347:62–78.

33. Erdle NJ, Verwiebe EG, Wenke JC, Smith CS. Debridement and irrigation: evolution and current recommendations. J Orthop Trauma. 2016;30(Suppl 3):S7–S10.

34. Morgan CG. AO principles of fracture management "Decision making in trauma surgery – timing of surgery.

35. Vaidya R, Waldron J, Scott A, Nasr K. Angiography and embolization in the management of bleeding pelvic fractures. J Am Acad Orthop Surg. 2018;26(4):e68–76.

36. Routt CML, Falicov A, Woodhouse E, Schildhauer TA. Circumferential pelvic antishock sheeting: a temporary resuscitation aid. J Orthop Trauma. 16(1):45–8.

37. Barei DP, Bellabarba C, Mills WJ, Routt ML Jr. Percutaneous management of unstable pelvic ring disruptions. Injury. 2001;32(Suppl 1):S-A33–44.

38. Burlew CC, Moore EE, Smith WR, Johnson JL, Biffl WL, Barnett CC, Stahel PF. Preperitoneal pelvic packing/external fixation with secondary angioembolization: optimal care for life-threatening hemorrhage from unstable pelvic fractures. J Am Col Surg. 2011;212(4):628–35.

39. Bone LB, Johnson KD, Weigelt J, Scheinberg R. Early versus delayed stabilization of femoral fractures. A prospective randomized study. J Bone Joint Surg Am. 1989;71(3):336–40.

40. Cothren CC, Osborn PM, Moore EE, Morgan SJ, Johnson JL, Smith WR. Preperitonal pelvic packing for hemodynamically unstable pelvic fractures: a paradigm shift. J Trauma. 2007;62:834–42.

Soft-Tissue Injury

8

Young Chul Suh, Hyunsuk Peter Suh,
and Joon Pio Hong

8.1 Introduction

A mangled extremity involves a combination of severe injuries to the bone, soft tissue, arteries, tendon, and/or nerve, resulting from a high-energy mechanism [1]. Seen in the civilian, or more frequently, military setting, a mangled extremity is associated with considerable early and long-term morbidity. According to the advanced trauma life support protocol, life-threatening injuries are addressed first and extremity injuries second. Evaluation of a severely injured extremity begins with assessing the viability of the extremity. Clinical examination continues to be of paramount importance and should include detailed evaluation of distal pulses, skin color, capillary refill, and sensory and motor function [2].

Once limb viability has been established, the assessment can be focused on the extent of the soft-tissue injuries. Size and depth of injured area should be measured, associated

fractures ruled out, mechanism of injury determined, and neurologic function examined in detail. Plastic surgery consultation regarding possible soft-tissue reconstruction options is appropriate. The management of a patient with lower extremity trauma involves a multidisciplinary approach. Following the initial provision of emergent trauma care and evaluation by orthopedic and general surgery/vascular surgery colleagues, the plastic surgeon is often involved in the management of extremity coverage and reconstruction of both salvaged and amputated limbs. This is often done in conjunction with orthopedics, thus emphasizing Levin's concept of the "orthoplastic approach" [3]. The importance of this team effort was highlighted in management guidelines published by the British Orthopaedic Association and the British Association of Plastic Surgeons [4]. Several studies have shown better functional outcomes in patients treated at trauma centers that have both orthopedic and plastic surgeons and higher rates of complications and revision surgeries at hospitals that do not combine orthopedic and plastic services [5–7].

The current literature is constantly evolving to reflect changes in practice regarding the criteria for limb salvage, timing of reconstruction, and appropriate supportive and adjunctive patient care (Fig. 8.1).

Y. C. Suh (✉) · H. P. Suh
Department of Plastic Surgery, Bucheon St. Mary
Hospital, The Catholic University,
Seoul, South Korea
e-mail: ycsuh@catholic.ac.kr

J. P. Hong
Department of Plastic Surgery, Asan Medical Center,
University of Ulsan College of Medicine,
Seoul, South Korea

© Springer Nature Singapore Pte Ltd. 2019
S.-K. Hong et al. (eds.), *Primary Management of Polytrauma*,
https://doi.org/10.1007/978-981-10-5529-4_8

Fig. 8.1 Decision making process for crushing injury of lower extremity

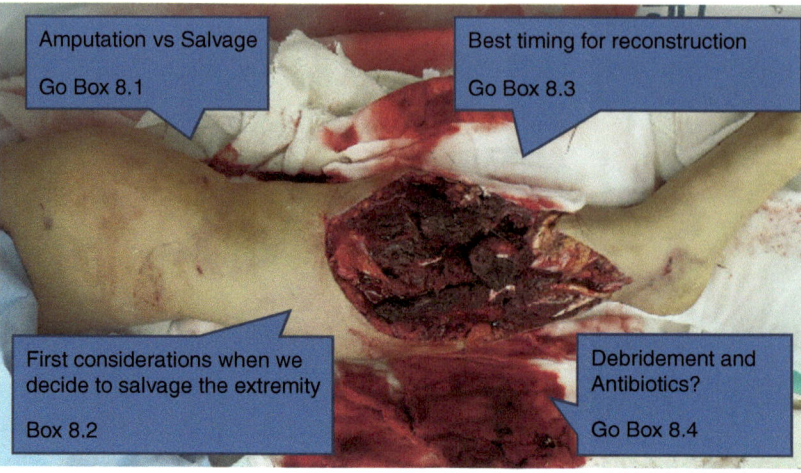

Amputation vs Salvage

Go Box 8.1

Best timing for reconstruction

Go Box 8.3

First considerations when we decide to salvage the extremity

Box 8.2

Debridement and Antibiotics?

Go Box 8.4

8.2 Amputation Versus Salvage

The 7-year follow-up of the LEAP trials showed no functional differences between patients who underwent amputation and those who underwent limb salvage. It was found that hospital stay was longer in the amputation group (63.7 versus 56.9 days), but this was nonsignificant. Of those initially reconstructed, the pooled secondary amputation rate was 5.1% in type IIIB fractures and 28.7% in type IIIC fractures [8–11]. When regressed against the year of study publication, the secondary amputation rate decreased – likely due to improved operative technique and increasing incidence of successful salvage [12]. Patient satisfaction did not correlate with either procedure; it correlated instead with physical function, ability to return to work, overall clinical recovery, pain level, and postinjury mental health [13].

A subset of the LEAP studies assessed several available clinical decision-making scores relating to injury severity. These include MESS, LSI, PSI, NISSSA score, and HFS-97. When applying these scores to the open tibial fracture group, MESS, PSI, and LSI demonstrated high specificity (91%, 87%, and 97%, respectively) but low sensitivity (46% each). Specificity is important to insure that a minimal number of salvageable limbs are incorrectly assigned to amputation, and sensitivity is important to guard against delay in amputation for limbs that are not salvageable. Discrimination was moderately good in assessing salvage versus amputation of the limb. Overall, the analysis did not validate the clinical utility of any of the lower extremity injury severity scores and advised for their cautious application when making decisions regarding limb salvage. Additionally, these scores are not predictive of functional recovery in patients who undergo successful limb reconstruction, as shown by Ly et al. [14].

Box 8.1
Risk factors that may contribute to or predict the need for amputation include:

- Gustilo IIIC tibial injuries
- Sciatic or tibial nerve injury
- Prolonged ischemia (>4–6 h)/muscle necrosis
- Crush or destructive soft-tissue injury
- Significant wound contamination
- Multiple/severely comminuted fractures and segmental bone loss
- Old age or severe comorbidity
- Apparent futility of revascularization or failed revascularization

Unfortunately, despite a number of studies, there are still no definite criteria for amputation. Several proposed criteria have since been refuted following proper outcome studies. For example, it is a widely held belief that tibial nerve injury or absence of plantar foot sensation is an indication for amputation. However, in a study by Bosse et al. [15] examining functional outcomes of patients with severe lower extremity injuries, they found that more than half of the patients who initially presented with an insensate foot that underwent salvage regained sensation by 2 years. The authors concluded that initial plantar sensation was not prognostic of long-term plantar sensation status or functional outcome and that this should therefore not be a criterion in limb salvage algorithms.

Risk factors that may contribute to or predict the need for amputation include:

- Gustilo IIIC tibial injuries
- Sciatic or tibial nerve injury
- Prolonged ischemia (>4–6 h)/muscle necrosis
- Crush or destructive soft-tissue injury
- Significant wound contamination
- Multiple/severely comminuted fractures and segmental bone loss
- Old age or severe comorbidity
- Apparent futility of revascularization or failed revascularization

In addition to these risk factors, several prognostic factors for limb salvage have been identified [16]. These include mechanism of injury, anatomy of injury (e.g., popliteal artery injury has worst prognosis), presence of associated injuries, age and physiologic health of the patient, and clinical presentation (e.g., shock, limb ischemia) [16]. The environmental circumstance may also play a role in determining salvage, with higher amputation rates in combat zones, austere environments, and multi-casualty events.

If early amputation is deemed necessary, it should be performed at an appropriate level above the destructive wound without attempting to close the wound at this time. Photographs may be useful to document severity of injury prior to amputation. Marginally viable soft tissue should be preserved and the open wound copiously irrigated and debrided of contaminating debris. The amputation stump should be dressed with a bulky absorbent dressing and protective splint if amputation is below the knee and/or elbow. Early return to the operating room for further wound

debridement and debridement and definitive management should be anticipated [16].

If the need for amputation is not clear on initial presentation, limb salvage should be attempted and the extremity observed carefully for the next 24–48 h for soft tissue viability, skeletal stability, and sensorimotor function.

8.3 Initial Assessment: CTA Versus Angioplasty

True vascular injury in the setting of lower extremity trauma is rare. Most definitive signs of vascular compromise can be attributed to soft-tissue and bone bleeding, traction of intact arteries with pulse loss (i.e., due to displaced fractures), or compartment syndrome. However, it is prudent to rule out vascular injury, and therefore liberal use of diagnostic tool should be carried out in the presence of hard signs (active hemorrhage; large, expanding, or pulsatile hematoma; Bruit or thrill over the wounds; absent palpable pulses distally; distal ischemic manifestations).

Box 8.2

The initial assessment

1. ABI
   - ABI lower than 0.90 has high possibility of having arterial injury that required surgical management.
2. Duplex Ultrasonography
   - Duplex ultrasonography can also be used when ABI is lower than 0.90 or when ABI is difficult to obtain.
3. Computed tomography angiography (CTA)
   - Computed tomography angiography (CTA) has recently become more popular in detecting vascular injury.

Multiple studies have shown that the ankle brachial index (ABI), when used in conjunction with the physical examination, is effective in assessing limb arterial viability [17–19]. Stannard et al.

demonstrated the usefulness of the physical examination in determining the need for selective arteriography in patients with knee dislocation [20]. Mills et al. prospectively evaluated 38 patients with knee dislocation. They used ABI and clinical pulse examination to evaluate the extremity for possible arterial injury. Eleven patients had ABI lower than 0.90, subsequently underwent arteriography, and had arterial injury that required surgical management (sensitivity, specificity, and positive predictive value were 100%). Twenty-seven patients had ABI of 0.90 or higher, were admitted and observed with serial physical examinations, and had no evidence of vascular injury on serial clinical examinations or duplex ultrasonography [21].

Duplex ultrasonography can also be used when ABI is lower than 0.90 or when ABI is difficult to obtain. Duplex ultrasonography is relatively inexpensive and is easy to perform in the emergency department. Fry et al. found 100% sensitivity and 97.3% specificity for this test, which was successfully used in detecting 18 vascular injuries in 225 cases [22].

Traditionally, the arteriogram was the gold standard in the diagnosis of vascular injuries. Schwartz et al. determined that pulse deficit and ABI lower than 1.00 were significant predictors of arterial injury, and they recommended arteriography for patients with these findings [23]. Although it is accurate in diagnosing vascular injury, it has several disadvantages, including cost, duration of procedure, and potential delay to repair, and need for a specialized team to perform it [24]. There is also an associated risk of morbidity in the form of contrast allergy and percutaneous vascular access-related complications. Computed tomography angiography (CTA) has recently become more popular in detecting vascular injury. Proponents of CTA argue that arteriography is expensive and invasive and delays definitive care [25]. CTA is considered safer, more cost-effective, and less time-consuming than arteriography and has excellent sensitivity and specificity in detecting vascular injury [26]. Seamon et al. prospectively used CTA to evaluate 22 extremities with potential vascular injury and found 100% sensitivity and specificity for clinically relevant vascular injury

detection [27]. Similarly, Inaba et al. found 100% sensitivity and specificity for the use of CTA in evaluating lower extremity vascular injury [28].

There is no doubt that "time is muscle," and prompt repair of any vascular injury should be carried out. Permanent ischemic injury may occur anywhere from 2 to 12 h postinjury according to the literature. This wide range may be due to variation in injury mechanism, presence of collateral flow, and level of injury. The decision to perform a definitive vascular repair in the setting of lower extremity trauma depends on the clinical circumstances [29].

In combined injuries involving bone and vascular disruption, the operative sequence of repair has been debated. In one systematic review, survival of the extremity was directly related to ischemic time, with a steep increase in incidence beyond 3–4 h of ischemic time [30]. Those favoring immediate vascular repair believe that the reversal of ischemia is most important, whereas those favoring skeletal fixation prior to vascular repair argue that stabilization of the bony fragments first will avoid disruption of a vascular repair during bony manipulation. There have been several reports of fracture fixation following vascular repair, with no disruption of the repair [31, 32]. A meta-analysis comparing the outcomes of surgical sequence in 14 published studies did not demonstrate a clear difference between groups regarding incidence of subsequent amputation [33].

8.4   Timing of Reconstruction

> **Box 8.3**
> **Best timing for reconstruction**
>   Acute coverage by days 5–7 is generally accepted as having a good prognosis in terms of decreased risk of infection, flap survival, and fracture healing.

Regardless of the degree of contamination and extent of injury when indicated for salvage, there is no need to delay definitive coverage provided that the general condition of the patient and the status of the wound allow it. General consensus favors early aggressive wound debridement and soft-tissue coverage. Byrd et al. described acute, subacute, and chronic phases of an open tibial fracture [34]. Ideally, the wound is covered in the first 5–6 days after injury at the acute phase of the wound. In severe Gustilo type IIIB and type IIIC injuries, free muscle transplantation obtained the best results. At 1–6 weeks, the wound enters the subacute phase where wounds had higher tendency of infections and flap failures. Between 4 and 6 weeks, the wound enters the chronic phase, and clear demarcation between the viable and nonviable bone becomes apparent. Godina further demonstrated that radical debridement and coverage within 72 h result in best outcome where only 0.75% of flap fails, 1.5% are infected, and 6.8 months are needed for union of the bone [35]. The failure rate compared remarkable to 12% when reconstructed from day 3 to 3 months and 10% when reconstructed after 3 months of injury. Yaremchuk et al. recommended early coverage between days 7 and 14 after several debridements allowing better identification of zone of injury [36]. The common idea behind early intervention is that it minimizes the risk for increasing bacterial colonization and inflammation leading to complications. Acute coverage by days 5–7 is generally accepted as having a good prognosis in terms of decreased risk of infection, flap survival, and fracture healing [35–37]. If patient condition does not allow prolonged surgical procedures, then the wound should be debrided as early as possible and maintain a clean and well-vascularized recipient bed till conditions allow definitive reconstruction [38].

8.5   Antibiotic Therapy

In 1974, Patzakis et al. were the first to demonstrate that early administration of antibiotics after open fractures is the most important determinant of infection prevention [39]. A 2004 Cochrane review concluded that antibiotic therapy reduces the incidence of early infection in open limb fractures [40]. Antibiotic therapy is now considered the standard of care for open fractures of all types. Although orthopedic surgeons agree that the use of antibiotics is effective and necessary for infection prophylaxis, they continue to debate the duration of antibiotic use, the need for Gram-negative organism coverage, and the appropriate route of administration.

There is general agreement that patients with Gustilo-Anderson type I, II, or III open fractures should be intravenously administered a first-generation cephalosporin for up to 48 h, as highlighted by the surgical infection guidelines of Hauser et al. [41]. It is also common practice to repeat 24-hour courses of perioperative antibiotic prophylaxis after repeated irrigation and debridement procedures. However, many studies have shown no superiority of multiple-dose antibiotics over single-dose antibiotics in preventing infection. Hauser et al. reviewed more than 100 studies and found no evidence supporting the prolonged use of antibiotics (>24 h), repeated short courses of antibiotics, or routine coverage extending to Gram-negative species [41].

> **Box 8.4**
> **Antibiotics for open fracture**
>   There is general agreement that patients with Gustilo-Anderson type I, II, or III open fractures should be intravenously administered a first-generation cephalosporin for up to 48 h
>
> **Debridement**
>   Recent literature suggests that, with proper use of prophylactic antibiotics, there is no obvious advantage in debriding within 6 h versus 6 to 24 h after injury. Efforts to debride wounds within 24 h after injury should be undertaken.

A role for extended Gram-negative coverage has been established as well. In the 1980s, Patzakis et al. reported a 4.5% infection rate when both Gram-positive and Gram-negative coverage were provided with cefamandole and tobramycin after open tibia fractures, compared with a 13% infection rate with the use of only cephalothin [42]. More recently, in 2000, Patzakis et al. demonstrated that patients who were treated with ciprofloxacin alone after type III open fractures were 5.33 times more likely to develop an infection than patients treated with cefamandole and gentamicin combined [43]. Gentamicin 80 mg was administered every 8 h as part of combined therapy. Although many authors report administering gentamicin every 8–12 h, the safety and efficacy of once-daily dosing have also been established in patients with open fractures. Sorger et al. randomized 76 patients with type II or III open fractures into two dosage groups: gentamicin 6 mg/kg once daily and gentamicin 5 mg/kg twice daily. These groups showed no statistical difference in infection rates [44]. Similarly, Russell et al. monitored gentamicin serum levels and clinical outcomes for 16 patients who sustained type II or III open tibial fractures and received gentamicin 5 mg/kg once daily. Mean time to fracture union was 8 months, no patient developed nephrotoxicity or ototoxicity, and only one superficial wound infection and two deep wound infections were recorded [45].

8.6   Debridement

After all life-threatening emergencies are addressed and the patient is medically stabilized, operative surgical debridement and irrigation can be initiated. Thorough removal of all nonviable skin, soft tissue, muscle, bone, and foreign bodies is crucial in obtaining a clean wound bed, reducing bacterial contamination, and preventing subsequent infection. Consistency, color, contractility, and circulation are used to determine muscle viability. The skin should be excised to leave a fresh-bleeding skin edge. It entails removal of dead and contaminated tissue that, if left, would become a medium for infection. For limb wounds, a pneumatic tourniquet and magnification in the form of loupes should be always used to reduce blood loss, distinguish surviving from devitalized tissue, and also prevent inadvertent iatrogenic trauma to vital structures. At the end of the procedure, the wound should be washed with copious quantities of saline, preferably as pulsed lavage and then soft-tissue coverage planned in the form of suturing, skin grafts, or flaps. The correct level to which necrotic tissue should be resected is based on two observations: the surrounding soft tissue must be adherent to live bone and live soft tissue and bone must bleed [35].

Controversy remains about the timing of wound debridement. Recent literature suggests that, with proper use of prophylactic antibiotics, there is no obvious advantage in debriding within 6 h versus 6–24 h after injury [46–48]. Werner et al. reviewed multiple studies and found no difference in infection rates when open fractures were debrided within 6 h or within 24 h. Ultimately, the surgeon, patient, and hospital all have a role in determining when to debride. Efforts to debride wounds within 24 h after injury should be undertaken [49].

The Versajet Hydrosurgery System (Smith & Nephew, Key Largo, Florida) offers a unique way of performing debridement: a high-pressure fluid jet running parallel to the surface draws devitalized soft tissues into a cutting chamber for excision and evacuation. It is highly suited to excising concave and convex surfaces. Its use as a debridement tool has been on the rise in recent years. Oosthuizen et al. demonstrated the value of the system for Gustilo & Anderson type III A and III B open tibia fractures through randomized controlled trial. There was significant evidence ($p < 0.001$) that VERSAJET patients required fewer debridement procedures than standard surgical debridement prior to wound closure [50]. However, the cost of a disposable handpiece is roughly $500. Further investigation is needed to determine the efficacy of this technique in orthopedic acute traumatic soft-tissue wound debridement and its cost-efficiency over standard methods.

The rate of osteomyelitis in limb salvage patients was variable, with a range of 4–56%. Complete flap loss was 5.8% (pooled result; range 0–15%). Overall, this study did not reveal a superior strategy in treating patients with lower limb-threatening injuries, as the outcomes were similar between groups.

8.7 Reconstructive Elevator

Once the wound is evaluated to have good vascular supply, stable skeletal structures and a relatively clean wound, soft-tissue coverage is then considered. The concept of reconstructive ladder was proposed to achieve wounds with adequate closure using a stepladder approach from simple to complex procedures (Fig. 8.2). Each line on the ladder represents a wound-closure option. The lowest rung is the simplest (i.e., primary closure) and the highest is the most complicated (i.e., free flap).

Surgeons are advised to choose the lowest rung that offers successful wound management and soft-tissue coverage. Although still valued and widely taught, the reconstructive ladder comes from the concept of wound-closure ladder dating back beyond the era of modern reconstructive surgery [51]. In the era of modern reconstructive surgery, one must consider not only adequate closures but form and function. A skin graft after mastectomy can still provide coverage but a pedicled TRAM (transverse rectus abdominis muscle) flap will provide superior results in addition to coverage.

Fig. 8.2 Reconstructive elevator

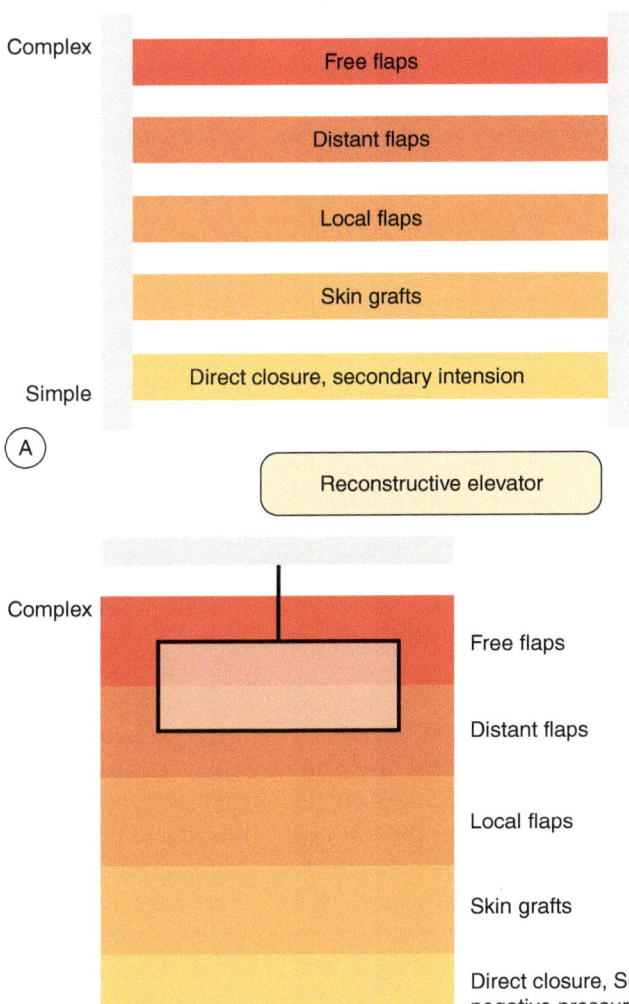

Reconstructive ladder

Complex

Free flaps

Distant flaps

Local flaps

Skin grafts

Direct closure, secondary intension

Simple

(A)

Reconstructive elevator

Complex

Free flaps

Distant flaps

Local flaps

Skin grafts

Direct closure, Secondary intension, negative pressure wound therapy

Simple

Now with introduction of DIEP (deep inferior epigastric perforator) flaps, the reconstructive ladder approach seems to show more flaws. Other techniques including tissue expansion, skin stretching, and vacuum-assisted closure have made new changes in approaching reconstructive options. A simpler reconstructive option may not necessarily produce optimal results. This is especially true for lower extremity coverage, where consequences of inadequate coverage will lead to complications such as additional soft tissue. Others have advocated a "revised reconstructive ladder" that incorporates, at the highest rung of the ladder, vacuum-assisted closure (VAC) therapy (V.A.C. Therapy System; Kinetic Concepts, San Antonio, Texas), acute bone shortening, and bone transport [52]. The increased use of VAC therapy has also resulted in the trend of moving down the reconstructive ladder to less use of skin flaps and more use of delayed primary closures and skin grafts [53].

The reconstructive elevator requires creative thoughts and considerations of multiple variables to achieve the best form and function rather than a sequential climb up the ladder. This paradigm of thought does not eliminate the concept of reconstructive ladder but replaces it as a ladder of wound closure and makes its mark in the field where variety of advanced reconstructive procedures and techniques are not readily available. Based on the reconstructive elevator, method of reconstruction should be chosen based on procedures that result in optimal function as well as appearance.

8.8 Vacuum-Assisted Closure Therapy

Since its introduction in 1997, VAC therapy has revolutionized initial management soft-tissue injuries [54]. VAC dressings are easily applied after initial debridement and irrigation. The VAC system mechanically induces negative pressure over the wound bed. Negative pressure removes fluid from the extravascular space, improves blood supply and oxygen delivery, and promotes formation of granulation tissue within the wound bed [55]. These combined effects improve wound healing

and decrease bacteria counts. Compared with a wet-to-dry dressing, VAC therapy showed a nearly 80% increase in granulation tissue formation [56]. The efficacy of VAC therapy in promoting granulation tissue formation has resulted in less need for free tissue transfers. With these wounds reduced in size, defects can be closed with delayed primary closure, split-thickness skin grafts (STSGs), or local flaps. VAC therapy led to successful primary closure of 71 of 75 lower extremity wounds with exposed tendon, bone, or orthopedic hardware and has become the cost-effective alternative to free tissue transfer. As VAC therapy reduces infection rates and the need for complex microsurgical procedures, its use has led to lowered hospital costs [57]. According to a recent study, between 1992 and 2003, the use of VAC therapy increased from 0% to 47% in the management of all open fractures and to 74% in the management of type III fractures [53].

VAC therapy has also lengthened the "critical period" for wound closure. There is no established period within which a wound managed with VAC therapy requires definitive closure. Conflicting studies have tried to establish a critical period of 7 days or less, but, with small retrospective studies, drawing definitive conclusions is difficult [58–60]. In a group of 38 patients with type IIIB open fractures, soft-tissue defects managed with VAC therapy and then closed within 7 days were associated with a significantly lower rate of infection (12.5%) than wounds closed after 7 days (57%) [61]. Steiert et al. showed that flap coverage delayed to a mean of 28 days after injury was associated with failure rates of 2.6% in free flaps and 25% in pedicle flaps, which compare favorably with reported flap-failure rates [60]. Rinker et al. showed that the use of VAC therapy as a bridge to free-flap reconstruction was associated with decreased infection and flap-related complications in patients with type IIIB or IIIC open tibia fractures [59].

Reported rates of infection after open fracture range from 25% to 66% [39, 40]. In a prospective randomized study, Stannard et al. found that high-energy trauma wounds managed with VAC therapy developed significantly fewer infections than did wounds managed with standard gauze dressing (5.4% vs 28%) [62]. A retrospective study of 50 type III open tibia fractures showed that the infection and nonunion rates associated with the use of VAC therapy as a temporizing measure were similar to the rates associated with the use of historical wound dressings [61]. The use of VAC therapy had no detrimental effects and had major potential benefits for soft-tissue closure. A recent study of injuries sustained in Iraq war showed that the use of VAC therapy protected wounds from the war environment and was associated with no reported infections or wound complications [63]. VAC therapy facilitated delayed primary closure and closure with local flaps or STSGs, a mean of 4.24 days after injury.

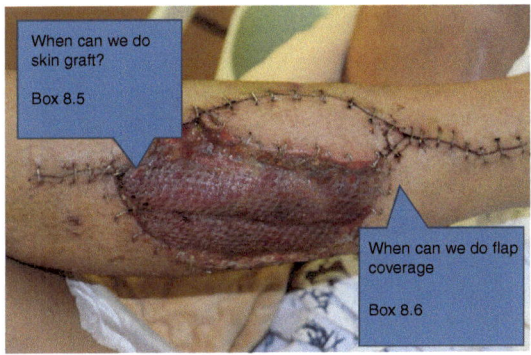

8.9   Skin Grafts and Substitutes

Autologous skin grafts are used in a variety of clinical situations. It can be full or partial thickness and requires a recipient bed that is well vascularized and free of bacterial contamination. The split-thickness grafts are usually used as the first line of treatment where wounds cannot be closed primarily or undue tension is suspected. In the extremity often with complex wounds, bone exposure and/or avascular beds, infected wounds, wound with dead space, and poorly coagulated beds, skin grafts should be avoided. Autologous cultured keratinocytes can be used where split-thickness donor sites are limited. However, the use of cultured epithelial autograft has been hampered by reports that show it to be more susceptible to bacterial contamination, has a variable take rate, and is costly [64].

Box 8.5
Autologous skin grafts are used in a variety of clinical situations. It can be full or partial thickness and requires a recipient bed that is well vascularized and free of bacterial contamination. The split-thickness grafts are usually used as the first line of treatment where wounds cannot be closed primarily or undue tension is suspected. In the extremity often with complex wounds, bone exposure and/or avascular beds, infected wounds, wound with dead space, and poorly coagulated beds, skin grafts should be avoided.

A skin substitute is defined as a naturally occurring or synthetic bioengineered product that is used to replace the skin in a temporary, semipermanent, or permanent fashion [65]. Temporary epidermal replacements may be beneficial in superficial to mid-dermal depth wounds. In deeper wounds, dermal replacements are of primary importance. Bioengineered products for superficial wounds are porcine products such as EZ-Derm and Mediskin (Brennen Medical-LLC, St Paul, MN), which help to close the wound, decrease pain, and improve rate of healing [65]. Biobrane (UDL Laboratories Inc, Rockford, Illinois) is a bilaminate skin substitute that is used temporarily. The outer layer is formed with thin silicone payer with pores that allow removal of exudates and penetration of antibiotics. The inner layer is composed of three-dimensional nylon filament weave impregnated with type I collagen to adhere to the wound. Bioengineered products that are used for deep wounds are Allograft, AlloDerm (Life Cell Corporation, Woodlands, TX), Integra (Integra Life Sciences, Plainsboro, NJ), and Apligraf (Organogenesis Inc., Canton, MA). The gold standard for temporary skin coverage is cadaver skin or allograft. Allograft is used to cover extensive partial- and full-thickness wounds. It prevents tissue desiccation; decreases pain; causes insensible loss of water, electrolytes, and protein; suppresses the proliferation of bacteria; and decreases the hypermetabolic component of thermal injuries [66, 67]. AlloDerm is an acellular dermal matrix engineered from banked, human cadaver skin. It can also provide single-stage reconstruction when used with a split-thickness skin graft [68]. AlloDerm is known to improve functional and cosmetic results in deep burn wounds [69]. Integra is an acellular collagen matrix composed of type I bovine collagen cross-linked with chondroitin-6-sulfate and covered by a thin silicone layer that serves as an epidermis [70]. It is readily available and does not require a donor site and coverts open to closed wound and decreases metabolic demand on the patient.

However, Integra must be used on clean wounds and requires a two-stage procedure later for the graft. Simultaneous use with negative wound pressure therapy may accelerate the vascularization. Apligraf is a bilaminate human epidermal and dermal analogue that can act as a permanent skin substitute. The epidermal layer is formed by human keratinocytes with a well-differentiated stratum corneum. The dermal layer is formed with bovine type I collagen lattice impregnated with human fibroblasts from neonatal foreskin. Apligraf is not antigenic and the dermal layer incorporates into the wound bed. Apligraf has been shown to significantly decrease the time of venous ulcer healing compared to compression [71].

8.10 Reconstructive Option

In patients with lower extremity trauma, it is important to consider all options for reconstruction and choose that which is most reliable or will provide the best functional outcome. The reconstructive ladder is often considered, but in major lower extremity trauma where soft-tissue damage is extensive and the zone of injury is wide, local options are often eliminated, emphasizing the need for free-flap coverage. When choosing a reconstructive option, consideration is given to the size and location of the defect, functional needs (i.e., innervated flap), zone of injury, proposed location of vascular anastomosis for free-flap reconstruction, and accordingly the length of vascular pedicle required to achieve this. Consideration should also be given to the need

for future operative interventions (e.g., tendon reconstruction, bony reconstruction), and flap choice should consider ease of re-elevation. Regardless of flap options chosen for reconstruction, adequate debridement of all nonviable tissue is imperative. High-energy trauma can result in significant soft-tissue destruction with a need for extensive debridement of nonviable tissue.

8.10.1 Local Flaps

The thigh can be divided into three parts: the proximal thigh, midthigh, and the distal thigh (supracondylar knee) regions. The proximal thigh wounds can result from various causes such as complications from hip fractures, infected bypass vascular graft, after tumor resection, and trauma. The medial portion of the proximal thigh can be especially challenging due to location of vital structures and the likely formation of dead space. Local lower extremity muscle or myocutaneous flap options include using the flaps based from the lateral circumflex femoral artery such as tensor fascia lata, vastus lateralis, and rectus femoris flaps. Vertical rectus abdominis muscle or myocutaneous flap using the deep inferior epigastric artery can allow stable coverage of the proximal thigh. The gracilis muscle or myocutaneous flap based on the medial femoral circumflex artery may lack muscle bulk but is a good option when the dead space is not extensive. Now with increased knowledge of perforator and perforator-based flaps, basically any perforator can be chosen as a source of vascular supply to the skin flap and be rotated to cover a defect [72, 73]. When the use of local flaps is not feasible due to the complexity of the wound, free tissue transfer is indicated. The midthigh wound, due to the anatomical character where femur is surrounded by a thick layer of soft tissue, rarely requires reconstruction using free tissue transfer and often is sufficiently reconstructed by skin graft or local flap. Local muscle or musculocutaneous flaps based on the lateral or medial femoral circumflex artery can be used when available. Also, any perforator can be chosen as a source of vascular supply to the skin flap and be rotated to cover a defect. However, if the patient has undergone massive resection or has special considerations such as postoperative radiation therapy, it may warrant free tissue coverage. The wounds of the distal thigh (supracondylar knee) can be very difficult due to the limit of rotation from previously described local muscle or musculocutaneous flaps from the thigh. Pedicled medial gastrocnemius muscle or musculocutaneous flap from the lower leg can be extended to cover this region. However, extensive or complex defects may require free tissue transfer or coverage using a perforator-based rotation/advancement skin flap.

The traditional planning for reconstruction of the lower extremity has been approached according to the location of the defect: divided into thirds, gastrocnemius muscle flap for proximal third, soleus muscle flap for middle third, and free flap transfer for the distal third of the leg. Like the reconstructive ladder concept, this traditional approach can be useful, but the surgeon must individualize each wound and choose the initial procedure that can yield the best chance of success and avoid morbidity.

Box 8.6

When choosing a reconstructive option, consideration is given to the size and location of the defect, functional needs (i.e., innervated flap), zone of injury, proposed location of vascular anastomosis for free-flap reconstruction, and accordingly the length of vascular pedicle required to achieve this. Consideration should also be given to the need for future operative interventions (e.g., tendon reconstruction, bony reconstruction), and flap choice should consider ease of re-elevation

---

8.10.2 Microvascular Free Tissue Transfer

The need for flap reconstruction in injuries with massive soft-tissue defects and exposed hardware persists particularly in the case of type IIIB and

IIIC open tibia fractures. Although size, location, and depth of soft-tissue injury all figure in determining the flap options for soft-tissue coverage, zone of injury is arguably the most important factor. Occasionally, zone of injury may include an area that involves components of a possible local flap, such as what occurs in some type IIIB and IIIC tibia fractures associated with severe damage to the gastrocnemius and soleus. Damage to these muscles generally precludes them from being used as flaps and may result to move up the reconstructive ladder to more complex coverage options.

One must choose a proper surgical plan to achieve optimal function and cosmesis. Flaps are selected based on accessibility of local tissue and donor morbidity. Frequently, the high-energy impact in lower extremity trauma results in extensive and complex wounds. Workhorse for soft-tissue coverage includes muscle or musculocutaneous flaps such as latissimus dorsi, rectus abdominis, and gracilis. The perforator flap, where a skin flap is based on a single or multiple perforators, such as the anterolateral thigh flap or thoracodorsal artery perforator flap has added on to the list. Whichever flap you select, the guideline for lower extremity reconstruction using free flaps remains the same: anastomose the vessel outside the zone of injury, make end-to-side arterial anastomosis and end-to-side or end-to-end venous anastomosis, and reconstruct the soft tissues first and then restore the skeletal support.

Many lower extremity wounds resulting from trauma are high-energy injuries with a substantial "zone of injury." This thrombogenic zone is known to extend beyond what is macroscopically evident, and failure to recognize the true extent of this zone is cited as a leading cause of microsurgical anastomotic failure. Within the zone, perivascular changes such as increased friability of vessels and increased perivascular scar tissue may lead to difficult dissection of recipient vessels and higher incidence of thrombosis after anastomosis [74]. How extensive it is clinically very difficult to realize. Thus, Isenberg and Sherman demonstrated that clinical presentation of recipient vessel (vessel wall pliability and the quality of blood from transected end of vessel) was more important than the distance from the wound [75]. Park et al. also concluded that the site of injury and vascular status of the lower extremity were the most important factor in choosing a recipient vessel [76]. This idea was further supported by successful anastomosis of perforator to perforator adjacent to or within zone of injury [77]. Based on these findings, one of the most important factors in selecting the recipient vessel may be the vascular quality itself.

Perforator flaps are based on musculocutaneous perforator arteries and are composed exclusively of skin and subcutaneous fat. They are being used more often, but little is known about their functional outcomes, compared with the outcomes of traditional muscle flaps. Compared with muscle flaps, perforator flaps, such as the deep inferior epigastric artery perforator flap, which preserves the rectus abdominus muscle, spare functional muscle units, and the loss of even one of these functional units may not be inconsequential in a trauma patient. Rodriguez et al. retrospectively reviewed 42 cases of lower extremity injuries managed with either free muscle flaps or perforator flaps [78]. The quality of life and functional outcomes did not differ between the two flap groups, and time to bony union, union rate in presence of infection, and rate of flap infection were not related to flap type.

8.10.3 Skeletal Reconstruction

Options for bony reconstruction of the lower extremity include autogenous bone graft, vascularized bone transfer, and distraction osteogenesis, including the Ilizarov technique. Autogenous cancellous bone grafts are typically used to fill small defects in bone. While it is possible to bridge larger gaps (8–10 cm) with autogenous bone, it is not the favored approach. In this situation, the use of vascularized bone transfer or distraction techniques may be preferred. The most commonly employed vascularized bone flap is the free fibula flap, based on

segmental and nutrient supply from the peroneal artery. Alternative flaps include the iliac crest vascularized bone flap (deep circumflex iliac artery) and the vascularized scapular flap (circumflex scapular artery). Bone flaps will hypertrophy over time, but this occurs over months to a few years. For defects over 10 cm, distraction osteogenesis is considered. This involves the division of cortical bone outside the zone of injury, preserving the medullary bone and blood supply. Pins are applied on either side of the bone ends, and a circumferential external distraction Ilizarov device is applied. Distraction starts 1 week later, with approximately 1 mm distraction carried out daily at the corticotomy sites. The process can take up to 1 year to allow adequate distraction followed by bony consolidation. It can be very arduous, with associated pin site infection and pain.

8.11 Complication

8.11.1 Wound Complication

The goal of reconstruction is to provide soft-tissue coverage that creates a closed wound, provides vascularized tissue, and prevents secondary complications of the injury, including late infection and nonunion. A subset of the LEAP study specifically examined wound complications as stratified by type of reconstruction. It was found that those reconstructed with free flaps were more likely to have multi-compartment functional compromise in the leg with more severe soft-tissue injury. Despite this, there was no overall difference in complication rates between patients reconstructed with local rotational flaps versus those reconstructed with free tissue transfer. However, when patients were further stratified by underlying osseous injury, regression analysis demonstrated that this was an important predictor of wound complication. In patients with American Society for Internal Fixation–Orthopaedic Trauma Association type C osseous injury, those with rotational flap reconstruction were 4.3 times more likely to have a wound complication requiring operative intervention than those with free-flap reconstruction [79]. Interestingly, there was not an increased rate of wound complications when the patients were stratified by time to reconstruction, suggesting that in this cohort, time to reconstruction was not an important predictor, as is suggested by Godina [35].

8.11.2 Osteomyelitis

It has been shown that the tibia is the most common site of infected nonunion and chronic post-traumatic osteomyelitis [80]. This is associated with morbidity and may be limb-threatening. In this regard, it is important to prevent the occurrence of osteomyelitis and treat it early and aggressively. The LEAP study had an incidence of 7.7% of osteomyelitis, with 84% of these patients requiring operative intervention and hospitalization [13]. It is thought that an aggregation of microbe colonies called "biofilm" is the key in the development and persistence of infection [81]. The most common organism in chronic osteomyelitis is *Staphylococcus aureus*, which may be combined with other pathogens, commonly including *Pseudomonas aeruginosa*.

Four anatomic types of osteomyelitis exist: [1] medullary (IM bone surface), [2] superficial (bone surface), [3] localized (full-thickness cortex extending into medullary canal), and [4] diffuse (circumferential bone involvement). Furthermore, the patient can be classified according to physiologic status: good systemic defenses (type A), systemic/local/combined deficiency in wound healing (type B), or severe local/systemic factors (type C). Infection may be clinically silent, emphasizing the need for a high index of suspicion. Diagnosis relies on clinical findings, laboratory tests (erythrocyte sedimentation rate, C-reactive protein), diagnostic imaging (X-ray, magnetic resonance imaging, technetium-99 m bone scan), and, the gold standard, bone culture. The management of osteomyelitis includes debridement and antibiotics, in conjunction with fracture stabilization. It is necessary to remove all operative hardware, debride infected bony sequestra aggressively, and ream out the IM canal if rod fixation was used. It cannot be emphasized enough how important it is to perform extensive bony debridement until viable bone with punctate bleeding is achieved. It is possible to use local antibiotic therapy in the form of antibiotic-impregnated beads, placed in the defect site following debridement. Systemic antibiotic therapy should be broad initially and tailored according to culture results. If internal fixation is removed and the fracture is not healed or in a state of nonunion, a temporary external fixator may be placed until the infection is eradicated. The secondary stages of reconstruction involve local or free tissue coverage (usually within 1 week of initial debridement), followed by management of bony defects or ununited fractures. Hong et al. reported that used with adequate debridement, bone reconstruction, and obliteration of dead space, a primary remission rate of 91.6% and a secondary remission rate of 98.3% were achieved using perforator flap. The predictors of chronic osteomyelitis recurrence were peripheral vascular disease and major vascular compromise [82].

Bone-grafting procedures are carried out once the soft-tissue envelope has healed and infection is under control, typically 6–8 weeks after soft-tissue coverage. In some situations, amputation may be required, including in those with extensive bone defects, poor soft-tissue coverage, neurovascular compromise of the extremity, anticipated poor function, and multiple comorbidities [81].

Summary

An algorithm for surgical management of lower extremity trauma patients

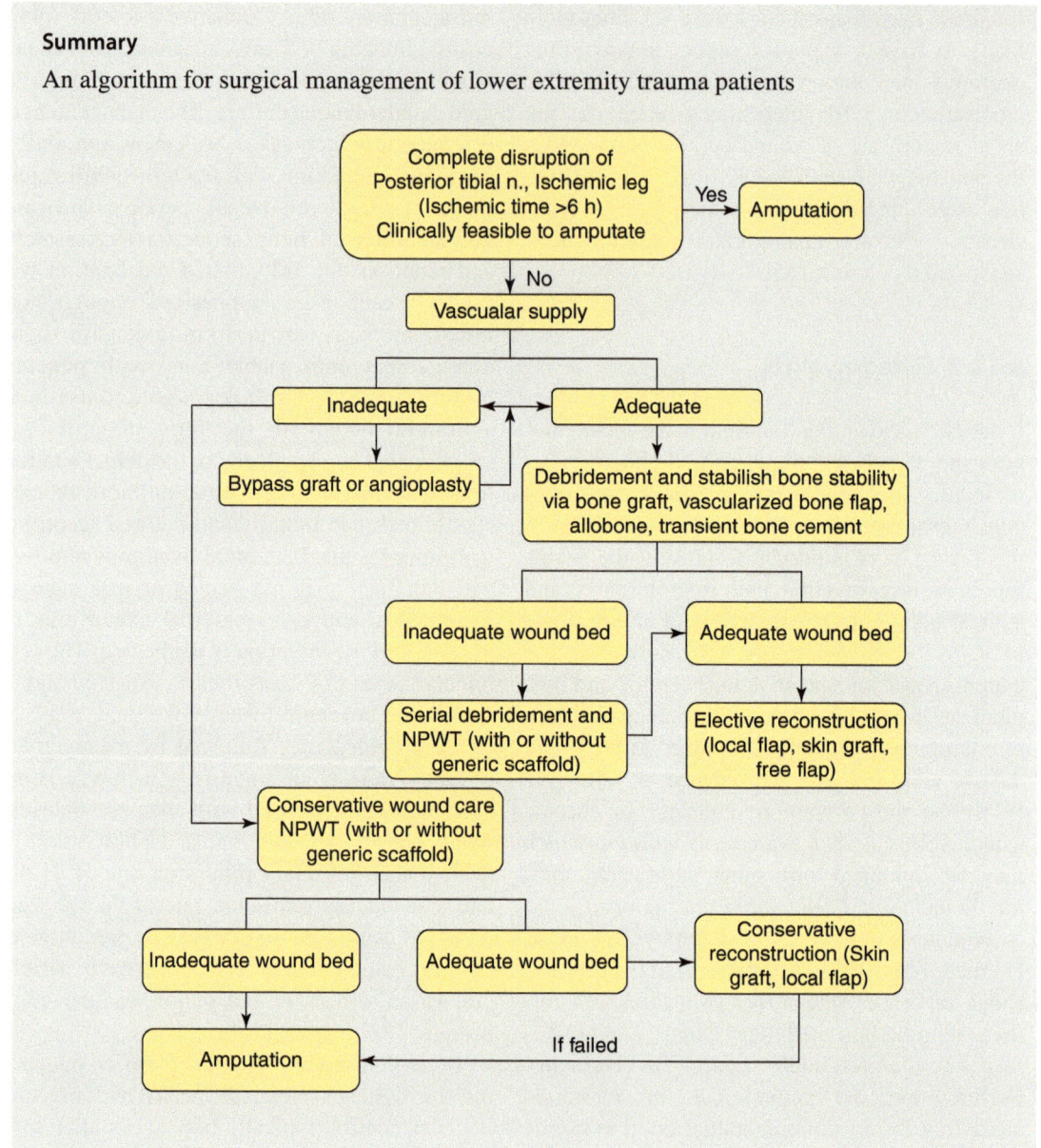

References

1. Langer V. Management of major limb injuries. Sci World J. 2014;2014:640430.
2. de Mestral C, Sharma S, Haas B, Gomez D, Nathens AB. A contemporary analysis of the management of the mangled lower extremity. J Trauma Acute Care Surg. 2013;74:597–603.
3. Levin LS. The reconstructive ladder. an orthoplastic approach. Orthop Clin North Am. 1993;24:393–409.
4. A report by the British Orthopaedic Association/ British Association of Plastic Surgeons Working Party on the management of open tibial fractures. September 1997. Br J Plast Surg. 1997;50:570–83.
5. Mackenzie EJ, Rivara FP, Jurkovich GJ, et al. The impact of trauma-center care on functional outcomes following major lower-limb trauma. J Bone Joint Surg Am. 2008;90:101–9.
6. MacKenzie EJ, Jones AS, Bosse MJ, et al. Health-care costs associated with amputation or reconstruc-

tion of a limb-threatening injury. J Bone Joint Surg Am. 2007;89:1685–92.

7. Naique SB, Pearse M, Nanchahal J. Management of severe open tibial fractures: the need for combined orthopaedic and plastic surgical treatment in specialist centres. J Bone Joint Surg Br. 2006;88:351–7.

8. Busse JW, Jacobs CL, Swiontkowski MF, Bosse MJ, Bhandari M. Complex limb salvage or early amputation for severe lower-limb injury: a meta-analysis of observational studies. J Orthop Trauma. 2007;21:70–6.

9. Giannoudis PV, Harwood PJ, Kontakis G, et al. Long-term quality of life in trauma patients following the full spectrum of tibial injury (fasciotomy, closed fracture, grade IIIB/IIIC open fracture and amputation). Injury. 2009;40:213–9.

10. MacKenzie EJ, Bosse MJ, Kellam JF, et al. Early predictors of long-term work disability after major limb trauma. J Trauma. 2006;61:688–94.

11. MacKenzie EJ, Bosse MJ, Pollak AN, et al. Long-term persistence of disability following severe lower-limb trauma. Results of a seven-year follow-up. J Bone Joint Surg Am. 2005;87:1801–9.

12. MacKenzie EJ, Bosse MJ, Castillo RC, et al. Functional outcomes following trauma-related lower-extremity amputation. J Bone Joint Surg Am. 2004;86-a:1636–45.

13. Harris AM, Althausen PL, Kellam J, Bosse MJ, Castillo R. Complications following limb-threatening lower extremity trauma. J Orthop Trauma. 2009;23: 1–6.

14. Ly TV, Travison TG, Castillo RC, Bosse MJ, MacKenzie EJ. Ability of lower-extremity injury severity scores to predict functional outcome after limb salvage. J Bone Joint Surg Am. 2008;90:1738–43.

15. Bosse MJ, McCarthy ML, Jones AL, et al. The insensate foot following severe lower extremity trauma: an indication for amputation? J Bone Joint Surg Am. 2005;87:2601–8.

16. American College of Surgeons Committee on Trauma. Management of complex extremity trauma. 2005.

17. Johansen K, Lynch K, Paun M, Copass M. Non-invasive vascular tests reliably exclude occult arterial trauma in injured extremities. J Trauma. 1991;31:515–9; discussion 9–22.

18. Levy BA, Zlowodzki MP, Graves M, Cole PA. Screening for extremity arterial injury with the arterial pressure index. Am J Emerg Med. 2005;23: 689–95.

19. Lynch K, Johansen K. Can Doppler pressure measurement replace "exclusion" arteriography in the diagnosis of occult extremity arterial trauma? Ann Surg. 1991;214:737–41.

20. Stannard JP, Sheils TM, Lopez-Ben RR, McGwin G Jr, Robinson JT, Volgas DA. Vascular injuries in knee dislocations: the role of physical examination in determining the need for arteriography. J Bone Joint Surg Am. 2004;86-a:910–5.

21. Mills WJ, Barei DP, McNair P. The value of the ankle-brachial index for diagnosing arterial injury after knee dislocation: a prospective study. J Trauma. 2004;56:1261–5.

22. Fry WR, Smith RS, Sayers DV, et al. The success of duplex ultrasonographic scanning in diagnosis of extremity vascular proximity trauma. Arch Surg. 1993;128:1368–72.

23. Schwartz MR, Weaver FA, Bauer M, Siegel A, Yellin AE. Refining the indications for arteriography in penetrating extremity trauma: a prospective analysis. J Vasc Surg. 1993;17:116–22; discussion 22–4.

24. Miller-Thomas MM, West OC, Cohen AM. Diagnosing traumatic arterial injury in the extremities with CT angiography: pearls and pitfalls. Radiographics. 2005;25(Suppl 1):S133–42.

25. Klineberg EO, Crites BM, Flinn WR, Archibald JD, Moorman CT 3rd. The role of arteriography in assessing popliteal artery injury in knee dislocations. J Trauma. 2004;56:786–90.

26. Redmond JM, Levy BA, Dajani KA, Cass JR, Cole PA. Detecting vascular injury in lower-extremity orthopedic trauma: the role of CT angiography. Orthopedics. 2008;31:761–7.

27. Seamon MJ, Smoger D, Torres DM, et al. A prospective validation of a current practice: the detection of extremity vascular injury with CT angiography. J Trauma. 2009;67:238–43; discussion 43–4.

28. Inaba K, Potzman J, Munera F, et al. Multi-slice CT angiography for arterial evaluation in the injured lower extremity. J Trauma. 2006;60:502–6; discussion 6–7.

29. Fitzgerald J, Michael E. Protocol for lower extremity trauma. J Foot Ankle Surg. 1995;34:2–11.

30. Glass GE, Pearse MF, Nanchahal J. Improving lower limb salvage following fractures with vascular injury: a systematic review and new management algorithm. J Plast Reconstr Aesthet Surg. 2009;62:571–9.

31. Ashworth EM, Dalsing MC, Glover JL, Reilly MK. Lower extremity vascular trauma: a comprehensive, aggressive approach. J Trauma. 1988;28:329–36.

32. Starr AJ, Hunt JL, Reinert CM. Treatment of femur fracture with associated vascular injury. J Trauma. 1996;40:17–21.

33. Fowler J, Macintyre N, Rehman S, Gaughan JP, Leslie S. The importance of surgical sequence in the treatment of lower extremity injuries with concomitant vascular injury: a meta-analysis. Injury. 2009;40:72–6.

34. Byrd HS, Cierny G 3rd, Tebbetts JB. The management of open tibial fractures with associated soft-tissue loss: external pin fixation with early flap coverage. Plast Reconstr Surg. 1981;68:73–82.

35. Godina M. Early microsurgical reconstruction of complex trauma of the extremities. Plast Reconstr Surg. 1986;78:285–92.

36. Yaremchuk MJ, Brumback RJ, Manson PN, Burgess AR, Poka A, Weiland AJ. Acute and definitive management of traumatic osteocutaneous defects of the lower extremity. Plast Reconstr Surg. 1987;80:1–14.

37. Heller L, Levin LS. Lower extremity microsurgical reconstruction. Plast Reconstr Surg. 2001;108:1029–41; quiz 42.
38. Guzman-Stein G, Fix RJ, Vasconez LO. Muscle flap coverage for the lower extremity. Clin Plast Surg. 1991;18:545–52.
39. Patzakis MJ, Harvey JP Jr, Ivler D. The role of antibiotics in the management of open fractures. J Bone Joint Surg Am. 1974;56:532–41.
40. Gosselin RA, Roberts I, Gillespie WJ. Antibiotics for preventing infection in open limb fractures. Cochrane Database Syst Rev. 2004:CD003764.
41. Hauser CJ, Adams CA Jr, Eachempati SR. Surgical infection society guideline: prophylactic antibiotic use in open fractures: an evidence-based guideline. Surg Infect (Larchmt). 2006;7:379–405.
42. Patzakis MJ, Wilkins J, Moore TM. Considerations in reducing the infection rate in open tibial fractures. Clin Orthop Relat Res. 1983:36–41.
43. Patzakis MJ, Bains RS, Lee J, et al. Prospective, randomized, double-blind study comparing single-agent antibiotic therapy, ciprofloxacin, to combination antibiotic therapy in open fracture wounds. J Orthop Trauma. 2000;14:529–33.
44. Sorger JI, Kirk PG, Ruhnke CJ, et al. Once daily, high dose versus divided, low dose gentamicin for open fractures. Clin Orthop Relat Res. 1999:197–204.
45. Russell GV Jr, King C, May CG, Pearsall AW 4th. Once daily high-dose gentamicin to prevent infection in open fractures of the tibial shaft: a preliminary investigation. South Med J. 2001;94:1185–91.
46. Merritt K. Factors increasing the risk of infection in patients with open fractures. J Trauma. 1988;28:823–7.
47. Skaggs DL, Friend L, Alman B, et al. The effect of surgical delay on acute infection following 554 open fractures in children. J Bone Joint Surg Am. 2005;87:8–12.
48. Spencer J, Smith A, Woods D. The effect of time delay on infection in open long-bone fractures: a 5-year prospective audit from a district general hospital. Ann R Coll Surg Engl. 2004;86:108–12.
49. Werner CM, Pierpont Y, Pollak AN. The urgency of surgical debridement in the management of open fractures. J Am Acad Orthop Surg. 2008;16:369–75.
50. Oosthuizen B, Mole T, Martin R, Myburgh JG. Comparison of standard surgical debridement versus the VERSAJET Plus Hydrosurgery system in the treatment of open tibia fractures: a prospective open label randomized controlled trial. Int J Burns Trauma. 2014;4:53–8.
51. Gottlieb LJ, Krieger LM. From the reconstructive ladder to the reconstructive elevator. Plast Reconstr Surg. 1994;93:1503–4.
52. Ullmann Y, Fodor L, Ramon Y, Soudry M, Lerner A. The revised "reconstructive ladder" and its applications for high-energy injuries to the extremities. Ann Plast Surg. 2006;56:401–5.
53. Parrett BM, Matros E, Pribaz JJ, Orgill DP. Lower extremity trauma: trends in the management of soft-tissue reconstruction of open tibia-fibula fractures. Plast Reconstr Surg. 2006;117:1315–22; discussion 23–4.
54. Morykwas MJ, Argenta LC, Shelton-Brown EI, McGuirt W. Vacuum-assisted closure: a new method for wound control and treatment: animal studies and basic foundation. Ann Plast Surg. 1997;38:553–62.
55. Scherer SS, Pietramaggiori G, Mathews JC, Prsa MJ, Huang S, Orgill DP. The mechanism of action of the vacuum-assisted closure device. Plast Reconstr Surg. 2008;122:786–97.
56. DeFranzo AJ, Argenta LC, Marks MW, et al. The use of vacuum-assisted closure therapy for the treatment of lower-extremity wounds with exposed bone. Plast Reconstr Surg. 2001;108:1184–91.
57. Herscovici D Jr, Sanders RW, Scaduto JM, Infante A, DiPasquale T. Vacuum-assisted wound closure (VAC therapy) for the management of patients with high-energy soft tissue injuries. J Orthop Trauma. 2003;17:683–8.
58. Bhattacharyya T, Mehta P, Smith M, Pomahac B. Routine use of wound vacuum-assisted closure does not allow coverage delay for open tibia fractures. Plast Reconstr Surg. 2008;121:1263–6.
59. Rinker B, Amspacher JC, Wilson PC, Vasconez HC. Subatmospheric pressure dressing as a bridge to free tissue transfer in the treatment of open tibia fractures. Plast Reconstr Surg. 2008;121:1664–73.
60. Steiert AE, Gohritz A, Schreiber TC, Krettek C, Vogt PM. Delayed flap coverage of open extremity fractures after previous vacuum-assisted closure (VAC) therapy - worse or worth? J Plast Reconstr Aesthet Surg. 2009;62:675–83.
61. Dedmond BT, Kortesis B, Punger K, et al. The use of negative-pressure wound therapy (NPWT) in the temporary treatment of soft-tissue injuries associated with high-energy open tibial shaft fractures. J Orthop Trauma. 2007;21:11–7.
62. Stannard JP, Volgas DA, Stewart R, McGwin G Jr, Alonso JE. Negative pressure wound therapy after severe open fractures: a prospective randomized study. J Orthop Trauma. 2009;23:552–7.
63. Leininger BE, Rasmussen TE, Smith DL, Jenkins DH, Coppola C. Experience with wound VAC and delayed primary closure of contaminated soft tissue injuries in Iraq. J Trauma. 2006;61:1207–11.
64. Meuli M, Raghunath M. Burns (part 2). Tops and flops using cultured epithelial autografts in children. Pediatr Surg Int. 1997;12:471–7.
65. Lou RB, Hickerson WL. The use of skin substitutes in hand burns. Hand Clin. 2009;25:497–509.
66. Burke JF, May JW Jr, Albright N, Quinby WC, Russell PS. Temporary skin transplantation and immunosuppression for extensive burns. N Engl J Med. 1974;290:269–71.
67. Delmonico FL, Cosimi AB, Russell PS. Temporary skin transplantation for the treatment of extensive burns. Ann Clin Res. 1981;13:373–81.

68. Kim EK, Hong JP. Efficacy of negative pressure therapy to enhance take of 1-stage allodermis and a split-thickness graft. Ann Plast Surg. 2007;58:536–40.

69. Callcut RA, Schurr MJ, Sloan M, Faucher LD. Clinical experience with Alloderm: a one-staged composite dermal/epidermal replacement utilizing processed cadaver dermis and thin autografts. Burns. 2006;32:583–8.

70. Burke JF, Yannas IV, Quinby WC Jr, Bondoc CC, Jung WK. Successful use of a physiologically acceptable artificial skin in the treatment of extensive burn injury. Ann Surg. 1981;194:413–28.

71. Kirsner RS. The use of Apligraf in acute wounds. J Dermatol. 1998;25:805–11.

72. Ali RS, Bluebond-Langner R, Rodriguez ED, Cheng MH. The versatility of the anterolateral thigh flap. Plast Reconstr Surg. 2009;124:e395–407.

73. Gravvanis AI, Tsoutsos DA, Karakitsos D, et al. Application of the pedicled anterolateral thigh flap to defects from the pelvis to the knee. Microsurgery. 2006;26:432–8.

74. Arnez ZM. Immediate reconstruction of the lower extremity--an update. Clin Plast Surg. 1991;18:449–57.

75. Isenberg JS, Sherman R. Zone of injury: a valid concept in microvascular reconstruction of the traumatized lower limb? Ann Plast Surg. 1996;36:270–2.

76. Park S, Han SH, Lee TJ. Algorithm for recipient vessel selection in free tissue transfer to the lower extremity. Plast Reconstr Surg. 1999;103:1937–48.

77. Hong JP. The use of supermicrosurgery in lower extremity reconstruction: the next step in evolution. Plast Reconstr Surg. 2009;123:230–5.

78. Rodriguez ED, Bluebond-Langner R, Copeland C, Grim TN, Singh NK, Scalea T. Functional outcomes of posttraumatic lower limb salvage: a pilot study of anterolateral thigh perforator flaps versus muscle flaps. J Trauma. 2009;66:1311–4.

79. Pollak AN, McCarthy ML, Burgess AR. Short-term wound complications after application of flaps for coverage of traumatic soft-tissue defects about the tibia. The Lower Extremity Assessment Project (LEAP) Study Group. J Bone Joint Surg Am. 2000;82-A:1681–91.

80. Patzakis MJ, Abdollahi K, Sherman R, Holtom PD, Wilkins J. Treatment of chronic osteomyelitis with muscle flaps. Orthop Clin North Am. 1993;24:505–9.

81. Patzakis MJ, Zalavras CG. Chronic posttraumatic osteomyelitis and infected nonunion of the tibia: current management concepts. J Am Acad Orthop Surg. 2005;13:417–27.

82. Hong JPJ, Goh TLH, Choi DH, Kim JJ, Suh HS. The efficacy of perforator flaps in the treatment of chronic osteomyelitis. Plast Reconstr Surg. 2017;140:179–88.

The Role of Radiology in Trauma Patients

9

Gil-Sun Hong and Choong Wook Lee

By providing rapid and broad surveys, radiologic imaging is an essential tool in modern medicine for the evaluation of trauma patients. Radiologic imaging may inform clinical diagnosis and the development of treatment strategies such as operation, angiointerventions, or conservative treatment.

Imaging modalities such as X-ray, ultrasonography (USG), computed tomography (CT), and magnetic resonance imaging (MRI) have unique advantages and disadvantages in the evaluation of trauma patients. Imaging strategies regarding when and which modalities are used depend on the proximity to the imaging facility, the availability of qualified imaging technicians to manage severely injured patients, and the presence of radiology experts to adjust imaging protocols according to individual cases, make interpretations, and provide reports. Generally, X-ray and USG can be used at the bedside of severely injured patients, even those with hemodynamically unstable conditions. CT offers objective findings of internal organ injury with a reasonable imaging acquisition time. MRI can be used for the evaluation of spinal cord, brain, or soft tissue injuries but is limited because of its long acquisition time and devices that can be affected by magnetic fields. Trauma clinicians should be aware of the merits and limitations of imaging modalities and provide proper imaging work-up.

This chapter discusses the general principals of radiologic imaging and the clinical application of each imaging modality based on the guidelines and recommendations.

9.1 General Principals of Imaging

1. Trauma surgeons need to know the merits and limitations of each radiologic imaging modality (Table 9.1).

Table 9.1 Characteristics of imaging modalities

	Accessibility	Sensitivity	Objectivity	Radiation	Time
X-ray	+++ (Portable)	+	++	++	Minutes
USG	+++ (Portable)	++	+	none	Variable*
CT	+	+++	+++	+++	< 10 min
MRI		+++	+++	none	> 20 min

*depend on operator

G.-S. Hong · C. W. Lee (✉)
Department of Radiology and Research Institute of
Radiology, Asan Medical Center, University of Ulsan
College of Medicine, Seoul, South Korea
e-mail: gshong@amc.seoul.kr; cwlee@amc.seoul.kr

© Springer Nature Singapore Pte Ltd. 2019
S.-K. Hong et al. (eds.), *Primary Management of Polytrauma*,
https://doi.org/10.1007/978-981-10-5529-4_9

2. Portable X-ray and USG should be available in the resuscitation room.
3. Patient stay in the CT room should be as short as possible.
   (a) The CT room must be located near the resuscitation room.
   (b) The CT room must be emptied before patient arrival.
   (c) Trauma surgeons and imaging technicians must be trained for the patient's safe movement to the CT table.
   (d) Radiologists have to manage the entire imaging process, from the individual patient-based protocol decision to the prompt interpretation.

9.2 Trauma Series of X-rays

X-ray is a useful tool for quick screening to assess the extent of traumatic injury. Even in unstable patients, portable X-ray can be used to exclude diseases that require immediate intervention such as tension pneumothorax, to diagnose injuries that may elicit life-threatening hemorrhage such as pelvic bone fracture, and to prevent further neurological deterioration such as C-spine dislocation. Therefore, a "trauma series of X-rays" comprising chest anteroposterior (AP), C-spine lateral, and pelvis AP is very useful for the initial evaluation of severely injured patients (Figs. 9.1, 9.2, 9.3, 9.4, 9.5, 9.6, and 9.7).

1. Chest radiography
   A. Diseases that can be diagnosed with chest radiography
      (i) Pneumothorax, tension pneumothorax, hemothorax
      (ii) Pneumomediastinum, pneumopericardium, hemomediastinum
      (iii) Pulmonary contusion, aspiration pneumonitis
      (iv) Rib fracture, flail chest
      (v) Diaphragmatic rupture
   B. Check list
      (i) Airway of trachea and main bronchus
      (ii) Position and route of tubes and lines

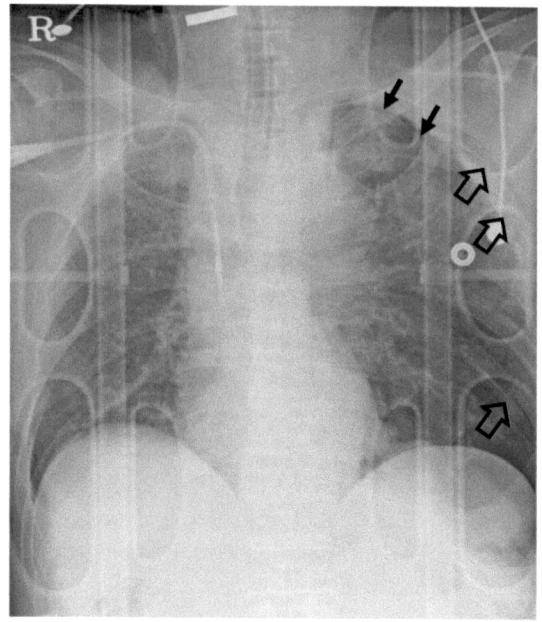

Fig. 9.1 Chest radiography of a severely injured patient. In severely injured patients, there are many limitations to the proper interpretation of radiography, including chest radiography being performed in the anteroposterior direction in a bed-ridden state with a portable machine, with low lung volumes and increased mediastinal width. These may lead to misinterpretation of lung or mediastinal injuries. Shadows from the spine board, tubes, and electrode wires may interfere with the normal lines of lung markings, visceral pleura, and bony thorax. In this patient, pneumothorax (arrows) and multiple rib fracture (open arrows) are present but are not easy to detect because of the overlying instrument

      (iii) Visceral pleural line
      (iv) Lung parenchymal opacities
      (v) Mediastinal width and position
      (vi) Rib contiguity

2. C-spine lateral radiography
   A. Diseases that can be diagnosed with C-spine lateral radiography
      (i) C-spine fracture and/or dislocation
      (ii) Hematoma in prevertebral space
      (iii) Airway compromise of upper airway
   B. Check list
      (i) C-spine alignment and bony integrity
      (ii) Width of retropharyngeal soft tissue
      (iii) Airway of larynx and upper trachea

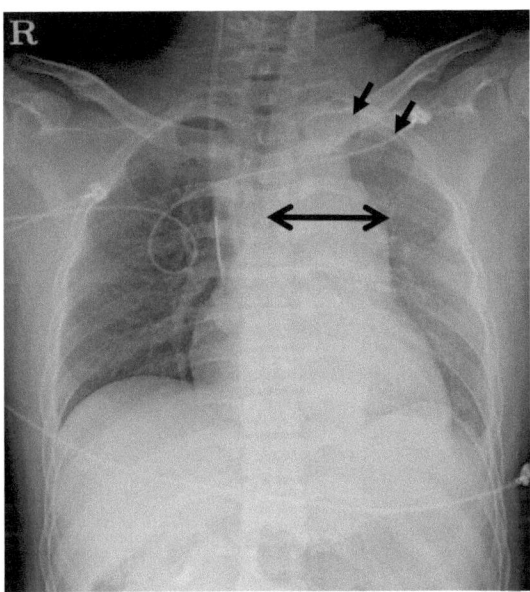

Fig. 9.2 Chest radiography of traumatic hemomediastinum and hemothorax. The chest radiography shows mediastinal widening (double-head arrow) that obscures the normal aortic knob contour and tracheal shifting to the right due to a mediastinal hematoma. The increased opacity of the left hemithorax with apical thickening (arrows) and left costophrenic angle blunting suggests hemothorax in this trauma patient

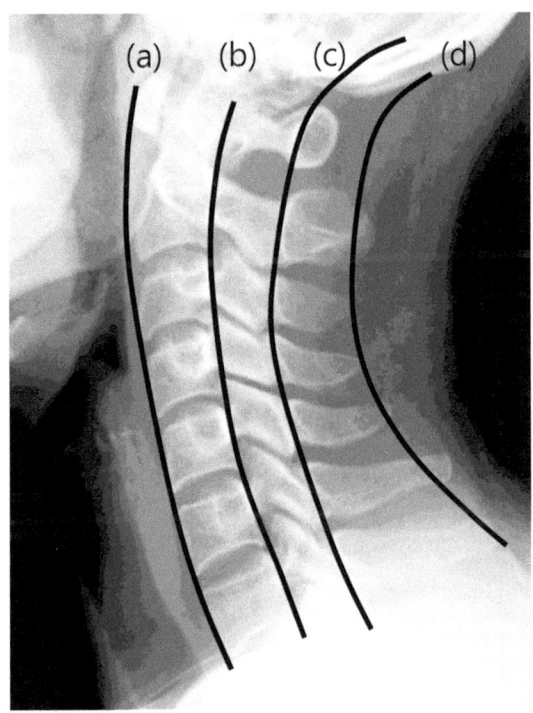

Fig. 9.4 In C-spine lateral imaging, assessment of the bony alignment is important, as well as bony integrity. The four imaginary lines—anterior vertebral line (**a**), posterior vertebral line (**b**), spinolaminar line (**c**), and posterior spinous line (**d**)—should be smoothly aligned

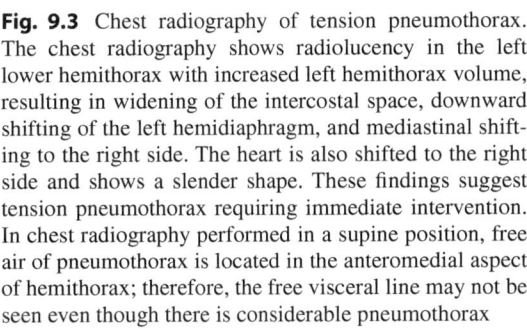

Fig. 9.3 Chest radiography of tension pneumothorax. The chest radiography shows radiolucency in the left lower hemithorax with increased left hemithorax volume, resulting in widening of the intercostal space, downward shifting of the left hemidiaphragm, and mediastinal shifting to the right side. The heart is also shifted to the right side and shows a slender shape. These findings suggest tension pneumothorax requiring immediate intervention. In chest radiography performed in a supine position, free air of pneumothorax is located in the anteromedial aspect of hemithorax; therefore, the free visceral line may not be seen even though there is considerable pneumothorax

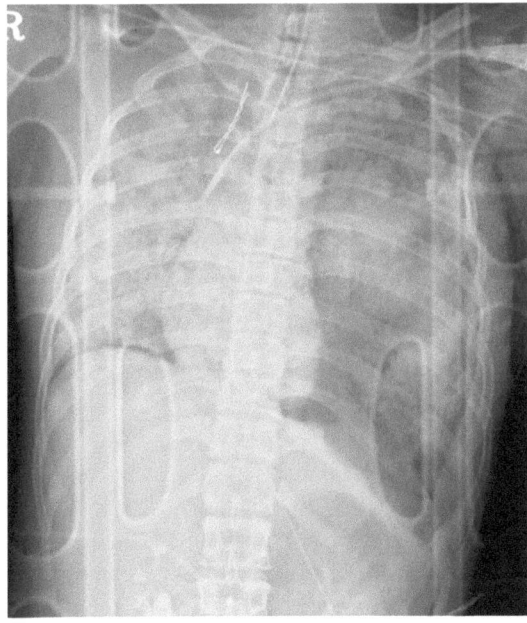

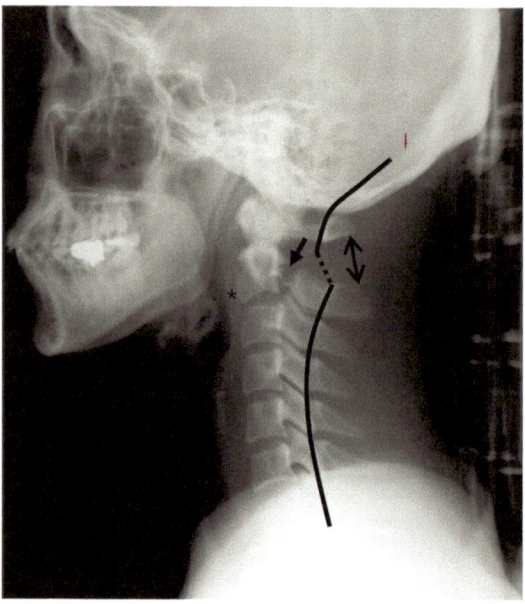

Fig. 9.5 Hangman's fracture of C2. There is a complete fracture of the pars interarticularis of C2 (arrow), with mild anterior dislocation of the C2 body. The imaginary spinolaminal line is disrupted (curved line), and the interspinous distance (double-head arrow) is increased. There is also widening of the retropharyngeal soft tissue shadow (asterisk) at the C2/C3 level due to a fracture-related hematoma

3. Pelvis AP radiography
   A. Disease that can be diagnosed with pelvis AP radiography
      (i) Pelvic bone fracture
      (ii) Prediction of bladder or urethral injury
   B. Check list
      (i) Bony integrity of sacrum and bilateral pelvic bones and femur
      (ii) Pelvic ring contiguity
      (iii) Hip joint and sacroiliac joint alignment

9.3 Ultrasonography

Severely injured patients can be evaluated at the bedside by USG, so-called focused assessment with sonography in trauma (FAST), during the initial resuscitation in the emergency room owing to the improved portability and image quality of

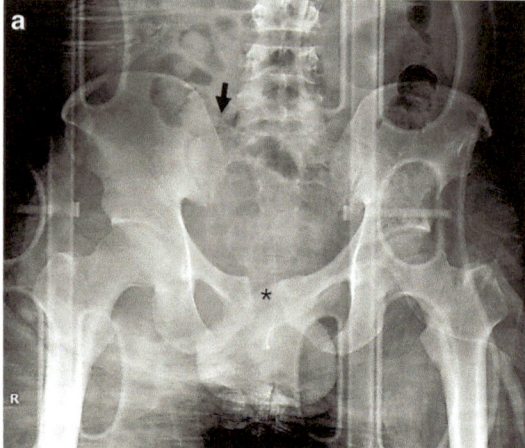

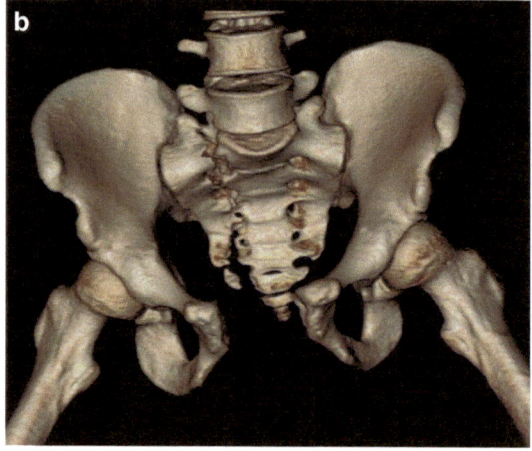

Fig. 9.6 Pelvic ring injury. (**a**) Pelvis AP images show diastasis of the pubic symphysis (asterisk) and a subtle fracture line in the right sacrum (arrow). (**b**) Three-dimensional volume rendering image of CT clearly demonstrates a vertical fracture of the right sacral ala and diastasis of the pubic symphysis

USG. Bedside USG can be easily performed anywhere and at any time and can provide critical real-time information about injured patients. In trauma situations, the role of FAST was initially confined to the detection of intraperitoneal (e.g., hemoperitoneum) and pericardial fluid, but its role has recently been extended to the evaluation of airway and thorax injuries (e.g., pneumothorax, hemothorax, etc.). Figure 9.7 illustrates the location of the standard FAST view. Originally, the standard view included four locations (the "four Ps"), namely, the pericardial, perihepatic (right upper quadrant), perisplenic (left upper quadrant), and pelvic areas (Fig. 9.8). These views allow the

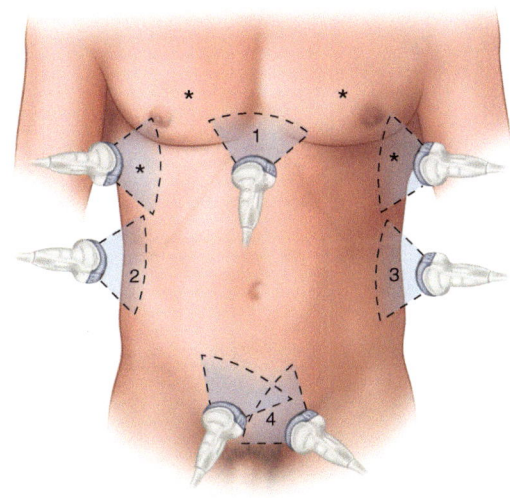

Fig. 9.7 Standard FAST views: (1) pericardial, (2) perihepatic, (3) perisplenic, and (4) pelvic. The additional thoracic views for E-FAST are also indicated (asterisks)

evaluation of sites where free fluid is more easily collected, identifying as little as 250 mL of free intraperitoneal fluid. USG can also be used to detect pneumothorax or hemothorax, referred to as extended FAST (E-FAST), by adding additional bilateral views of both hemithoraces (Fig. 9.9).

- General Principles
  - FAST must be available 24 h a day in the resuscitation room.
  - Trauma surgeons, emergency medicine physicians, and radiologists must be trained to perform FAST appropriately.
- Merits
  - Accessibility: bedside examination with portable USG
  - Real-time imaging with high temporal resolution
  - Non-radiation, noninvasive examination
  - Serial imaging for patient monitoring
- Pitfalls
  - Dependent on operator skill and patient habitus.
  - Limited for solid organ and gastrointestinal tract, retroperitoneal, and diaphragm injuries.
    - Negative FAST results do not exclude the presence of intra-abdominal injury.

- Interference due to intraperitoneal air.
- False-positive results from nonhemorrhagic intraperitoneal fluid such as ascites secondary to other medical conditions (e.g., liver cirrhosis, renal failure, etc.) or urine due to urinary bladder rupture.

9.4 CT and MRI Work-Up in Trauma Patients

Trauma surgeons and emergency medicine physicians should determine the severity of trauma on the basis of initial imaging (X-ray, FAST), physical examination, and trauma mechanisms. According to this severity, selective CT, limiting the extent of CT exposure in the suspected anatomical region, or whole-body CT (WBCT) is performed selectively in trauma patients. However, the use of selective CT requires attention because of the limited reliability of physical examination in patients with low levels of consciousness or other significant injuries. There is also a risk of unnoticed injuries, particularly in seriously injured elderly patients with traumatic brain injury or visible vascular damage. Therefore, trauma clinicians should be aware of the indication and limitation of CT and MRI to avoid missing critical trauma and unnecessary testing that may delay appropriate treatment in trauma patients.

- General Principles
  - CT scans should be performed only in hemodynamically stable patients. Trauma patients should be stabilized prior to radiographic studies, and clinicians should pay attention to potential spinal cord injuries and prevent further injuries during patient positioning and transfer for radiographic studies. Clinicians familiar with trauma care should accompany the patient to the CT room, as the patient may deteriorate rapidly.
  - CT scans of trauma patients should be completed at once, avoiding additional transfer and CT scans.

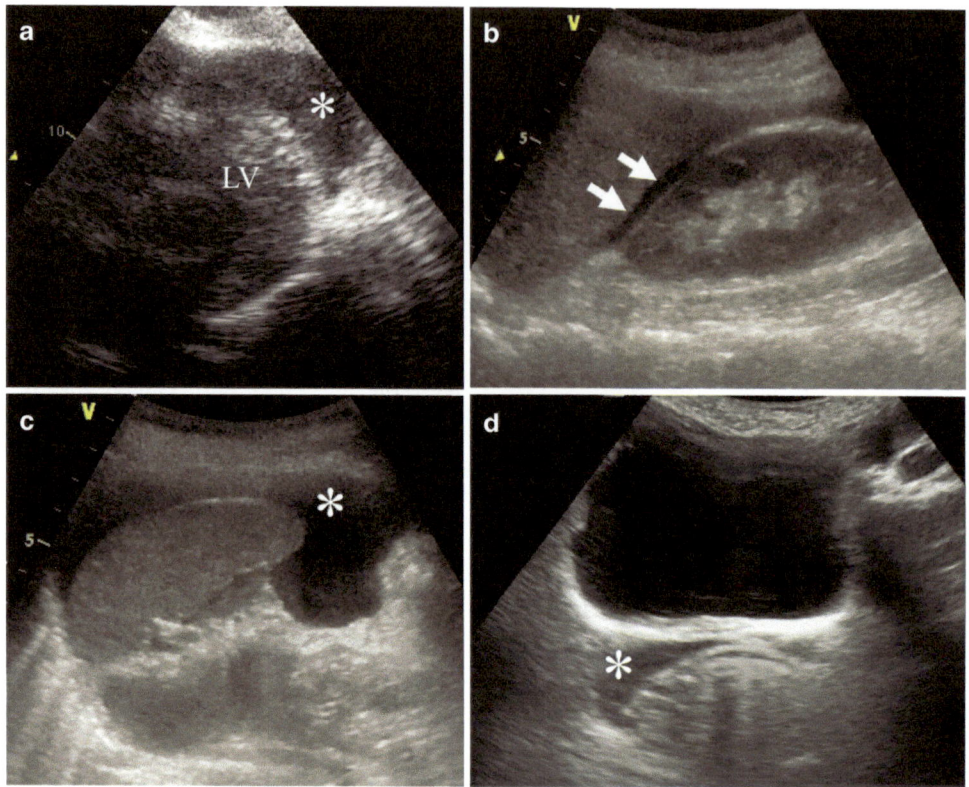

Fig. 9.8 Four standard focused assessment with sonography in trauma (FAST) views. (**a**) *Pericardial view* can be obtained by placing a transducer at the subxiphoid position pointing toward the left shoulder. Anechoic pericardial fluid (*) is observed in the periphery of the left ventricle (LV) wall. (**b**) *Prehepatic view* at the right mid- to posterior axillary line of the intercostal space between the 11th and 12th ribs showing a small amount of anechoic fluid (arrows) in the Morrison's pouch between the liver and right kidney. This location is the most common location of free fluid. (**c**) *Perisplenic view* at the left posterior axillary line of the intercostal space between the 10th and 11th ribs showing a large amount of free fluid (asterisk) around the spleen. (**d**) *Pelvic view* can be obtained by placing a transducer just superior to the symphysis pubis. This view allows the identification of the free fluid in the rectovesical (asterisk) and retrouterine spaces, the second most common locations of free fluid

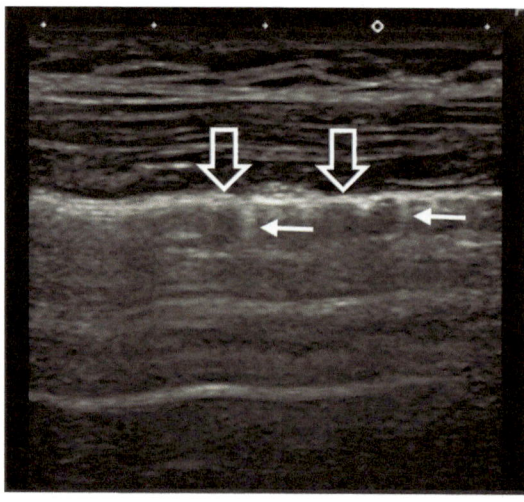

Fig. 9.9 Bilateral thoracic view for extended FAST (E-FAST). The thoracic view is usually obtained by placing a higher-frequency transducer in the 3rd or 4th intercostal space. In the normal thorax, "pleural sliding" and "comet-tail artifact" can be identified. "Pleural sliding" is the sliding motion of the visceral pleura (open arrows) against the inner margin of the thoracic wall (parietal pleura). A "comet-tail artifact" (arrows) is a hyperechogenic narrow-based reverberation artifact. If these findings are absent, pneumothorax should be considered

- CT should be performed without performing X-rays if the X-rays might delay CT
  scans or operation in trauma patients.
- The application of MRI to the investigation
  of trauma patients is limited because of the
  long image acquisition time and the difficulty in removing ferromagnetic material
  (i.e., foreign bodies and the use of life support devices) prior to testing.

9.4.1   Whole-Body CT for Severe Trauma Patients

9.4.1.1 Patient Selection Criteria for WBCT

Patient section criteria that requires WBCT in severe trauma patients [1]
1. High-risk injury mechanism
Traffic accidents
Pedestrian/cyclist/motorcyclist hit by a vehicle
Prolonged patient extrication (>15 min)
Death of another passenger
Ejection from the vehicle
High-speed automobile collision
Motorcycle accident
Fall from >3 m, unknown height, stairs
2. Evidence of anatomical injuries
Visible injuries in two anatomical regions (head/neck/thorax/abdomen/pelvis/long bones)
Sign of vascular damage (expansive hematoma, deep wound in arterial trajectory)
Signs of spinal cord damage
Unstable pelvic fracture
Fractures of more than one long bone
3. Vital signs
Glasgow score < 12, intubated
Systolic blood pressure < 100 mmHg
Respiratory frequency: <10 or >30 rpm
Pulse >120 bpm
$SatO_2 < 90\%$
Age > 65 years
Anticoagulation

- General Principles
  - The British Royal College of Radiologists
    (RCR) has restricted the use of WBCT in
    severe trauma patients with an Injury
    Severity Score (ISS) > 15 [2]
  - WBCT quickly identifies life-threatening
    trauma lesions, including the presence of
    active bleeding and unexpected injuries,
    and can be used to assess the overall inju-
    ries of the trauma patient simultaneously.
  - WBCT is useful in severely injured
    patients with changes in mental status.
  - In comparison to conventional imaging in
    severe trauma patients, WBCT takes about
    one-quarter of the time to scan and reduces
    about half of the patient transfer [3].
  - WBCT results in more radiation expo-
    sure compared to that of selective CT,
    limiting the extent of radiation exposure
    in the suspected anatomical region in
    mild trauma patients, which can be an
    important consideration, especially in
    younger patients.
  - In the case of WBCT, one report indi-
    cated that traumatic injury was not iden-
    tified in 30% of cases [4]; therefore,
    appropriate selection of trauma patients
    who require WBCT is needed.

9.4.1.2 Controversy Regarding the Application of WBCT

There is still some debate about the usefulness
of WBCT. WBCT has the advantage of reducing the duration of intensive care unit (ICU)
admission, reducing the duration of ventilation, decreasing the percentage of organ failure
[5], inducing rapid discharge [6], and minimiz-
ing unrecognized damage at the beginning [7].
Some researchers claim that WBCT is useful in
severely injured patients with changes in mental status. A retrospective database analysis of
5208 patients in Japan with Glasgow Coma
Scale (GCS) scores ranging from 3 to 12 noted
decreased mortality in patients who received
WBCT scans [8]. However, an international,
multicenter trial reported that in-hospital mortality did not differ between WBCT and conventional imaging work-up or between patients
with polytrauma and those with traumatic brain
injury [9]. Therefore, additional studies on the
usefulness and cost-effectiveness of WBCT are
needed.

9.4.2 Selective CT for Trauma Patients

9.4.2.1 Head Trauma

Patient section criteria that requires head CT [10–12]
1. GCS < 15 two hours post injury
2. Suspected open skull fracture
3. Sign of skull base fracture Hemotympanum Raccoon eyes (intraorbital bruising) Battle sign (retroauricular bruising) Cerebrospinal fluid leak, oto- or rhinorrhea
4. Vomiting more than twice
5. Age ≥ 60 years
6. Amnesia post event >30 min
7. Dangerous mechanism of injury Pedestrian struck by motor vehicle Occupant ejected from motor vehicle Fall from >3 feet or 5 stairs
8. Neurological deficit
9. Seizure
10. Blood thinner (oral anticoagulant use or bleeding diathesis)
11. Return visit for reassessment of a head injury

The clinical criteria were based on clinical criteria validated in three prospective studies: the Canadian CT head rule (CCHR) [10], the New Orleans Criteria (NOC) [11], and the National Emergency X-Radiography Utilization Study II (NEXUS II) [12]. These three clinical criteria have high sensitivity for patients with clinically significant CT findings and have the effect of reducing the number of CT examinations performed.

The sensitivities of the three clinical criteria for the identification of brain damage requiring neurological intervention were 100% (NOC), 100% (CCHR), and 95% (NEXUS II). The sensitivities of these clinical criteria for the identification of clinically significant brain injury without neurological intervention were 92%, 79%, and 89%, respectively. The sensitivity to clinical outcomes was highest in the NOC. However, the specificity of these criteria was very low, at less than 50%, and lowest in the NOC (<25%) [13].

9.4.2.2 Blunt Cerebrovascular Injury (BCVI)

Patient section criteria that requires CTA for screening BCVI [14–16]
1. Unexplained neurological sign and symptom Arterial hemorrhage from the neck, mouth, nose, or ear Cervical hematoma Cervical bruit in a patient younger (<50 years) Focal or lateralizing neurological deficit
2. Injury mechanism (severe cervical hyperextension/rotation or hyperflexion)
3. Severe facial trauma (bilateral facial fractures, complex midface, subcondylar fractures)
4. Basilar skull fracture involving carotid canal
5. Cervical vertebral body fracture, transverse foramen fracture, subluxation, or ligamentous injury at any level or any fracture at the level of C1–C3
6. Diffuse axonal brain injury (closed head injury with GCS < 6)
7. Near-hanging resulting in cerebral anoxia
8. Clothesline-type injury or seat belt abrasion with significant cervical pain, swelling, or altered mental status

These criteria have clinical signs, symptoms, or risk factors that suggest BCVI. The risk factors listed above are based on the Eastern and Western Trauma Associations of the United States, which are used to screen for patients with no symptoms [14–16]. Computed tomographic angiography (CTA) is the screening test of choice in patients with suspected BCVI in an emergency. The sensitivity and specificity of CTA vary depending on the CT equipment. A study using four- and eight-slice scanners showed 83–92% sensitivity and 88–92% specificity for blunt carotid injuries and 50–60% sensitivity and 90–97% specificity for blunt vertebral injury [17]. A 16-slice scanner study showed lesion detection equivalent to that of digital subtraction angiography [18]. A recent study showed that WBCT with a single dose of contrast agent may be as accurate as CTA for the diagnosis of BCVI [19].

- General Principles
  - Patients with BCVI initially have no symptoms but develop stroke symptoms about one day later [20].

- BCVI occurs in 30–37% of patients with multiple trauma who do not meet the BCVI screening criteria [21]. Therefore, it is necessary to carefully evaluate WBCT images in severe trauma patients, always considering the possibility of BCVI, even if it is not the case for these indications.
- Bilateral cerebrovascular injuries are common, occurring in 18–25% of patients [22].
- Carotid injuries occur more frequently than vertebral injuries [23].
- BCVI may occur in the contralateral vessel as well as in the ipsilateral vessel in the injured area of the head and neck due to vessel sharing injuries, requiring caution in image analysis [23]. Therefore, in patients with BCVI or blunt neck trauma, it is necessary to carefully evaluate both vessels of the neck (Figs. 9.10 and 9.11).

9.4.2.3 Cervical Spine Injury

Patient section criteria that requires cervical spinal CT [24, 25]
1. Dangerous mechanism of injury (high-speed motor vehicle collision, fall from height including diving, rollover motor accident, bicycle collision)
2. Death at scene of motor vehicle crash
3. Significant closed head injury or intracranial hemorrhage seen on CT
4. Neurologic symptoms or sign referred to the cervical spine
5. Pelvic or multiple extremity fractures
6. Multi-region trauma
7. Technically inadequate plain X-ray
8. Suspicious or definitely abnormal plain X-ray
9. Age ≥ 60 years

- General Principles
  - Cervical spinal CT should be performed in patients with severe trauma, those at high risk, or those with changes in mental status.
  - There is insufficient evidence to replace plain radiography with CT as the initial screening method in lower-risk patients.

- It may be necessary to perform cervical spinal CT if it is difficult to obtain a technically appropriate image by plain radiography. A retrospective study of blunt trauma patients showed that 72% of plain radiography images were inadequate to view the entire cervical spine [26]. In addition, insufficient images are often obtained in severe trauma patients due to blunt trauma, and misdiagnosis of cervical spinal fractures are reported in up to 16% of cases [27].
- It may be preferable to perform cervical spinal CT in elderly patients because the interpretation of plain radiography may be difficult in elder trauma patients [28].

9.4.2.4 Thoracic, Lumbar, and Sacral (TLS) Spinal Injury

Patient section criteria that requires TLS spinal CT [29–32]
1. Suspicious or definitely abnormal plain X-ray
2. Signs of injury or neurological deficit in the thoracic or lumbosacral regions
3. New another spine injury, particularly a known cervical fracture
4. High-energy mechanism (fall ≥3 m, ejection from a vehicle, motor vehicle rack, forceful direct blow)
5. Patient (age ≥ 60 years) with sign/symptom or mechanism causing TLS spine injury
6. Depressed metal status (GCS < 15 or signs of intoxication) with sign/symptom or mechanism causing TLS spine injury

- General Principles
  - According to the Eastern Association for the Surgery of Trauma practice guidelines, there is no need to perform an imaging test on the TLS spine in blunt trauma patients with normal mental status and no risks [31].
  - In addition to physical examination, it is necessary to consider the traumatic mechanism when selecting patients who require CT examination because there are limitations in the physical examinations. In one large prospective study, TLS spine injuries

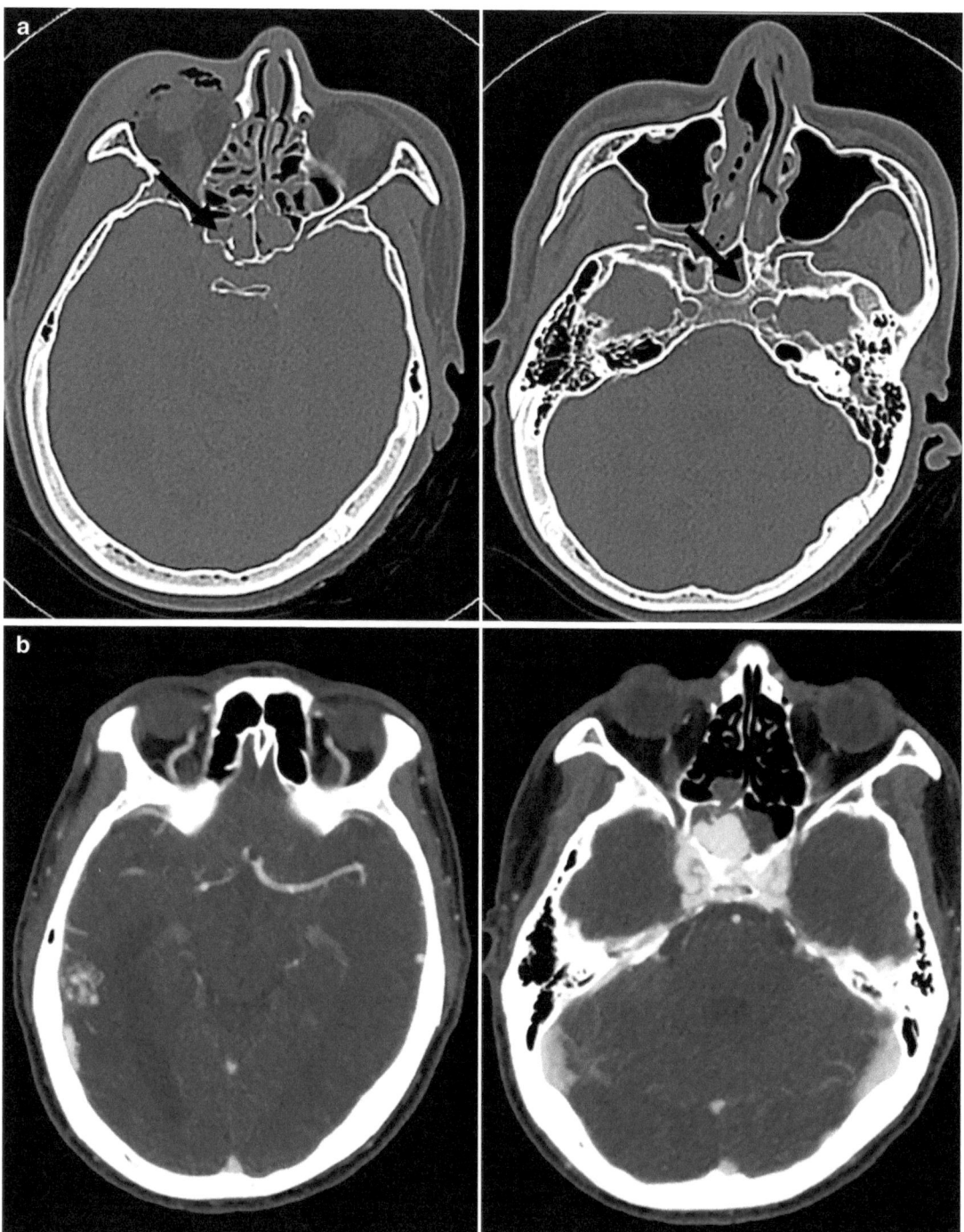

Fig. 9.10 Carotid cavernous fistula in a major trauma patient with skull base fracture. (**a**) Brain CT shows a fracture that obliquely crosses the skull base. (**b**) CT angi-ography shows a carotid-cavernous fistula with an engorged ophthalmic vein and pseudoaneurysm

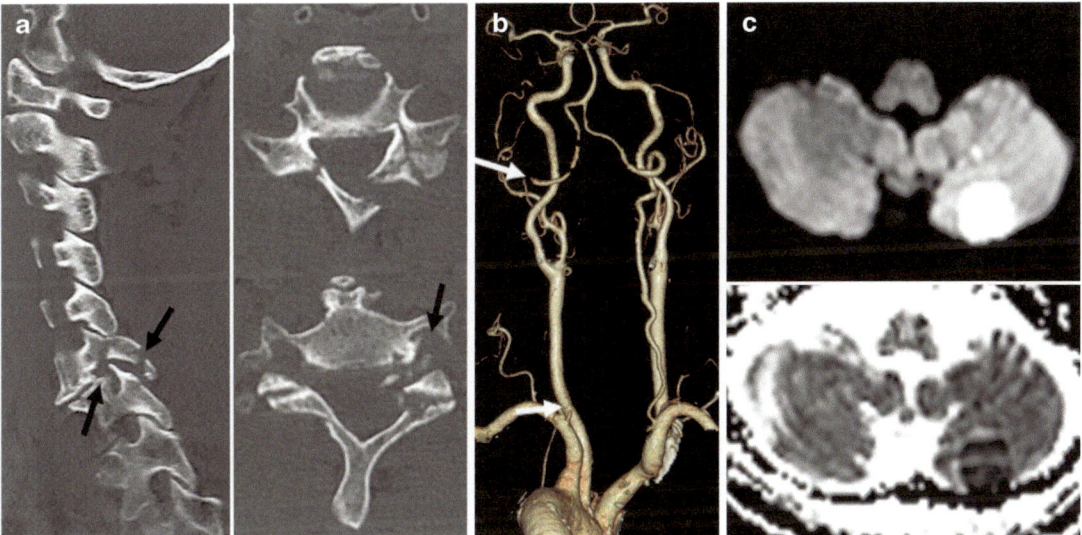

Fig. 9.11 BCVI (blunt cerebrovascular injury) in a major trauma patient. (**a**) Cervical spinal CT shows a fracture of the cervical spine across the left transverse foramen. (**b**) CT angiography shows a left vertebral artery occlusion. (**c**) Diffusion-weighted images show acute infarct in the left cerebellar hemisphere

requiring surgical treatment were found in more than 20% of patients with normal physical examinations [32].

- TLS spinal CT may still be required despite an unremarkable physical examination.
- However, reformatted thoracic and abdominal CT images in severe trauma patients may be sufficient to assess most TLS spine injuries and do not require additional TL spine administration [33].

9.4.2.5 Thoracic Injury

Patient section criteria that requires thoracic CT
1. Severe trauma patients
2. Mild trauma patient with following risk factors Abnormal plain chest radiograph despite the absence of obvious clinical signs of injury
Concerning clinical findings (e.g., severe pain or marked chest tenderness, hypoxia, dyspnea, tachypnea) with normal chest radiography
High-energy mechanism

Generally, chest CT is unnecessary in trauma patients with low-energy mechanisms of injury, minimal injury on physical examination, and nor-

mal chest radiography findings [34]. However, observational studies have shown clinically significant chest trauma on chest CT in trauma patients with normal chest radiography, although these studies included only a small number of patients [35]. Conversely, abnormal findings in simple chest radiography suggest clinically significant chest trauma [36].

There is conflicting evidence regarding the need for chest CT in trauma patients with high-energy mechanisms of injury; however, chest CT is generally preferred. In one prospective study, although there was no external sign of thoracic injury in 592 hemodynamically stable patients with a significant injury mechanism, clinically significant findings were found in 19.6% of chest CTs [37]. In a prospective study of 609 blunt trauma patients, clinically significant findings were found in 11% of chest CT cases in which emergency physicians determined that CT was unnecessary [38].

The NEXUS is a prospectively validated decision instrument to determine the need for chest CT in trauma patients [39, 40].

Types	Criteria factors	Accuracy
NEXUS decision instrument (earlier iteration) [39]	Age > 60 years Chest pain Intoxication Abnormal alertness or mental status Chest wall tenderness Distracting painful injury Rapid deceleration mechanism	Sensitivity (98.8%) and specificity (13.3%) percent for any thoracic injury seen on chest imaging (If all criteria are absent, the patient has a very low risk for intrathoracic injury and chest imaging is not indicated)
NEXUS decision instrument (Chest CT-All) [40]	Chest wall tenderness Distracting painful injury Rapid deceleration mechanism Abnormal plain chest radiograph Sternal tenderness Thoracic spine tenderness Scapular tenderness	Sensitivity (99.2%), specificity (20.8%), and negative predictive value (NPV) (99.8%) for major injury Sensitivity (95.4%), specificity (25.5%), and a NPV (93.9%) for either major or minor injury
NEXUS decision instrument (chest CT-major[a]) [40]	Chest wall tenderness Distracting painful injury Abnormal plain chest radiograph Sternal tenderness Thoracic spine tenderness Scapular tenderness	Sensitivity (99.2%), specificity (31.7%), and a NPV (99.9%) for major injury

[a]Major injuries included aortic or great vessel injury; diaphragm rupture; pneumothorax or hemothorax requiring thoracostomy; spine or other major fracture requiring surgical repair; esophageal, tracheal, or bronchial injury requiring surgical intervention; pulmonary contusion requiring ventilatory support; and several others.

The application of these criteria would reduce unnecessary chest CT. However, when applying the NEXUS criteria to trauma patients, it is important to note the presence of any one criteria factor represents a low rate of major clinical injury, so clinicians should discuss the potential risks and benefit of chest CT in these cases. However, in the patient with an abnormal chest X-ray, the risks of major clinical injury and minor injury are considerably higher than with the other criteria [36].

- General Principales
  - Chest CT should be performed in cases of abnormal chest radiography findings in mild trauma patients and clinically suspicious cases with normal chest radiography findings.
  - Chest CT should be performed if the clinician suspects chest injury regardless of the criteria. The clinician should lower the threshold for performing an imaging test for a chest injury.

9.4.2.6 Abdominal Injury

Patient section criteria that requires abdominal CT [41, 42]

1. Physical examination findings
   Seat belt sign
   Rebound tenderness
   Hypotension
   Abdominal distension
   Abdominal guarding
   Severe distracting injury (e.g., femur fracture)
2. The presence of an altered sensorium or painful extra-abdominal injuries, even in the absence of suggestive symptoms or signs
3. Abnormal chest radiograph suggesting intra-abdominal injury (lower rib fractures, diaphragmatic hernia, free air under the diaphragm)
4. Fracture involving the pelvic ring
5. History features
   Fatality at the scene
   Vehicle type and velocity
   Whether the vehicle rolled over
   Patient's location within the vehicle
   Extent of intrusion into the passenger compartment
   Extent of damage to the vehicle; steering wheel deformity
   Whether seat belts were used and what type (unrestrained victims are at higher risk of injury); whether air bags deployed
6. Age > 60

Emergency and trauma clinicians managing blunt trauma should maintain a high clinical suspicion of intra-abdominal injuries, especially in patients with suggestive trauma mechanisms, signs of external trauma, and altered sensorium due to head injury and intoxication. Up to 10% of isolated head injury patients may have an intra-abdominal injury [43]. According to one prospective observational study, approximately 7% of blunt trauma patients with distracting extra-abdominal injuries have intra-abdominal injuries despite the absence of signs or symptoms suggestive of abdominal injuries [44]. Patients with fractures of the pelvic ring should also be suspected of intra-abdominal injury. Abdominal injuries are observed in up to 16.5% of patients with pelvic bone fractures [45]. Both visceral organs (i.e., liver and spleen) and the bowels can be involved in the damage [42, 45].

- General Principles
  - Abdominal pain and tenderness increase the likelihood of intra-abdominal injuries; however, the negative likelihood ratio for each is low, and the absence of these findings cannot exclude abdominal injuries.
  - Clinicians should maintain a high index of suspicion for intra-abdominal injuries especially in those patients older than 60 years of age since the signs and symptoms of abdominal injuries often appear to be weakened.
  - Altered sensorium or painful extra-abdominal injuries increase the likelihood of intra-abdominal injuries even in the absence of symptoms or signs suggestive of abdominal injuries.

9.4.3 MRI Work-Up for Trauma Patients

9.4.3.1 MRI for Head Trauma

MRI is not a first-line imaging study in the initial examination of patients with head trauma. It is difficult to perform MRI in emergency situations. Long scan times and multiple devices are limiting factors in performing MRI. MRI is more sensitive than CT for the detection of parenchymal, subdural, and epidural hemorrhages, as well as contusion, brainstem injury including posterior fossa, and diffusion axonal injury [46, 47]. In acute mild traumatic brain injury patients, abnormal MRI findings are reported in 30% of normal CT patients [46, 47]. Most of these findings were axonal injuries but also included small contusions and subarachnoid hemorrhage. Both brain contusion and hemorrhagic axonal injury are associated with poor 3-month outcomes [47]. In head trauma patients, selective MRI is useful in patients with unexplained neurological deficits or in patients who do not recover as expected.

- General Principle
  - If the trauma patient has a severe neurologic abnormality with normal CT findings at the initial examination, the patient is judged to have an axonal or brainstem injury, and MRI should be performed after emergency operation and treatment.

9.4.3.2 MRI for Spinal Column Injury

MRI is more useful than CT for the evaluation of spinal cord integrity, intervertebral discs, soft tissues, and ligamentous structures around the vertebra and is more sensitive to the detection of epidural hematoma than CT [48]. Traumatic spinal cord injury (TSCI) is found in MRI scans in 5.8% of cases with negative CT scans [49]. However, it is difficult to perform MRI in the initial examination of trauma patients because of metallic foreign bodies and lift-supporting equipment as well as cardiac pacemakers in trauma patients. In addition, it may be difficult to monitor patient vital signs during MRI.

- General Principles
  - MRI should be performed when the clinical condition of the patient is suitable for performing MRI, if spinal cord injury is suspected or occult spinal injury is suspected in patients with normal CT findings.
  - The high incidence of multiple vertebral injuries means that whole-spine MRI scans should be performed [50].

9.5   Summary

1. Trauma clinicians should aware of the merits, limitations, and indications for imaging.
2. Portable X-ray and USG should be available in the resuscitation room.
3. A "trauma series of X-rays" comprising chest AP (anteroposterior), C-spine lateral, and pelvis AP views is very useful for the initial evaluation of severely injured patients.

4. Trauma clinicians can skip X-rays if it might delay the CT scan or operation in trauma patients.

5. CT scans should be performed only in hemodynamically stable patients.

6. CT scans of trauma patients should be completed all at once to avoid additional transfer and CT scans.

7. WBCT quickly identifies life-threatening trauma lesions in severe trauma patient all at once.

8. The application of MRI for the initial evaluation of trauma patients is limited because of the long image acquisition time and the difficulty of removing ferromagnetic material.

9. Discrepancies between the neurologic abnormalities and head CT findings in trauma patients suggest axonal injury and follow-up MRI of the brain should be performed after emergency operation.

10. The high incidence of multiple vertebral injuries means that whole-spine scans should be performed.

References

1. Artigas Martin JM, Marti de Gracia M, Claraco Vega LM, Parrilla Herranz P. Radiology and imaging techniques in severe trauma. Med Intensiva. 2015;39(1):49–59.
2. RCR. Standards of practice and guidance for trauma radiology in severely injured patient. London: Royal College of Radiologist; 2011.
3. Saltzherr TP, Bakker FC, Beenen LF, Dijkgraaf MG, Reitsma JB, Goslings JC. Randomized clinical trial comparing the effect of computed tomography in the trauma room versus the radiology department on injury outcomes. Br J Surg. 2012;99(Suppl 1):105–13.
4. Harvey JJ, West AT. The right scan, for the right patient, at the right time: the reorganization of major trauma service provision in England and its implications for radiologists. Clin Radiol. 2013;68(9):871–86.
5. Weninger P, Mauritz W, Fridrich P, et al. Emergency room management of patients with blunt major trauma: evaluation of the multislice computed tomography protocol exemplified by an urban trauma center. J Trauma. 2007;62(3):584–91.
6. Livingston DH, Lavery RF, Passannante MR, et al. Admission or observation is not necessary after a negative abdominal computed tomographic scan in patients with suspected blunt abdominal trauma:

results of a prospective, multi-institutional trial. J Trauma. 1998;44(2):273–80; discussion 80–2.
7. Geyer LL, Korner M, Linsenmaier U, et al. Incidence of delayed and missed diagnoses in whole-body multidetector CT in patients with multiple injuries after trauma. Acta Radiol. 2013;54(5):592–8.
8. Kimura A, Tanaka N. Whole-body computed tomography is associated with decreased mortality in blunt trauma patients with moderate-to-severe consciousness disturbance: a multicenter, retrospective study. J Trauma Acute Care Surg. 2013;75(2):202–6.
9. Sierink JC, Treskes K, Edwards MJ, et al. Immediate total-body CT scanning versus conventional imaging and selective CT scanning in patients with severe trauma (REACT-2): a randomised controlled trial. Lancet. 2016;388(10045):673–83.
10. Stiell IG, Wells GA, Vandemheen K, et al. The Canadian CT head rule for patients with minor head injury. Lancet. 2001;357(9266):1391–6.
11. Haydel MJ, Preston CA, Mills TJ, Luber S, Blaudeau E, DeBlieux PM. Indications for computed tomography in patients with minor head injury. N Engl J Med. 2000;343(2):100–5.
12. Mower WR, Hoffman JR, Herbert M, Wolfson AB, Pollack CV Jr, Zucker MI. Developing a decision instrument to guide computed tomographic imaging of blunt head injury patients. J Trauma. 2005;59(4):954–9.
13. Ro YS, Shin SD, Holmes JF, et al. Comparison of clinical performance of cranial computed tomography rules in patients with minor head injury: a multicenter prospective study. Acad Emerg Med. 2011;18(6):597–604.
14. Biffl WL, Cothren CC, Moore EE, et al. Western Trauma Association critical decisions in trauma: screening for and treatment of blunt cerebrovascular injuries. J Trauma. 2009;67(6):1150–3.
15. Bromberg WJ, Collier BC, Diebel LN, et al. Blunt cerebrovascular injury practice management guidelines: the eastern Association for the Surgery of trauma. J Trauma. 2010;68(2):471–7.
16. Mundinger GS, Dorafshar AH, Gilson MM, Mithani SK, Manson PN, Rodriguez ED. Blunt-mechanism facial fracture patterns associated with internal carotid artery injuries: recommendations for additional screening criteria based on analysis of 4,398 patients. J Oral Maxillofacial Surg. 2013;71(12):2092–100.
17. Bub LD, Hollingworth W, Jarvik JG, Hallam DK. Screening for blunt cerebrovascular injury: evaluating the accuracy of multidetector computed tomographic angiography. J Trauma. 2005;59(3):691–7.
18. Berne JD, Reuland KS, Villarreal DH, McGovern TM, Rowe SA, Norwood SH. Sixteen-slice multidetector computed tomographic angiography improves the accuracy of screening for blunt cerebrovascular injury. J Trauma. 2006;60(6):1204–9; discussion 1209–10.
19. Sliker CW, Shanmuganathan K, Mirvis SE. Diagnosis of blunt cerebrovascular injuries with 16-MDCT: accuracy of whole-body MDCT compared with

neck MDCT angiography. AJR Am J Roentgenol. 2008;190(3):790–9.

20. Cothren CC, Moore EE, Ray CE, et al. Screening for blunt cerebrovascular injuries is cost-effective. Am J Surg. 2005;190(6):849–54.

21. Jacobson LE, Ziemba-Davis M, Herrera AJ. The limitations of using risk factors to screen for blunt cerebrovascular injuries: the harder you look, the more you find. World J Emerg Surg. 2015;10:46.

22. Edwards NM, Fabian TC, Claridge JA, Timmons SD, Fischer PE, Croce MA. Antithrombotic therapy and endovascular stents are effective treatment for blunt carotid injuries: results from long-term follow-up. J Am Coll Surg. 2007;204(5):1007–13.

23. Biffl WL, Ray CE Jr, Moore EE, et al. Treatment-related outcomes from blunt cerebrovascular injuries: importance of routine follow-up arteriography. Ann Surg. 2002;235(5):699.

24. Hanson JA, Blackmore CC, Mann FA, Wilson AJ. Cervical spine injury: a clinical decision rule to identify high-risk patients for helical CT screening. AJR Am J Roentgenol. 2000;174(3):713–7.

25. Amy Kaji RSH. Evaluation and acute management of cervical spinal column injuries in adults. UpToDate; 2017.

26. Gale SC, Gracias VH, Reilly PM, Schwab CW. The inefficiency of plain radiography to evaluate the cervical spine after blunt trauma. J Trauma Acute Care Surg. 2005;59(5):1121–5.

27. Widder S, Doig C, Burrowes P, Larsen G, Hurlbert RJ, Kortbeek JB. Prospective evaluation of computed tomographic scanning for the spinal clearance of obtunded trauma patients: preliminary results. J Trauma Acute Care Surg. 2004;56(6):1179–84.

28. Greenbaum J, Walters N, Levy PD. An evidenced-based approach to radiographic assessment of cervical spine injuries in the emergency department. J Emerg Med. 2009;36(1):64–71.

29. Hsu JM, Joseph T, Ellis AM. Thoracolumbar fracture in blunt trauma patients: guidelines for diagnosis and imaging. Injury. 2003;34(6):426–33.

30. O'Connor E, Walsham J. Review article: indications for thoracolumbar imaging in blunt trauma patients: a review of current literature. Emerg Med Australas. 2009;21(2):94–101.

31. Sixta S, Moore FO, Ditillo MF, et al. Screening for thoracolumbar spinal injuries in blunt trauma: an Eastern Association for the Surgery of Trauma practice management guideline. J Trauma Acute Care Surg. 2012;73(5 Suppl 4):S326–32.

32. Inaba K, Nosanov L, Menaker J, et al. Prospective derivation of a clinical decision rule for thoracolumbar spine evaluation after blunt trauma: an American Association for the Surgery of Trauma Multi-Institutional Trials Group Study. J Trauma Acute Care Surg. 2015;78(3):459–65; discussion 65–7.

33. Kim S, Yoon CS, Ryu JA, et al. A comparison of the diagnostic performances of visceral organ-targeted versus spine-targeted protocols for the evaluation of spinal fractures using sixteen-channel multidetec-tor row computed tomography: is additional spine-targeted computed tomography necessary to evaluate thoracolumbar spinal fractures in blunt trauma victims? J Trauma. 2010;69(2):437–46.

34. Kea B, Gamarallage R, Vairamuthu H, et al. What is the clinical significance of chest CT when the chest x-ray result is normal in patients with blunt trauma? Am J Emerg Med. 2013;31(8):1268–73.

35. Brink M, Deunk J, Dekker HM, et al. Added value of routine chest MDCT after blunt trauma: evaluation of additional findings and impact on patient management. AJR Am J Roentgenol. 2008;190(6):1591–8.

36. Raja AS, Mower WR, Nishijima DK, et al. Prevalence and diagnostic performance of isolated and combined NEXUS chest CT decision criteria. Acad Emerg Med. 2016;23(8):863–9.

37. Salim A, Sangthong B, Martin M, Brown C, Plurad D, Demetriades D. Whole body imaging in blunt multisystem trauma patients without obvious signs of injury: results of a prospective study. Arch Surg. 2006;141(5):468–75.

38. Gupta M, Schriger DL, Hiatt JR, et al. Selective use of computed tomography compared with routine whole body imaging in patients with blunt trauma. Ann Emerg Med. 2011;58(5):407–16.e15.

39. Rodriguez RM, Anglin D, Langdorf MI, et al. NEXUS chest: validation of a decision instrument for selective chest imaging in blunt trauma. JAMA Surg. 2013;148(10):940–6.

40. Rodriguez RM, Langdorf MI, Nishijima D, et al. Derivation and validation of two decision instruments for selective chest CT in blunt trauma: a multicenter prospective observational study (NEXUS Chest CT). PLoS Med. 2015;12(10):e1001883.

41. Nishijima DK, Simel DL, Wisner DH, Holmes JF. Does this adult patient have a blunt intra-abdominal injury? JAMA. 2012;307(14):1517–27.

42. Cannada LK, Taylor RM, Reddix R, Mullis B, Moghadamian E, Erickson M. The Jones-Powell classification of open pelvic fractures: a multicenter study evaluating mortality rates. J Trauma Acute Care Surg. 2013;74(3):901–6.

43. Schurink G, Bode P, Van Luijt P, Van Vugt A. The value of physical examination in the diagnosis of patients with blunt abdominal trauma: a retrospective study. Injury. 1997;28(4):261–5.

44. Ferrera PC, Verdile VP, Bartfield JM, Snyder HS, Salluzzo RF. Injuries distracting from intraabdominal injuries after blunt trauma. Am J Emerg Med. 1998;16(2):145–9.

45. Demetriades D, Karaiskakis M, Toutouzas K, Alo K, Velmahos G, Chan L. Pelvic fractures: epidemiology and predictors of associated abdominal injuries and outcomes. J Am Coll Surg. 2002;195(1):1–10.

46. Hughes DG, Jackson A, Mason DL, Berry E, Hollis S, Yates DW. Abnormalities on magnetic resonance imaging seen acutely following mild traumatic brain injury: correlation with neuropsychologi-

cal tests and delayed recovery. Neuroradiology. 2004;46(7):550–8.

47. Yuh EL, Mukherjee P, Lingsma HF, et al. Magnetic resonance imaging improves 3-month outcome prediction in mild traumatic brain injury. Ann Neurol. 2013;73(2):224–35.

48. Goldberg AL, Kershah SM. Advances in imaging of vertebral and spinal cord injury. J Spinal Cord Med. 2010;33(2):105–16.

49. Schoenfeld AJ, Bono CM, McGuire KJ, Warholic N, Harris MB. Computed tomography alone versus computed tomography and magnetic resonance imaging in the identification of occult injuries to the cervical spine: a meta-analysis. J Trauma Acute Care Surg. 2010;68(1):109–14.

50. Barron D. (ii) Polytrauma imaging–the role of integrated imaging. Orthop Trauma. 2011;25(2):83–90.

Interventional Radiology

Jong Woo Kim and Ji Hoon Shin

10.1 The Role of Interventional Radiology in Trauma

Along with the development of imaging modalities and endovascular techniques, interventional radiology (IR) has played an important role in the management of trauma patients. Interventional radiologist, as a physician who received broad-based multimodality imaging training, can easily interpret findings from preprocedural imaging studies to optimize diagnosis and treatment of trauma patients in the emergency setting. IR management is now regarded as well-accepted treatment option for various kinds of trauma which could cause massive hemorrhage, including large vessel trauma such as the aorta, abdominal solid organ trauma, and pelvic trauma [1–3]. IR management provides minimally invasive approach and frequently offers the benefit of a focused definitive therapy, even in the presence of massive hemorrhage that allows for preservation of major vessels or injured solid organs and serves as an alternative to an open surgical treatment [4].

Above all things, treatment of trauma as a multidisciplinary approach requires efficient use of resources as well as cooperation and communication among all medical persons involved in the treatment of trauma patients. Patients need to be rapidly and accurately assessed to determine the nature of their injuries with treatments prioritized by injury severity. This chapter reviews the role, outcomes, and relevant issues linked to IR management in the trauma setting.

10.1.1 Why Is Early IR Management Necessary?

In trauma patients, to stem active hemorrhage is the most pressing concern of any trauma team, although severe injuries often require complex reconstruction and rehabilitation. Blood loss triggers a downward spiral of decreasing blood pressure, hypothermia, and acidosis. Early resolution of this lethal triad is vital because, once developed, it can form a vicious result that may not be able to overcome. Among them, coagulopathy could be the most influential factor for trauma-related mortality. This coagulopathy could be initiated by tissue trauma and systemic hypoperfusion and then be exacerbated by consumption, dysfunction, or hemodilution of hemostatic factors and platelets. Therefore, establishing rapid hemostasis is crucial for improving survivability in acute trauma setting with massive hemorrhage.

J. W. Kim (✉) · J. H. Shin
Department of Radiology and Research Institute of Radiology, Asan Medical Center, University of Ulsan, College of Medicine, Seoul, South Korea
e-mail: ewooya@empas.com

© Springer Nature Singapore Pte Ltd. 2019
S.-K. Hong et al. (eds.), *Primary Management of Polytrauma*,
https://doi.org/10.1007/978-981-10-5529-4_10

10.1.2 Interventional Management Modalities

The following IR management modalities are commonly utilized in the trauma patients.

10.1.2.1 Balloon Occlusion

Balloon occlusion is a temporary method to control life-threatening bleeding and divert blood to coronary and cerebral perfusion and thereby to stabilize the trauma patients in hemorrhagic shock by inflating an angioplasty balloon or an occlusion balloon proximal to or at a major arterial injury.

10.1.2.2 Embolization

Embolization could rapidly diagnose and treat massive hemorrhage even in multiple and anatomically distant bleeding sites and could reduce the risk of trauma-related coagulopathy as well as need for blood transfusion. Thus, early embolization is very important for improving clinical outcome in heavily injured trauma victims, especially combined with massive hemorrhage. Embolization is also suitable for surgically precluded injuries, such as blush-bleeding of the liver or kidney, and for locating and treating intimal vessel tears, and is useful for treating retroperitoneal and pelvic hemorrhage, both of which are difficult to access surgically. The choice of embolic agent will vary based on the site and nature of the injury, the desire to preserve collateral flow, and operator preference.

10.1.2.3 Stent Grafting

Penetrating or blunt trauma can cause the aorta and peripheral vessels to be punctured, or dissected, and stent grafts can be deployed via catheter delivery to stop life-threatening hemorrhage, reestablish tissue perfusion, and prevent delayed hemorrhage. Stent grafting could replace the need for surgical treatment for traumatic injury and reduce mortality related to surgery. Emergent thoracic endovascular aortic repair (TEVAR) for trauma-related thoracic aorta injury has become the treatment of choice, with favorable results. While open repair for trauma-related thoracic aorta injury is associated with an operative mortality of up to 28%, mortality rate of TEVAR for trauma-related thoracic aorta injury is 9%, and TEVAR is associated with decreased risk of complication. Recently, peripheral arterial injuries in a variety of anatomic locations have also been increasingly treated using stent grafts. However, the criteria used to choose the best method must be individualized. These considerations must be weighed against the long-term sequelae of device implantation, which are largely unknown.

10.2 Interventional Radiology in Aortic Trauma

Blunt traumatic aortic injury (BTAI) is a life-threatening condition from blunt trauma, behind only to intracranial hemorrhage as the primary cause of death [5, 6]. Historically, most patients die before reaching the hospital. Of those who survive, 50% of patients die within 24 h of admission to the hospital. The mortality gets higher to 100%, if the contained rupture converts to free rupture while awaiting treatment [7–10]. Indeed, quicker diagnosis and better emergency management has led to improvements in overall survival [11].

The mechanism of BTAI is complex. BTAIs after rapid deceleration accidents such as motor vehicle collisions, falls from a height, and crush injuries are thought to result from a number of different mechanical factors, which all contribute to injury [6]. Until now, several mechanisms have been suggested to explain these injuries: rapid deceleration, shearing forces, osseous pinch, and hydrostatic forces or water hammer phenomenon [6, 12–16]. Most injuries involve partial or full-thickness disruptions of the aortic wall. BTAIs most commonly occur at sites of aortic tethering: aortic root, the isthmus, and at the diaphragmatic hiatus. Approximately 90% of BTAIs occur at the anteromedial aspect of the aortic isthmus distal to the origin of the left subclavian artery. In less than 8%, BTAIs are located in the aortic root and are often associated with aortic valve tears, cardiac contusions or ruptures, coronary artery tears, and/or hemopericardium with cardiac tamponade.

In nearly 2%, BTAIs occur at the level of the diaphragm [8, 14, 15, 17].

Careful initial evaluation with a high degree of suspicion is necessary for diagnosing BTAI. Computed tomography angiography (CTA) has proven utility in evaluation of patients with suspected BTAI and has shown sensitivity, specificity, and accuracy similar to conventional angiography [18, 19]. Identifying the class for grading the severity of BTAI based on CT images is important because the classification scheme allows a suitable treatment to be chosen, whether emergent or deferred. According to the Society for Vascular Surgery (SVS) guidelines, BTAI is graded as follows [20, 21]:

- Grade 1—intimal tear or flap
- Grade 2—intramural hematoma without significant change in the external contour of the aorta
- Grade 3—pseudoaneurysm with extension beyond the normal contours of the aorta
- Grade 4—rupture; full-thickness aortic injury with extravasation

The most accepted and widely established grading system proposed by the SVS, while straightforward and descriptive, does not guide treatment. Several alternate algorithms have been proposed to assist in making decisions about treatment. Starnes et al. have proposed a new classification scheme based on the presence or absence of an external contour abnormality [22]. This group has promoted the importance of aortic lesion dimension measurements, parameters not specifically included in SVS criteria, as crucial to determining the need for TEVAR. Rabin et al. suggested incorporating into this classification the following parameters for serious injury: significant mediastinal hematoma, extent of left hemothorax, and the presence of pseudocoarctation [23]. Specifically, this group has highlighted that the presence of extensive mediastinal hematoma and large left hemothorax may prove important hallmarks of impending aortic rupture. More recently, Heneghan et al. proposed a simplification of the SVS grading criteria of BTAI into minimal, moderate, and severe injury based on

Table 10.1 New Harborview classification scheme

Classification	Description	Notes
Minimal (grades 1 and 2)	No external contour abnormality Intimal tear/thrombus <10 mm	Optimal follow-up imaging
Moderate (grade 3)	External contour abnormality or intimal tear >10 mm	Semi-elective repair: stabilize concomitant injuries, impulse control
Severe (grade 4)	Active extravasation Left subclavian artery hematoma >15 mm	Immediate repair: ATAI takes first priority

treatment differences among the three groups (Table 10.1) [24].

Aortography is still considered the reference test for BTAI and is used when the results from other modalities are inconclusive. Aortographic findings of the BTAI include an abnormality or outpouching of the aortic contour, an intimal flap or dissection, retention of contrast in a pseudoaneurysm sac, and/or, rarely, the appearance of a coarctation.

The management approach to the patient with BTAI depends upon the hemodynamic status of the patient, grade of aortic injury, and presence of other injuries and medical comorbidities. Although prospective randomized trials have not been published to date, TEVAR is the primary and preferred treatment option for the treatment of BTAI, which is associated with significantly lower mortality, paraplegia, and procedural morbidity rates than open repair [9, 25–38]. SVS guidelines recommend TEVAR for grade 2 through 4 BTAIs, given that grade 1 injuries typically heal spontaneously [21]. Given the mounting evidences [24, 39, 40], conservative management of minimal aortic injuries is recommended with appropriate observation and follow-up imaging. The optimal timing of aortic repair has continued to evolve as the treatment of BTAI has shifted from open aortic repair to TEVAR. The SVS suggested urgent repair (<24 h) in the absence of other serious concomitant injuries or repair immediately after other injuries have been treated, but at the latest, prior to hospital discharge [21]. Delayed management of BTAI until life-threatening nonaortic injuries have been treated has been shown to be a safe and beneficial approach [29, 41].

Case Scenario

Case: A 22-year-old man involved in a high-speed motor vehicle collision with a typical acute posttraumatic aortic pseudoaneurysm

(a, b) Contrast-enhanced axial (a) and sagittal (b) CT images demonstrate the typical location and appearance of an acute aortic injury. The pseudoaneurysm (arrow) projects from the anteromedial aorta at the level of the left main stem bronchus and distal to the left subclavian artery.

Note the associated hemomediastinum and hemothorax (asterisk).

(c, d) Digital subtraction aortogram before placement (c) and after deployment (d) of the stent graft. Note the proximal bare portion of the stent graft only across the origin of the left subclavian artery.

(e) Contrast-enhanced sagittal CT image 6 months after thoracic endovascular aortic repair (TEVAR) shows patent stent graft without endoleak.

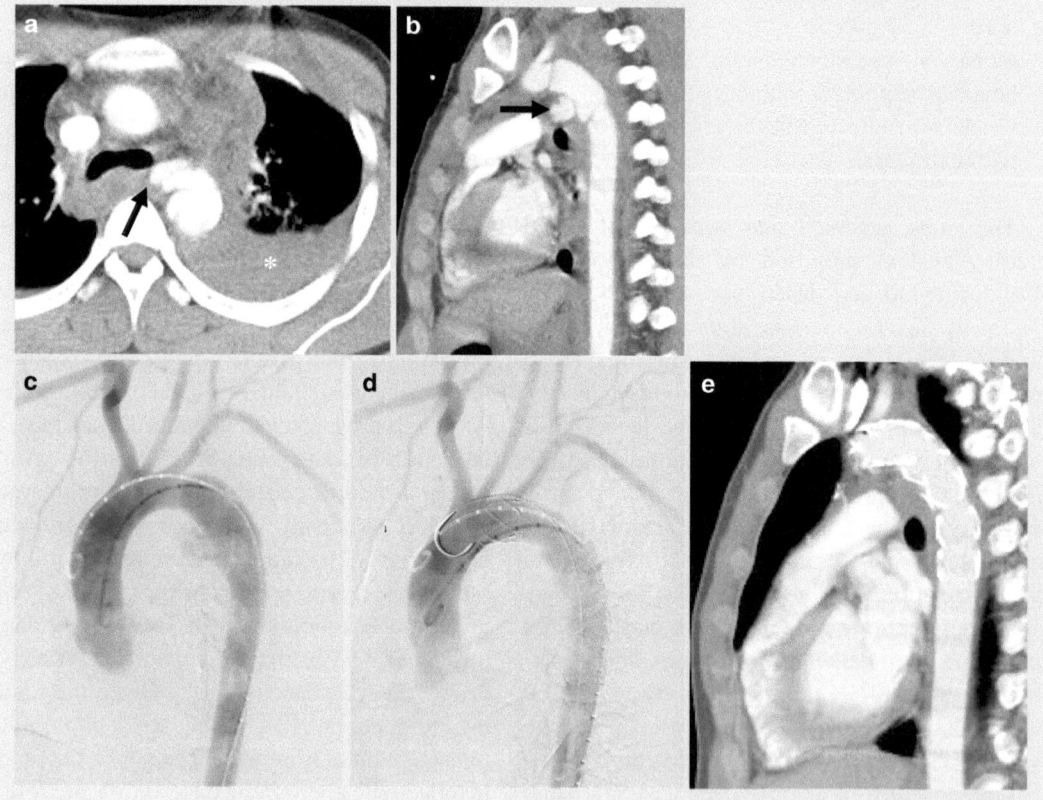

Summary

- BTAIs have a high mortality rate and a high index of suspicion and careful evaluation is necessary for accurate diagnosis.
- Aortic injuries can be graded based upon CT findings as follows: grade 1 (intimal tear), grade 2 (intramural hematoma), grade 3 (pseudoaneurysm), and grade 4 (rupture).
- With the growing shift from open repair to TEVAR as the primary treatment in patients with BTAI, outcomes have improved with significantly reduced mortality and morbidity.
- SVS guidelines recommend TEVAR for grade 2 through 4 BTAIs, given that grade 1 injuries typically heal spontaneously.
- Open repair is reserved for patients who are not suitable for TEVAR.

10.3 Interventional Radiology in Abdominal Trauma

10.3.1 Spleen

The spleen is the most commonly injured intra-abdominal organ in blunt trauma [42]. The management of splenic injuries is continuously evolving. Until recently, the preferred management of splenic trauma was surgery, but nonoperative management (NOM) for splenic salvage is increasingly preferred owing to preserving patients' immunity to infection [43–47]. Clearly, NOM has become the standard of care for the hemodynamically stable patient with a blunt splenic injury [48, 49]. The merits of NOM include earlier discharge, lower hospital cost, fewer intra-abdominal complications, and reduced transfusion requirement associated with

Table 10.2 Multidetector CT-based splenic injury grading system

Injury grade	Description of injury
I	Subcapsular hematoma <1 cm thick; laceration <1 cm parenchymal depth; parenchymal hematoma <1 cm diameter
II	Subcapsular hematoma 1–3 cm thick; laceration 1–3 cm parenchymal depth; parenchymal hematoma 1–3 cm diameter
III	Splenic capsular disruption; subcapsular hematoma >3 cm thick; laceration >3 cm parenchymal depth; parenchymal hematoma >3 cm diameter
IVA	Active intraparenchymal or subcapsular splenic bleeding; splenic vascular injury (pseudoaneurysm or arteriovenous fistula); shattered spleen
IVB	Active intraperitoneal bleeding

Source: Ref. [53]

an overall improvement in mortality of these injuries [50, 51]. Meanwhile, patients who have peritonitis or those who are hemodynamically unstable should be taken urgently for explorative laparotomy [49, 52]. Management decisions in cases of acute splenic injury are based on patient demographics and clinical signs and symptoms and often rely on the splenic injury grade as determined on the basis of CT results [53].

Splenic injuries are commonly classified according to the American Association for the Surgery of Trauma (AAST) Splenic Injury Scale (Table 10.2) [54]. This uses five grades to describe the degree of laceration or hematoma in the spleen following injury (grade 1, hematoma <10% or laceration <1 cm; grade 2, hematoma 10–50% or laceration 1–3 cm; grade 3, hematoma >50% or laceration >3 cm with devascularization <25%; grade 4, major laceration with devascularization >25%; and grade 5, comminuted fracture or complete devascularization). Higher grades correlate with increasing anatomic splenic injury. However, the AAST grading scale is limited at predicting outcome with NOM because it does not take into account evidence of vascular injury, degree of hemoperitoneum, and the patient's clinical situation [44, 55, 56].

Recently, a modified grading system has been proposed by Marmery et al. in 2007 [57], taking into account the presence of splenic vascular injury (pseudoaneurysm or arteriovenous fistula) and active bleeding (intraparenchymal, subcapsular, or intraperitoneal). The modified CT grading scale can improve the accuracy of predicting the need for intervention, as compared with the traditional AAST scale.

Embolization can expand the territory of NOM, but the role of embolization as an adjunct to NOM of blunt splenic injuries remains controversial. Multiple studies have shown that embolization may increase the nonoperative salvage rate for patients with blunt splenic injuries [45, 58–64], while other studies showed no improvement in their splenic salvage rate [65–69]. This was because of the lack of clear indication or optimal protocol for embolization, variability in physician practice, and questionable clinical decision-making [58, 68]. However, Requarth et al. in a 2011 systemic review concluded that embolization significantly reduced failure rates of NOM in grade 4 and grade 5 injuries [70]. A recent prospective data by Miller et al. recommended angiography and embolization as an adjunct to NOM for all grade III to V splenic injuries [71]. Another meta-analysis by Crichton et al. concluded that embolization should be strongly considered as an adjunct to NOM in patients with grade 4 and grade 5 splenic injuries [72].

Although there is no clear indication for embolization, it is important to define which patients are likely to benefit from embolization, as it is also risky than observation. To date, in many studies, specific indications for angiography and embolization were included as follows [58, 59, 64, 73–77]: a vascular injury (contrast leak/blush, pseudoaneurysm, arteriovenous fistula) regardless of the AAST scale; grade 4 or 5 splenic injury; and a grade 3 splenic injury associated with a large hemoperitoneum (injury involving the perisplenic space, Morrison's space, the two paracolic gutters, and the pelvis). In the Eastern Association for the Surgery of Trauma (EAST) guideline [49], angiography with embolization should be considered for patients with AAST grade greater than three injuries, presence of a contrast blush, moderate hemoperitoneum, or clinical evidence of ongoing splenic bleeding.

Embolization may be performed proximally, distally, or the combination of both techniques. There is also much debate regarding whether the spleen should be embolized proximally or distally and what material should be used to embolize the spleen [59, 76]. Proximal embolization in the main splenic artery using a coil or vascular plug reduces pulse pressure to the spleen, promoting native hemostasis, but preserves flow to the spleen through collaterals. Proximal embolization may be feasible when multiple inaccessible or excessive numbers of vascular abnormalities were present [45, 59]. Distal embolization in the small arterial branches within the splenic parenchyma is worthwhile to achieve hemostatic control if there is extrasplenic hemorrhage or pseudoaneurysms or intrasplenic arteriovenous fistula. The success of embolization after splenic injuries is almost 90%, with rebleeding being the most common reason for failure [78]. Both techniques have an equivalent rate of major infarctions and infections requiring splenectomy. Minor complications not requiring splenectomy occur more often after distal than after proximal embolization [78]. Combined embolization can be performed in isolated instances of diffuse splenic injury combined with a rapid peripheral bleeding vessel, but complication rates are much higher in these circumstances and should only be used on a case-by-case basis.

Complications after splenic embolization were reported variably; some studies reported no complications at all, while others describe serious complications [58, 63, 67, 74, 75, 79]. The complications attributed to embolization are generally minor like fever or pain requiring analgesics. Infarcts may occur in up to 20% of patients but usually resolve without clinical sequelae [58].

Case Scenario

Case: A 23-year-old man involved in a motor vehicle collision

(a, b) Axial contrast-enhanced CT images demonstrate multifocal low attenuation areas (arrowheads) representing splenic lacerations with or without hematoma and a small contrast-filling pseudoaneurysm (arrow) inside the low attenuation area. Also, note hemoperitoneum in the perisplenic space.

(c) Splenic arteriogram shows multiple pseudoaneurysms with contrast blush and throughout the spleen.

(d) Splenic arteriogram after selective embolization using a microcoil and gelatin sponge particles shows disappeared splenic pseudoaneurysms.

(e, f) Axial contrast-enhanced CT images one month after embolization show decreased low attenuation areas throughout the spleen. No splenic pseudoaneurysms are seen.

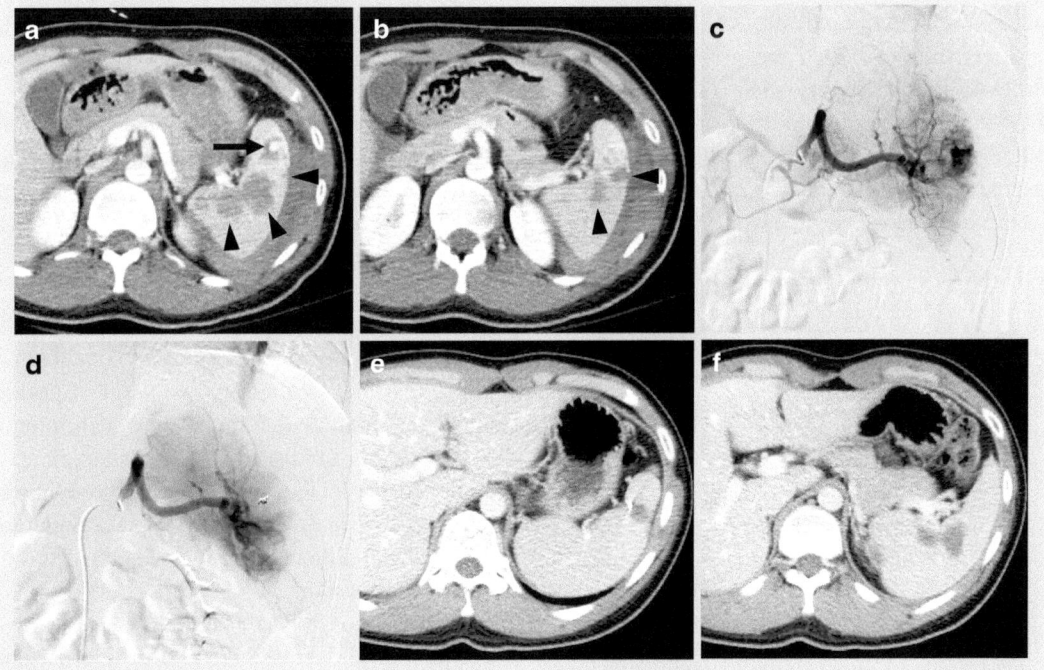

Summary

- Splenic embolization improves the success rate of NOM of higher blunt splenic injuries.
- The indications for splenic angiography and embolization are as follows: a vascular injury (contrast leak/blush, pseudoaneurysm, arteriovenous fistula) regardless of the AAST scale; grade 4 or 5 splenic injury; and a grade 3 splenic injury associated with moderate hemoperitoneum (injury involving the perisplenic space, Morrison's space, the two paracolic gutters, and the pelvis).

10.3.2 Liver

The liver is a frequently injured organ in patients suffering blunt abdominal trauma [80]. Similar to the spleen, integration of CT in early trauma management and shift to NOM in hemodynamically stable patients resulted in improved survival and has become a mainstay in the management for liver trauma [81–84]. These dramatic changes in the way that liver injuries are handled are due to marked improvements in diagnostic imaging, the widespread availability and performance of angiography and embolization, and the use of noninvasive interventional techniques for the management of complications [85].

Liver injuries on CT are graded according to the AAST organ injury scale (Table 10.3). The AAST scale is similar to that for splenic injuries but uses six rather than five grades to describe the degree of laceration, hematoma, or vascular injury to the liver. However, there are shortcomings to

Table 10.3 AAST liver injury scale (1994 revision)

Grade and type of injury	Description of injury
I	
Hematoma	Subcapsular, <10% surface area
Laceration	<1 cm in depth
II	
Hematoma	Subcapsular, 10–50% of surface area; intraparenchymal hematoma <10 cm in diameter
Laceration	1–3 cm in depth or <10 cm in diameter
III	
Hematoma	Subcapsular, >50% surface area or expanding; ruptured subcapsular or parenchymal hematoma; intraparenchymal hematoma >10 cm or expanding
Laceration	>3 cm parenchymal depth
IV	
Laceration	Parenchymal disruption involving 25–75% of hepatic lobe or one to three Couinaud segments in a single lobe
V	
Laceration	Parenchymal disruption involving >75% of hepatic lobe or more than three Couinaud segments in a single lobe
Vascular	Juxtahepatic venous injuries (i.e., retrohepatic vena cava and/or central major hepatic veins)
VI	
Vascular	Hepatic avulsion

this grading scale, as in other grading scales, in that it does not determine the need for operative intervention. There may be major discrepancies between CT grading and the operative grading, and it does not incorporate the CT finding of active contrast extravasation, an important feature in predicting failure of NOM and an indication for angiography and embolization [86, 87]. Ultimately, hemodynamic stability is the only determining factor for NOM, rather than AAST grade [86–89].

Hepatic angiography with embolization is a beneficial adjunct and enhances the success of NOM in liver injuries [89–91]. In the hemodynamic stable patients, indications for angiography include active contrast extravasation on CT, decreasing hemoglobin levels, and high-grade (IV or V) liver injuries [89, 92]. By a study by Misselbeck et al., patients with active contrast extravasation on CT have a 20 times greater need for embolization than those without contrast extravasation [89]. Embolization may prevent progression of arterial injuries and delayed hemodynamic compromise when done early. All the hemodynamically unstable patients, having intraoperative liver bleeding of presumed arterial origin resistant to well-applied surgical packing, mandates immediate angiography with intention to treat, as it will improve the overall clinical outcome [91, 93]. Decision to proceed to angiography with embolization involves collaboration between trauma surgeon, interventional radiologist, and intensivist.

Generally, it is best to embolize as selectively as possible to decrease the risk of liver ischemia and to preserve uninjured tissue. Nonselective embolization of an entire hepatic lobe or segment may be performed using gelfoam or glue to treat multiple sites of injury simultaneously or to get prompt cessation of hemorrhage. An injury to the common or proper hepatic arteries can be embolized proximally and distally by the so-called "sandwich" technique; however, stent grafting using a covered stent may be beneficial, if technically possible, to spare the arterial supply to the liver (figure). The technical success rate of hepatic embolization ranges from 88% to 100%, but it drops to 60–70% due to distorted anatomy and manipulation following surgical packing [94].

Conversely, angiography and embolization are not risk-free procedures and are associated with serious consequences and complications [94–96]. As the grade of liver injury increases, so does the rate of complications with embolization [95, 96]. Some of the complications are major hepatic necrosis and biliary complications such as biliary leaks, gallbladder necrosis, biliary stricture, biloma or abscess, cholecystitis, and aneurysms and pseudoaneurysms. Interventional radiology also has a significant role in the management of complications related to the liver injury itself, as well as the surgical and postembolization complications.

Case Scenario

Case 1: A 36-year-old female with blunt abdominal trauma

(a) Grade III subcapsular hepatic hematomas (asterisk) compressing liver parenchyma with a small pseudoaneurysm at the medial capsular margin in the right hemiliver are obvious on the contrast-enhanced CT.

(b) Hepatic arteriogram shows multiple small pseudoaneurysms at the periphery of the right hepatic artery and active contrast extravasation (arrow) from one of the pseudoaneurysms.

(c) After embolization with particles, there are no longer pseudoaneurysms.

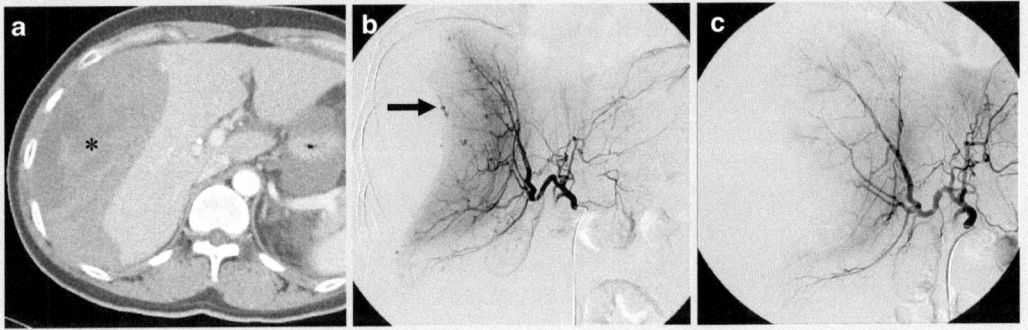

Case Scenario

Case 2: A 42-year-old male with abdominal trauma in a vehicle rollover accident

(a) Contrast-enhanced CT image shows a pseudoaneurysm (arrow) from the proper hepatic artery.

(b) Hepatic arteriogram shows a pseudoaneurysm (arrow) from the proper hepatic artery just proximal to the left hepatic artery.

(c) After a stent graft deployment and coil embolization of the proximal left hepatic artery, hepatic arteriogram shows spared right hepatic artery.

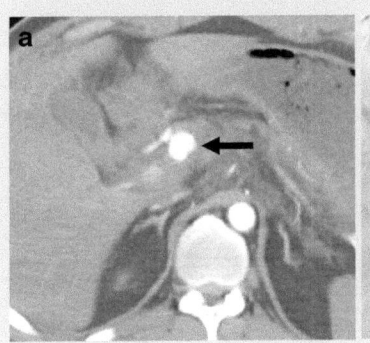 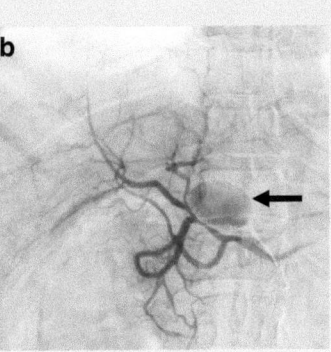 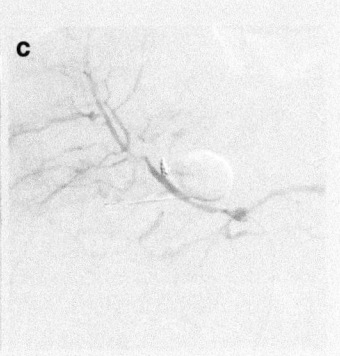

Case Scenario

Case 3: A 55-year-old male patient with blunt force trauma by a metal pipe

(a, b) Contrast-enhanced CT images show extensive lacerations of the right liver and the medial section with large amount of hemorrhagic ascites (asterisk) and active contrast extravasations (arrows) within the intraparenchymal hematoma (grade V injury).

(c) Immediate postop celiac angiogram after emergent surgical packing shows multiple active contrast extravasations (arrows) from the right anterior sectional artery and the left medial sectional artery.

(d) After embolization of the right hepatic artery, massive active bleeding (arrow) from the left medial sectional arterial bleeding is seen, although it was invisi-

ble on the first celiac angiogram due to vascular spasm related to hypotension.

(e) After rapid embolization with gelatin sponge particles and coils, the bleeding is no longer seen.

(f, g) Follow-up CT images eight days (f) and three weeks (g) after the hepatic arterial embolization show hepatic necrosis and infected biloma in the right liver and segment 4.

(h–j) Significant bile leaks (arrow), managed with stenting through the endoscopic retrograde cholangiopancreatography (ERCP) (h), percutaneous drainage (i), and percutaneous transhepatic biliary drainage (PTBD) (j).

(k) Follow-up CT 13 months after embolization shows small amount of fluid (arrow) in the atrophied right liver and compensatory hypertrophy of the left liver.

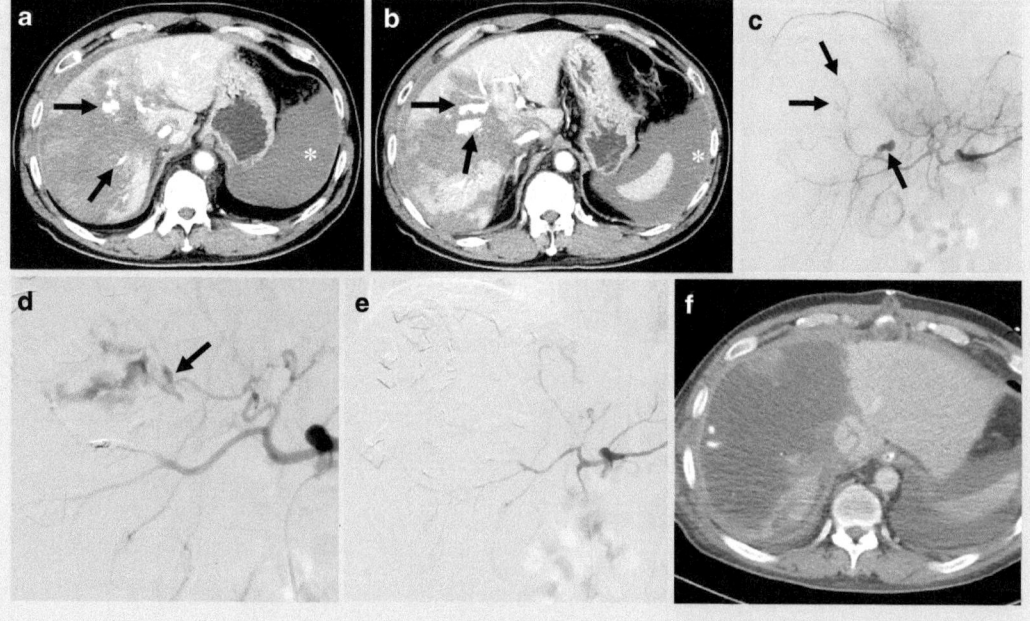

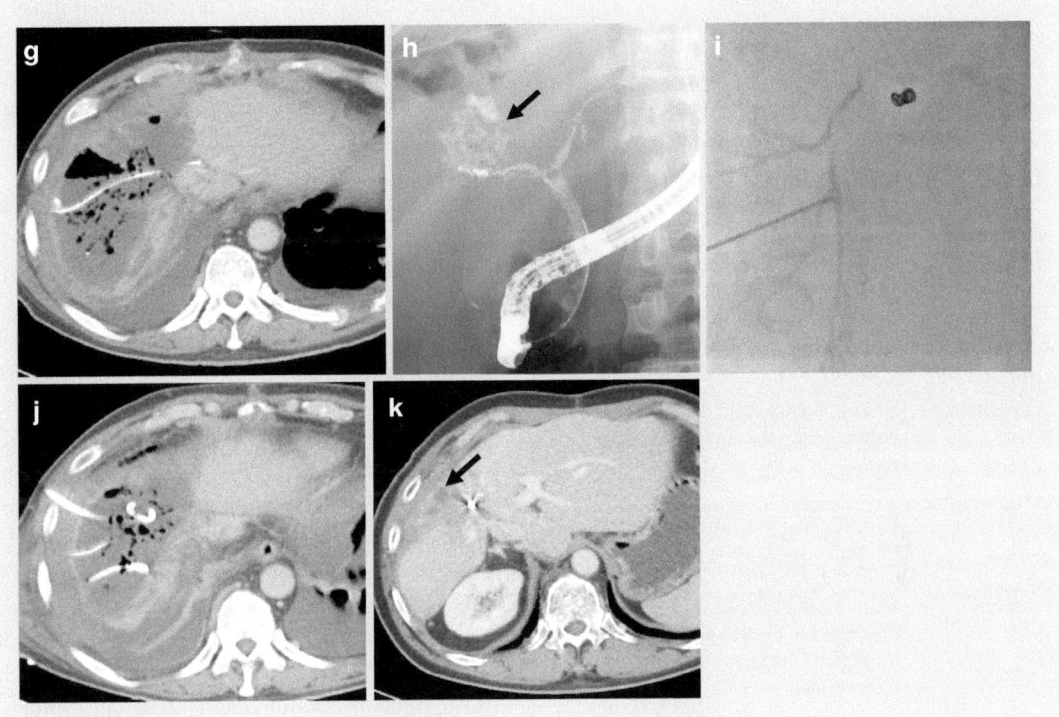

Summary

- The clinical and hemodynamic status of the patient is the most important factor for guiding trauma management.
- Indication for open surgical intervention for blunt hepatic trauma is most accurately predicted by an abnormal or unstable hemodynamic status, rather than the AAST grade of injury on CT.
- In the hemodynamic stable patients, indications for angiography include active contrast extravasation on CT, decreasing hemoglobin levels, and high-grade (IV or V) liver injuries
- Interventional radiology also has a significant role in the management of complications related to the liver injury itself, as well as the surgical and postembolization complications.
- Multidisciplinary approach is necessary for management of high-grade liver injuries.

10.3.3 Kidney

The kidney is the third most commonly injured abdominal solid organ after the spleen and liver, representing approximately 10% of those injuries [97]. Unlike the spleen and liver, renal trauma is recognized as commonly being relatively minor, because the kidneys have anatomical benefits protected by retroperitoneal space and having the Gerota fascia as an envelope of tissue to tamponade bleeding. However, most significant renal trauma is associated with injury to other major organs [98].

CT has a valuable role in the assessment of renal injuries. Similar to what exists for the spleen and liver, AAST grading scale is applied to classify the severity of renal trauma, taking into account the size and location of renal hematomas and lacerations and the presence of vascular injuries (Table 10.4) [99].

Similar to NOM of spleen and hepatic injuries, NOM has become the standard approach for renal injuries in the absence of hemodynamic instability. Recently, many studies have shown

Table 10.4 AAST kidney injury scale

Grade and type of injury	Description of injury
I	
Contusion	Microscopic or gross hematuria, with normal urologic studies
Hematoma	Subcapsular nonexpanding, without parenchymal laceration
II	
Hematoma	Nonexpanding perirenal hematoma confined to renal retroperitoneum
Laceration	<1 cm parenchymal depth of renal cortex, without urinary extravasation
III	
Laceration	>1 cm parenchymal depth of renal cortex, without collecting system rupture or urinary extravasation
IV	
Laceration	Parenchymal laceration extending through renal cortex, medulla, and collecting system
Vascular	Main renal artery or vein injury, with contained hemorrhage, segmental infarctions without associated lacerations
V	
Laceration	Completely shattered kidney or ureteropelvic junction avulsion
Vascular	Avulsion of renal hilum or thrombosis of main renal artery or vein with renal devascularization

Note: Advance one grade for bilateral injuries up to grade III

improved outcomes for the NOM of even higher-grade injuries [100–102]. Embolization is a useful adjunct in management of grades 3–5 renal injuries and in those patients who present hemodynamically compromised but respond to initial resuscitation [103].

Currently accepted indications for angiography in renal injuries are as follows [104–106]: [1] recurrent hemodynamic lability despite resuscitation (i.e., four units of packed red blood cell (PRBC) transfusion requirements in 24 h); [2] large subcapsular hematoma, active contrast extravasation, or absence of visualization of the kidney on contrast-enhanced CT, suggestive of a renovascular injury; [3] an abnormal bruit or thrill, suggesting an arteriovenous fistula; and [4] unrelenting gross hematuria and/or severe unremitting urinary colic, suggesting an arteriocalyceal fistula. Angiographic findings include contrast extravasation, occlusion, arteriovenous fistula, arteriocalyceal fistula, intimal tear, and pseudoaneurysm. Each abnormality requires a specific IR management [107]. A recent 10-year review of the use of intervention in renal vascular injury showed a success rate of over 94% in patients undergoing angiography and embolization as primary management [108].

IR techniques, such as percutaneous nephrostomy, percutaneous drainage of an abscess or urinoma, or other fluid collections, are also valuable as strategies for the nonoperative approach to blunt and isolated penetrating renal trauma [109]. The management of renal artery occlusion or thrombosis remains controversial. The diagnosis of renal artery occlusion is seldom made within warm renal ischemia time (<2 h), an indication for arterial reconstruction, and outcomes tend to be poor. The nature of the underlying arterial occlusion should be understood. The occlusion may be the result of an intimal tear, a laceration, or complete avulsion of the artery. Endovascular recanalization and stent treatment in cases of short-segment dissections of the renal artery can be successful [110, 111]. However, when there is a laceration or avulsion of the renal artery, attempts at endovascular recanalization may result in major bleeding, and rapid embolization of the stump of the renal artery may be required. The long-term results of stent placement are not always favorable.

Despite the advances of NOM, persistent hemorrhages from the kidney, pulsatile perirenal hematomas, and renal pedicle avulsion remain indications for surgical exploration. Ureteral and renal pelvic injuries associated with urinary extravasation and nonviable parenchyma are relative indications for surgery but may be repaired in a delayed fashion [99, 100].

Case Scenario

Case 1: A 45-year-old male patient involved in a motorcycle traffic accident

(a) Contrast-enhanced CT image shows active contrast extravasation (arrow), large perirenal hematoma, and multiple fractures (arrowheads) of the right kidney showing discontinuity of the Gerota fascia.

(b) Selective left renal arteriogram shows active contrast extravasation from branches of the left renal artery.

(c) After embolization, the pseudoaneurysm with contrast extravasation disappeared on the left renal arteriogram.

(d) Contrast-enhanced CT image three weeks after embolization demonstrates embolic materials (arrow) in the left renal artery without evidence of bleeding and subacute perirenal hematoma.

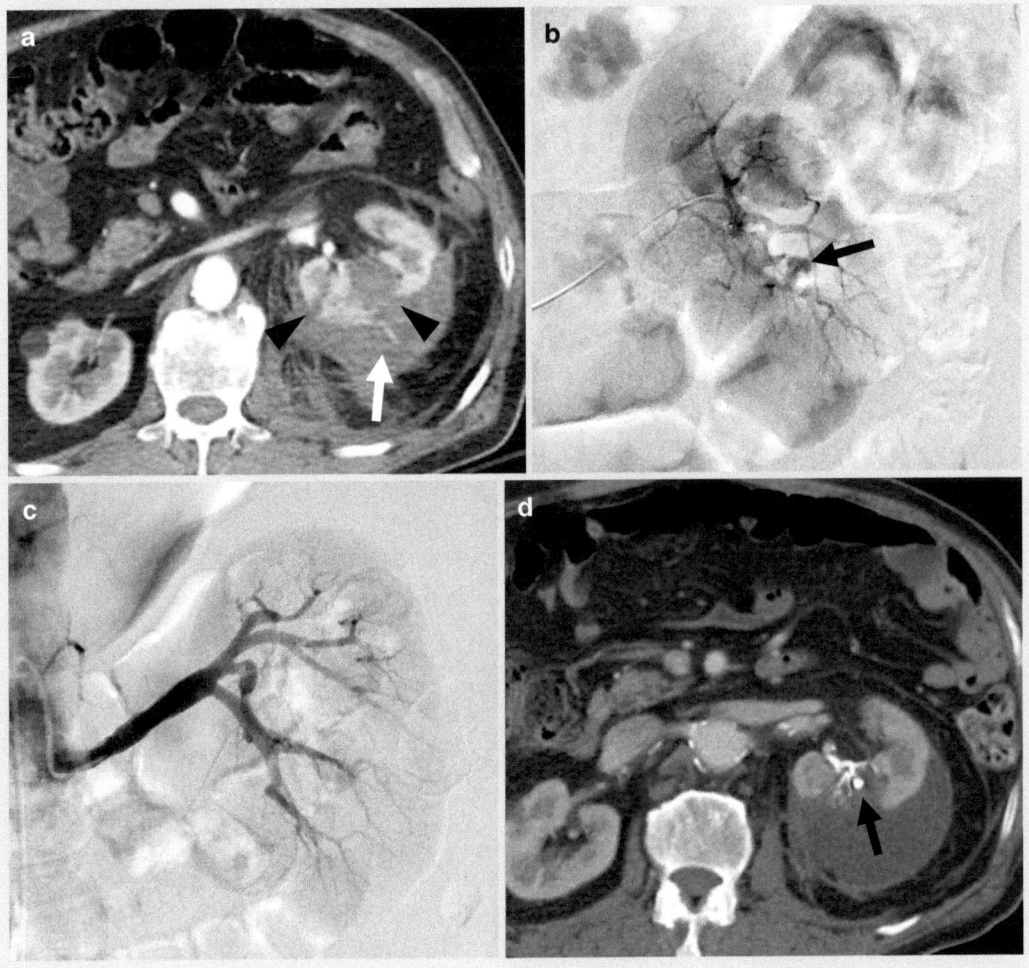

Case Scenario

Case 2: A 57-year-old male patient who suffered severe blunt trauma to his back

(a, b) Contrast-enhanced CT images show multifocal active bleeding foci (arrows) with perirenal hemorrhage.

   (c) Right renal arteriogram shows multifocal bleeding (arrows) from the left renal arteries.

(d) Selective right renal arteriogram shows active contrast extravasation (arrow) from an inferior segmental branch of the left kidney.

(e) Selective right renal capsular arteriogram shows active contrast extravasation (arrow) at the inferior polar area of the left kidney.

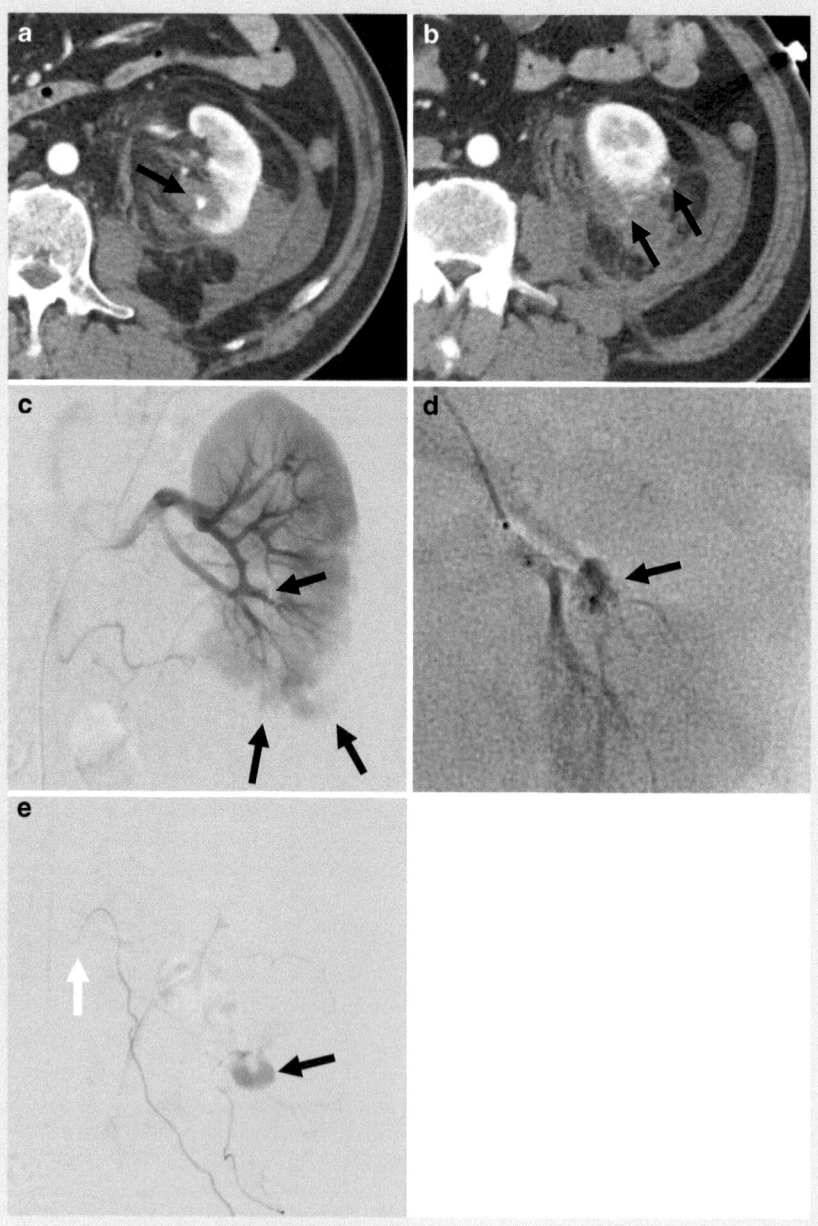

Case Scenario

Case 3: A 39-year-old female patient who had traumatic occlusion and dissection of the right main renal artery

(a) Contrast-enhanced CT shows poor enhancement (arrowhead) of the right kidney with a short-segment occlusion (arrow) of the right renal artery.

(b) Right renal arteriogram shows the occlusion (arrow) of the right renal artery.

(c) Right renal arteriogram after a stent placement (arrow) shows the recanalized right renal artery.

(d) Follow-up contrast-enhanced CT five months after stent graft placement shows resumption of the right renal enhancement (asterisk) with a patent stent (arrow).

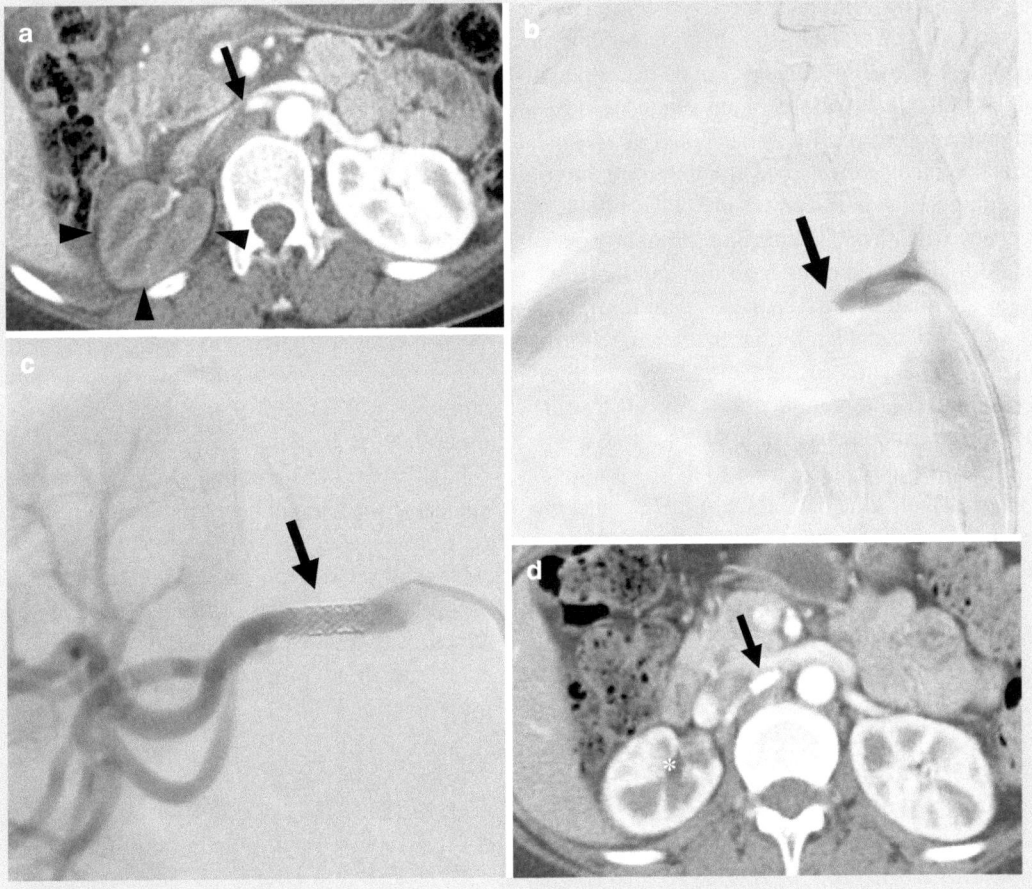

Summary
- Embolization is a useful adjunct in management of grades 3–5 renal injuries and in those patients who present hemodynamically compromised but respond to initial resuscitation.
- IR techniques are also valuable in managing complications of renal trauma.
- Persistent hemorrhages from the kidney, pulsatile perirenal hematomas, and renal pedicle avulsion remain indications for surgical exploration.

10.4 Interventional Radiology in Pelvic Trauma

Pelvic fractures are associated with mortality rates of 5.6–15% [112–116], but the addition of hemorrhagic shock raises rates to 36.4–54% [117, 118]. Associated organ injuries have been found in 11–20.3%, injuries that can increase morbidity and mortality [113]. Bleeding related to pelvic fractures may originate from arteries, veins, cancellous bone, or crushed soft tissue. Pelvic bleeding caused by veins and fractured bone can be controlled with fracture stabilization by external fixation, but arterial bleeding can be life-threatening [115]. Urgent angiography and subsequent embolization are currently accepted as the most effective methods for controlling ongoing arterial bleeding in pelvic fractures [112, 115, 119–124].

Patient death due to bleeding frequently occurs in the first 24 h, and the mortality rate rises with delays in treatment. Thus, the early or optimal triage of patients who might be beneficial from angiographic embolization could reduce blood loss, prevent late complications related to transfusion, and improve outcome [125].

Several authors have tried to define predictors to determine which patients with pelvic fractures are at high risk of arterial bleeding and thus might be candidates for angiography and embolization: a lack of response to initial resuscitation [118], the pelvic fracture pattern [117], the amount and location of pelvic hematoma [126, 127], and active contrast extravasation on enhanced CT

[128, 129] were associated with arterial bleeding. Based on the 2011 EAST guideline [124], pelvic angiography and embolization in patients with pelvic fractures are recommended as follows: [1] patients with hemodynamic instability or signs of ongoing bleeding without nonpelvic sources of blood loss (Level I); [2] patients with evidence of contrast extravasation on CT regardless of hemodynamic status (Level I); [3] patients who have signs of ongoing bleeding without nonpelvic sources of blood loss, after previous angiography (Level II); and [4] age >60 years with major pelvic fracture (open book, butterfly segment, or vertical shear) regardless of hemodynamic status (Level II). The success rates of pelvic embolization range from 85% to 100% with mortality rates of 17.6–47% despite successful embolization [116]. Lower mortality rates have been associated with early embolization [112]. Higher mortality has been seen in older patients and patients with greater hemodynamic compromise [112, 115].

The safety of pelvic angiography and embolization seems to be well established in several studies [122, 130]. Complications of pelvic embolization include those that are access site-related as well as nontarget embolization and tissue necrosis. Gluteal necrosis seems to be related to primary trauma to the gluteal region along with protracted hypotension rather than a direct complication of embolization [131, 132]. Sexual function in male patients does not seem to be impaired after bilateral internal iliac arterial embolization [133].

Case Scenario

Case: A 94-year-old female patient with traumatic pelvic bone fracture

(a) Axial contrast-enhanced CT image demonstrates an extravasation of contrast material (arrow) with acute hematoma (asterisk) in the prevesical and perivesical spaces.
(b) Left external iliac arteriogram shows an extravasation of contrast material from the inferior epigastric arterial branch.
(c) A 2-F microcatheter approaches from the left external iliac artery and has been placed in the branch of the inferior epi-

gastric artery. N-butyl cyanoacrylate (NBCA) was administered from this location to control the active bleeding (arrow).
(d) Left external iliac arteriogram after embolization demonstrates no further extravasation or bleeding.
(e) Right internal iliac arteriogram shows multiple active bleeding foci (arrows) from the obturator and internal pudendal arteries.
(f) After embolization with use of gelatin sponge particles, right iliac arteriogram demonstrates no further extravasation or bleeding.

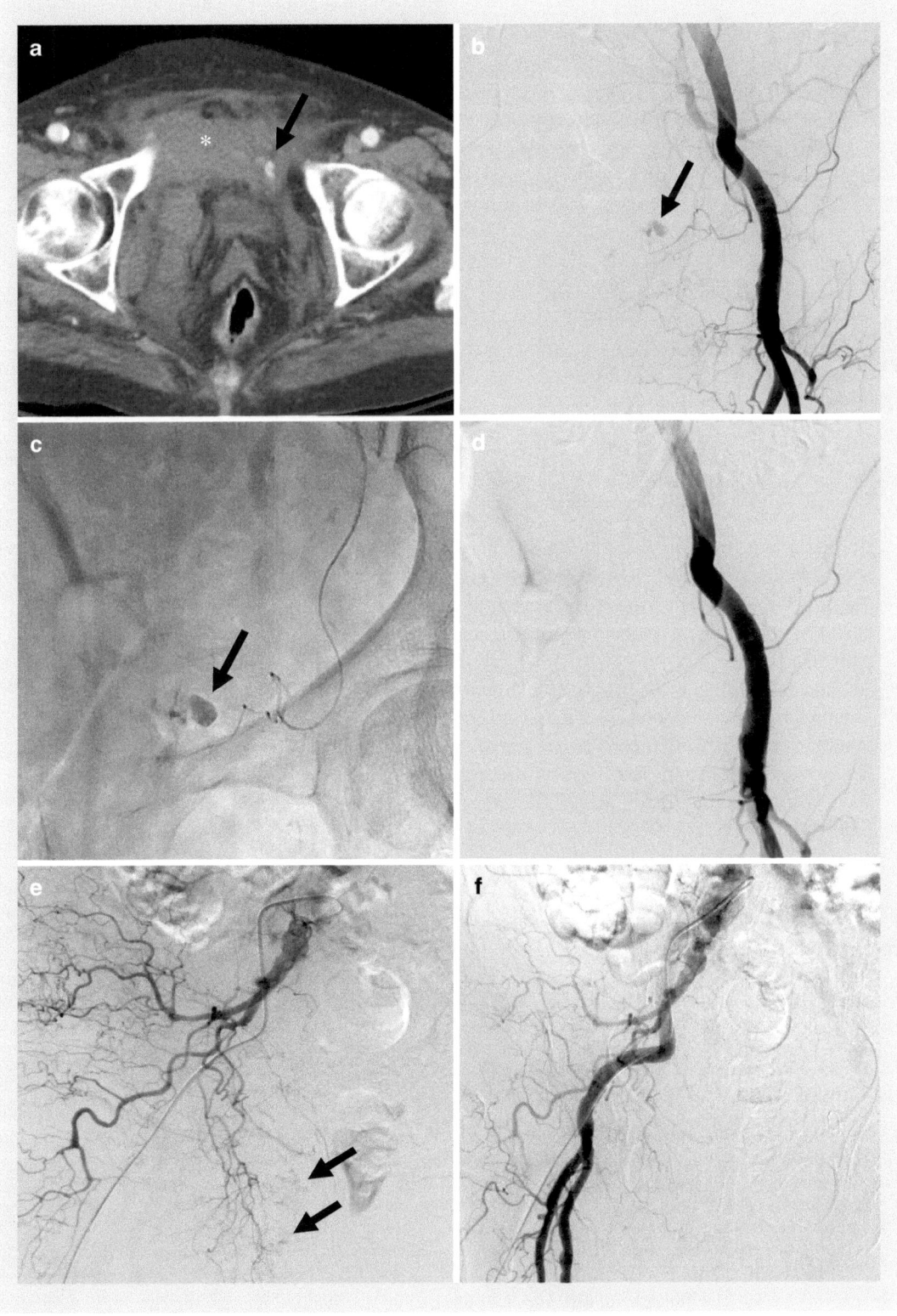

Summary

- The treatment for acute hemorrhage after an unstable pelvic fracture involves close coordination between the trauma, orthopedic, vascular, and IR services and includes control of hypotension and coagulopathy, pelvic stabilization, and percutaneous pelvic arterial embolization.
- When pelvic hemorrhage is the main issue, the faster the patient can be mobilized to the IR suite for embolization the better, regardless of stability.

10.5 Conclusions

- IR has a vital role in the multidisciplinary approach to trauma management and provides a significant contribution toward achieving the best possible clinical outcomes for trauma patients.
- IR management is now regarded as well-accepted treatment option for various kinds of vascular trauma which can cause massive hemorrhage, including large vessel trauma such as the aorta, abdominal solid organ trauma, and pelvic trauma.

References

1. Gould JE, Vedantham S. The role of interventional radiology in trauma. Semin Intervent Radiol. 2006;23:270–8.
2. Starnes BW, Arthurs ZM. Endovascular management of vascular trauma. Perspect Vasc Surg Endovasc Ther. 2006;18:114–29.
3. Tanizaki S, Maeda S, Hayashi H, Matano H, Ishida H, Yoshikawa J, et al. Early embolization without external fixation in pelvic trauma. Am J Emerg Med. 2012;30:342–6.
4. Salazar GM, Walker TG. Evaluation and management of acute vascular trauma. Tech Vasc Interv Radiol. 2009;12:102–16.
5. Clancy TV, Gary Maxwell J, Covington DL, Brinker CC, Blackman D. A statewide analysis of level I and II trauma centers for patients with major injuries. J Trauma. 2001;51:346–51.
6. Richens D, Field M, Neale M, Oakley C. The mechanism of injury in blunt traumatic rupture of the aorta. Eur J Cardiothorac Surg. 2002;21:288–93.
7. Mattox KL, Wall MJ Jr. Historical review of blunt injury to the thoracic aorta. Chest Surg Clin N Am. 2000;10:167–82, x.
8. Wintermark M, Wicky S, Schnyder P. Imaging of acute traumatic injuries of the thoracic aorta. Eur Radiol. 2002;12:431–42.
9. Fabian TC, Richardson JD, Croce MA, Smith JS Jr, Rodman G Jr, Kearney PA, et al. Prospective study of blunt aortic injury: multicenter Trial of the American Association for the Surgery of Trauma. J Trauma. 1997;42:374–80; discussion 380–373.
10. Jamieson WR, Janusz MT, Gudas VM, Burr LH, Fradet GJ, Henderson C. Traumatic rupture of the thoracic aorta: third decade of experience. Am J Surg. 2002;183:571–5.
11. Cullen EL, Lantz EJ, Johnson CM, Young PM. Traumatic aortic injury: CT findings, mimics, and therapeutic options. Cardiovasc Diagn Ther. 2014;4:238–44.
12. Cohen AM, Crass JR, Thomas HA, Fisher RG, Jacobs DG. CT evidence for the "osseous pinch" mechanism of traumatic aortic injury. AJR Am J Roentgenol. 1992;159:271–4.
13. Crass JR, Cohen AM, Motta AO, Tomashefski JF Jr, Wiesen EJ. A proposed new mechanism of traumatic aortic rupture: the osseous pinch. Radiology. 1990;176:645–9.
14. Creasy JD, Chiles C, Routh WD, Dyer RB. Overview of traumatic injury of the thoracic aorta. Radiographics. 1997;17:27–45.
15. Feczko JD, Lynch L, Pless JE, Clark MA, McClain J, Hawley DA. An autopsy case review of 142 non-penetrating (blunt) injuries of the aorta. J Trauma. 1992;33:846–9.
16. Macura KJ, Corl FM, Fishman EK, Bluemke DA. Pathogenesis in acute aortic syndromes: aortic aneurysm leak and rupture and traumatic aortic transection. AJR Am J Roentgenol. 2003;181:303–7.
17. Ben-Menachem Y. Rupture of the thoracic aorta by broadside impacts in road traffic and other collisions: further angiographic observations and preliminary autopsy findings. J Trauma. 1993;35:363–7.
18. Alkadhi H, Wildermuth S, Desbiolles L, Schertler T, Crook D, Marincek B, et al. Vascular emergencies of the thorax after blunt and iatrogenic trauma: multidetector row CT and three-dimensional imaging. Radiographics. 2004;24:1239–55.
19. Patterson BO, Holt PJ, Cleanthis M, Tai N, Carrell T, Loosemore TM. Imaging vascular trauma. Br J Surg. 2012;99:494–505.
20. Azizzadeh A, Keyhani K, Miller CC 3rd, Coogan SM, Safi HJ, Estrera AL. Blunt traumatic aortic injury: initial experience with endovascular repair. J Vasc Surg. 2009;49:1403–8.

21. Lee WA, Matsumura JS, Mitchell RS, Farber MA, Greenberg RK, Azizzadeh A, et al. Endovascular repair of traumatic thoracic aortic injury: clinical practice guidelines of the Society for Vascular Surgery. J Vasc Surg. 2011;53:187–92.

22. Starnes BW, Lundgren RS, Gunn M, Quade S, Hatsukami TS, Tran NT, et al. A new classification scheme for treating blunt aortic injury. J Vasc Surg. 2012;55:47–54.

23. Rabin J, DuBose J, Sliker CW, O'Connor JV, Scalea TM, Griffith BP. Parameters for successful nonoperative management of traumatic aortic injury. J Thorac Cardiovasc Surg. 2014;147:143–9.

24. Heneghan RE, Aarabi S, Quiroga E, Gunn ML, Singh N, Starnes BW. Call for a new classification system and treatment strategy in blunt aortic injury. J Vasc Surg. 2016;64:171–6.

25. Arthurs ZM, Starnes BW, Sohn VY, Singh N, Martin MJ, Andersen CA. Functional and survival outcomes in traumatic blunt thoracic aortic injuries: an analysis of the National Trauma Databank. J Vasc Surg. 2009;49:988–94.

26. Azizzadeh A, Charlton-Ouw KM, Chen Z, Rahbar MH, Estrera AL, Amer H, et al. An outcome analysis of endovascular versus open repair of blunt traumatic aortic injuries. J Vasc Surg. 2013;57:108–14; discussion 115.

27. de Mestral C, Dueck A, Sharma SS, Haas B, Gomez D, Hsiao M, et al. Evolution of the incidence, management, and mortality of blunt thoracic aortic injury: a population-based analysis. J Am Coll Surg. 2013;216:1110–5.

28. Demetriades D. Blunt thoracic aortic injuries: crossing the Rubicon. J Am Coll Surg. 2012;214:247–59.

29. Di Eusanio M, Folesani G, Berretta P, Petridis FD, Pantaleo A, Russo V, et al. Delayed management of blunt traumatic aortic injury: open surgical versus endovascular repair. Ann Thorac Surg. 2013;95:1591–7.

30. Dubose JJ, Azizzadeh A, Estrera AL, Safi HJ. Contemporary management of blunt aortic trauma. J Cardiovasc Surg (Torino). 2015;56:751–62.

31. Estrera AL, Miller CC 3rd, Guajardo-Salinas G, Coogan S, Charlton-Ouw K, Safi HJ, et al. Update on blunt thoracic aortic injury: fifteen-year single-institution experience. J Thorac Cardiovasc Surg. 2013;145:S154–8.

32. Jonker FH, Giacovelli JK, Muhs BE, Sosa JA, Indes JE. Trends and outcomes of endovascular and open treatment for traumatic thoracic aortic injury. J Vasc Surg. 2010;51:565–71.

33. Karmy-Jones R, Ferrigno L, Teso D, Long WB 3rd, Shackford S. Endovascular repair compared with operative repair of traumatic rupture of the thoracic aorta: a nonsystematic review and a plea for trauma-specific reporting guidelines. J Trauma. 2011;71:1059–72.

34. Murad MH, Rizvi AZ, Malgor R, Carey J, Alkatib AA, Erwin PJ, et al. Comparative effectiveness of the treatments for thoracic aortic transection [corrected]. J Vasc Surg. 2011;53:193–199.e1–21.

35. Patel HJ, Hemmila MR, Williams DM, Diener AC, Deeb GM. Late outcomes following open and endovascular repair of blunt thoracic aortic injury. J Vasc Surg. 2011;53:615–20. discussion 621

36. Takagi H, Kawai N, Umemoto T. A meta-analysis of comparative studies of endovascular versus open repair for blunt thoracic aortic injury. J Thorac Cardiovasc Surg. 2008;135:1392–4.

37. Tang GL, Tehrani HY, Usman A, Katariya K, Otero C, Perez E, et al. Reduced mortality, paraplegia, and stroke with stent graft repair of blunt aortic transections: a modern meta-analysis. J Vasc Surg. 2008;47:671–5.

38. Xenos ES, Minion DJ, Davenport DL, Hamdallah O, Abedi NN, Sorial EE, et al. Endovascular versus open repair for descending thoracic aortic rupture: institutional experience and meta-analysis. Eur J Cardiothorac Surg. 2009;35:282–6.

39. Paul JS, Neideen T, Tutton S, Milia D, Tolat P, Foley D, et al. Minimal aortic injury after blunt trauma: selective nonoperative management is safe. J Trauma. 2011;71:1519–23.

40. Osgood MJ, Heck JM, Rellinger EJ, Doran SL, Garrard CL 3rd, Guzman RJ, et al. Natural history of grade I-II blunt traumatic aortic injury. J Vasc Surg. 2014;59:334–41.

41. Demetriades D, Velmahos GC, Scalea TM, Jurkovich GJ, Karmy-Jones R, Teixeira PG, et al. Blunt traumatic thoracic aortic injuries: early or delayed repair-results of an American Association for the Surgery of Trauma prospective study. J Trauma. 2009;66:967–73.

42. Costa G, Tierno SM, Tomassini F, Venturini L, Frezza B, Cancrini G, et al. The epidemiology and clinical evaluation of abdominal trauma. An analysis of a multidisciplinary trauma registry. Ann Ital Chir. 2010;81:95–102.

43. King H, Shumacker HB Jr. Splenic studies. I. Susceptibility to infection after splenectomy performed in infancy. Ann Surg. 1952;136:239–42.

44. Becker CD, Spring P, Glattli A, Schweizer W. Blunt splenic trauma in adults: can CT findings be used to determine the need for surgery? AJR Am J Roentgenol. 1994;162:343–7.

45. Davis KA, Fabian TC, Croce MA, Gavant ML, Flick PA, Minard G, et al. Improved success in nonoperative management of blunt splenic injuries: embolization of splenic artery pseudoaneurysms. J Trauma. 1998;44:1008–13; discussion 1013–1005.

46. Gavant ML, Schurr M, Flick PA, Croce MA, Fabian TC, Gold RE. Predicting clinical outcome of nonsurgical management of blunt splenic injury: using CT to reveal abnormalities of splenic vasculature. AJR Am J Roentgenol. 1997;168:207–12.

47. Killeen KL, Shanmuganathan K, Boyd-Kranis R, Scalea TM, Mirvis SE. CT findings after embolization for blunt splenic trauma. J Vasc Interv Radiol. 2001;12:209–14.

48. Clancy TV, Ramshaw DG, Maxwell JG, Covington DL, Churchill MP, Rutledge R, et al. Management outcomes in splenic injury: a statewide trauma center review. Ann Surg. 1997;226:17–24.

49. Stassen NA, Bhullar I, Cheng JD, Crandall ML, Friese RS, Guillamondegui OD, et al. Selective non-operative management of blunt splenic injury: an Eastern Association for the Surgery of Trauma practice management guideline. J Trauma Acute Care Surg. 2012;73:S294–300.

50. Pachter HL, Guth AA, Hofstetter SR, Spencer FC. Changing patterns in the management of splenic trauma: the impact of nonoperative management. Ann Surg. 1998;227:708–17; discussion 717–709.

51. Sartorelli KH, Frumiento C, Rogers FB, Osler TM. Nonoperative management of hepatic, splenic, and renal injuries in adults with multiple injuries. J Trauma. 2000;49:56–61; discussion 61–52.

52. Wallis A, Kelly MD, Jones L. Angiography and embolisation for solid abdominal organ injury in adults – a current perspective. World J Emerg Surg. 2010;5:18.

53. Soto JA, Anderson SW. Multidetector CT of blunt abdominal trauma. Radiology. 2012;265:678–93.

54. Moore EE, Cogbill TH, Jurkovich GJ, Shackford SR, Malangoni MA, Champion HR. Organ injury scaling: spleen and liver (1994 revision). J Trauma. 1995;38:323–4.

55. Kohn JS, Clark DE, Isler RJ, Pope CF. Is computed tomographic grading of splenic injury useful in the nonsurgical management of blunt trauma? J Trauma. 1994;36:385–9; discussion 390.

56. Sutyak JP, Chiu WC, D'Amelio LF, Amorosa JK, Hammond JS. Computed tomography is inaccurate in estimating the severity of adult splenic injury. J Trauma. 1995;39:514–8.

57. Marmery H, Shanmuganathan K, Alexander MT, Mirvis SE. Optimization of selection for nonoperative management of blunt splenic injury: comparison of MDCT grading systems. AJR Am J Roentgenol. 2007;189:1421–7.

58. Haan JM, Biffl W, Knudson MM, Davis KA, Oka T, Majercik S, et al. Splenic embolization revisited: a multicenter review. J Trauma. 2004;56:542–7.

59. Haan JM, Bochicchio GV, Kramer N, Scalea TM. Nonoperative management of blunt splenic injury: a 5-year experience. J Trauma. 2005;58:492–8.

60. Haan JM, Marmery H, Shanmuganathan K, Mirvis SE, Scalea TM. Experience with splenic main coil embolization and significance of new or persistent pseudoaneurym: reembolize, operate, or observe. J Trauma. 2007;63:615–9.

61. Rajani RR, Claridge JA, Yowler CJ, Patrick P, Wiant A, Summers JI, et al. Improved outcome of adult blunt splenic injury: a cohort analysis. Surgery. 2006;140:625–31; discussion 631–622.

62. Wei B, Hemmila MR, Arbabi S, Taheri PA, Wahl WL. Angioembolization reduces operative intervention for blunt splenic injury. J Trauma. 2008;64:1472–7.

63. Wu SC, Chow KC, Lee KH, Tung CC, Yang AD, Lo CJ. Early selective angioembolization improves success of nonoperative management of blunt splenic injury. Am Surg. 2007;73:897–902.

64. Dent D, Alsabrook G, Erickson BA, Myers J, Wholey M, Stewart R, et al. Blunt splenic injuries: high non-operative management rate can be achieved with selective embolization. J Trauma. 2004;56:1063–7.

65. Harbrecht BG, Ko SH, Watson GA, Forsythe RM, Rosengart MR, Peitzman AB. Angiography for blunt splenic trauma does not improve the success rate of nonoperative management. J Trauma. 2007;63:44–9.

66. Duchesne JC, Simmons JD, Schmieg RE Jr, McSwain NE Jr, Bellows CF. Proximal splenic angioembolization does not improve outcomes in treating blunt splenic injuries compared with splenectomy: a cohort analysis. J Trauma. 2008;65:1346–51; discussion 1351–1343.

67. Smith HE, Biffl WL, Majercik SD, Jednacz J, Lambiase R, Cioffi WG. Splenic artery embolization: have we gone too far? J Trauma. 2006;61:541–4; discussion 545–546.

68. Cooney R, Ku J, Cherry R, Maish GO 3rd, Carney D, Scorza LB, et al. Limitations of splenic angioembolization in treating blunt splenic injury. J Trauma. 2005;59:926–32; discussion 932.

69. Zarzaur BL, Kozar R, Myers JG, Claridge JA, Scalea TM, Neideen TA, et al. The splenic injury outcomes trial: an American Association for the Surgery of Trauma multi-institutional study. J Trauma Acute Care Surg. 2015;79:335–42.

70. Requarth JA, D'Agostino RB Jr, Miller PR. Nonoperative management of adult blunt splenic injury with and without splenic artery embolotherapy: a meta-analysis. J Trauma. 2011;71:898–903; discussion 903.

71. Miller PR, Chang MC, Hoth JJ, Mowery NT, Hildreth AN, Martin RS, et al. Prospective trial of angiography and embolization for all grade III to V blunt splenic injuries: nonoperative management success rate is significantly improved. J Am Coll Surg. 2014;218:644–8.

72. Crichton JCI, Naidoo K, Yet B, Brundage SI, Perkins Z. The role of splenic angioembolization as an adjunct to nonoperative management of blunt splenic injuries: a systematic review and meta-analysis. J Trauma Acute Care Surg. 2017;83:934–43.

73. Omert LA, Salyer D, Dunham CM, Porter J, Silva A, Protetch J. Implications of the "contrast blush" finding on computed tomographic scan of the spleen in trauma. J Trauma. 2001;51:272–7; discussion 277–278.

74. Frandon J, Rodiere M, Arvieux C, Michoud M, Vendrell A, Broux C, et al. Blunt splenic injury: outcomes of proximal versus distal and combined splenic artery embolization. Diagn Interv Imaging. 2014;95:825–31.

75. Bessoud B, Denys A, Calmes JM, Madoff D, Qanadli S, Schnyder P, et al. Nonoperative management of traumatic splenic injuries: is there a role for proximal

splenic artery embolization? AJR Am J Roentgenol. 2006;186:779–85.

76. Bessoud B, Duchosal MA, Siegrist CA, Schlegel S, Doenz F, Calmes JM, et al. Proximal splenic artery embolization for blunt splenic injury: clinical, immunologic, and ultrasound-Doppler follow-up. J Trauma. 2007;62:1481–6.

77. Haan J, Scott J, Boyd-Kranis RL, Ho S, Kramer M, Scalea TM. Admission angiography for blunt splenic injury: advantages and pitfalls. J Trauma. 2001;51:1161–5.

78. Schnuriger B, Inaba K, Konstantinidis A, Lustenberger T, Chan LS, Demetriades D. Outcomes of proximal versus distal splenic artery embolization after trauma: a systematic review and meta-analysis. J Trauma. 2011;70:252–60.

79. Ekeh AP, McCarthy MC, Woods RJ, Haley E. Complications arising from splenic embolization after blunt splenic trauma. Am J Surg. 2005;189:335–9.

80. Croce MA, Fabian TC, Menke PG, Waddle-Smith L, Minard G, Kudsk KA, et al. Nonoperative management of blunt hepatic trauma is the treatment of choice for hemodynamically stable patients. Results of a prospective trial. Ann Surg. 1995;221:744–53; discussion 753–745.

81. Velmahos GC, Toutouzas KG, Radin R, Chan L, Demetriades D. Nonoperative treatment of blunt injury to solid abdominal organs: a prospective study. Arch Surg. 2003;138:844–51.

82. Pachter HL, Knudson MM, Esrig B, Ross S, Hoyt D, Cogbill T, et al. Status of nonoperative management of blunt hepatic injuries in 1995: a multicenter experience with 404 patients. J Trauma. 1996;40:31–8.

83. Saltzherr TP, van der Vlies CH, van Lienden KP, Beenen LF, Ponsen KJ, van Gulik TM, et al. Improved outcomes in the non-operative management of liver injuries. HPB (Oxford). 2011;13:350–5.

84. Lee SK, Carrillo EH. Advances and changes in the management of liver injuries. Am Surg. 2007;73:201–6.

85. Goffette PP, Laterre PF. Traumatic injuries: imaging and intervention in post-traumatic complications (delayed intervention). Eur Radiol. 2002;12:994–1021.

86. Yoon W, Jeong YY, Kim JK, Seo JJ, Lim HS, Shin SS, et al. CT in blunt liver trauma. Radiographics. 2005;25:87–104.

87. Fang JF, Wong YC, Lin BC, Hsu YP, Chen MF. The CT risk factors for the need of operative treatment in initially hemodynamically stable patients after blunt hepatic trauma. J Trauma. 2006;61:547–53; discussion 553–544.

88. Piper GL, Peitzman AB. Current management of hepatic trauma. Surg Clin North Am. 2010;90:775–85.

89. Misselbeck TS, Teicher EJ, Cipolle MD, Pasquale MD, Shah KT, Dangleben DA, et al. Hepatic angioembolization in trauma patients: indications and complications. J Trauma. 2009;67:769–73.

90. Carrillo EH, Spain DA, Wohltmann CD, Schmieg RE, Boaz PW, Miller FB, et al. Interventional techniques are useful adjuncts in nonoperative management of hepatic injuries. J Trauma. 1999;46:619–22; discussion 622–614.

91. Letoublon C, Morra I, Chen Y, Monnin V, Voirin D, Arvieux C. Hepatic arterial embolization in the management of blunt hepatic trauma: indications and complications. J Trauma. 2011;70:1032–6; discussion 1036–1037.

92. Sriussadaporn S, Pak-art R, Tharavej C, Sirichindakul B, Chiamananthapong S. A multidisciplinary approach in the management of hepatic injuries. Injury. 2002;33:309–15.

93. Gamanagatti S, Rangarajan K, Kumar A, Jineesh. Blunt abdominal trauma: imaging and intervention. Curr Probl Diagn Radiol. 2015;44:321–36.

94. Monnin V, Sengel C, Thony F, Bricault I, Voirin D, Letoublon C, et al. Place of arterial embolization in severe blunt hepatic trauma: a multidisciplinary approach. Cardiovasc Intervent Radiol. 2008;31:875–82.

95. Mohr AM, Lavery RF, Barone A, Bahramipour P, Magnotti LJ, Osband AJ, et al. Angiographic embolization for liver injuries: low mortality, high morbidity. J Trauma. 2003;55:1077–81; discussion 1081–1072.

96. Dabbs DN, Stein DM, Scalea TM. Major hepatic necrosis: a common complication after angioembolization for treatment of high-grade liver injuries. J Trauma. 2009;66:621–7; discussion 627–629.

97. Baverstock R, Simons R, McLoughlin M. Severe blunt renal trauma: a 7-year retrospective review from a provincial trauma centre. Can J Urol. 2001;8:1372–6.

98. Kawashima A, Sandler CM, Corl FM, West OC, Tamm EP, Fishman EK, et al. Imaging of renal trauma: a comprehensive review. Radiographics. 2001;21:557–74.

99. Santucci RA, McAninch JW, Safir M, Mario LA, Service S, Segal MR. Validation of the American Association for the surgery of trauma organ injury severity scale for the kidney. J Trauma. 2001;50:195–200.

100. Santucci RA, Fisher MB. The literature increasingly supports expectant (conservative) management of renal trauma--a systematic review. J Trauma. 2005;59:493–503.

101. Burns J, Brown M, Assi ZI, Ferguson EJ. Five-year retrospective review of blunt renal injuries at a level I trauma center. Am Surg. 2017;83:148–56.

102. Sujenthiran A, Elshout PJ, Veskimae E, MacLennan S, Yuan Y, Serafetinidis E, et al. Is nonoperative management the best first-line option for high-grade renal trauma? A systematic review. Eur Urol Focus 2017, pii: S2405–4569:30117.

103. van der Vlies CH, Olthof DC, van Delden OM, Ponsen KJ, de la Rosette JJ, de Reijke TM, et al. Management of blunt renal injury in a level 1 trauma

centre in view of the European guidelines. Injury. 2012;43:1816–20.

104. Nuss GR, Morey AF, Jenkins AC, Pruitt JH, Dugi DD 3rd, Morse B, et al. Radiographic predictors of need for angiographic embolization after traumatic renal injury. J Trauma. 2009;67:578–82; discussion 582.

105. Charbit J, Manzanera J, Millet I, Roustan JP, Chardon P, Taourel P, et al. What are the specific computed tomography scan criteria that can predict or exclude the need for renal angioembolization after high-grade renal trauma in a conservative management strategy? J Trauma. 2011;70:1219–27; discussion 1227–1218.

106. Fu CY, Wu SC, Chen RJ, Chen YF, Wang YC, Chung PK, et al. Evaluation of need for angioembolization in blunt renal injury: discontinuity of Gerota's fascia has an increased probability of requiring angioembolization. Am J Surg. 2010;199:154–9.

107. Sofocleous CT, Hinrichs C, Hubbi B, Brountzos E, Kaul S, Kannarkat G, et al. Angiographic findings and embolotherapy in renal arterial trauma. Cardiovasc Intervent Radiol. 2005;28:39–47.

108. Chow SJ, Thompson KJ, Hartman JF, Wright ML. A 10-year review of blunt renal artery injuries at an urban level I trauma centre. Injury. 2009;40:844–50.

109. Broghammer JA, Fisher MB, Santucci RA. Conservative management of renal trauma: a review. Urology. 2007;70:623–9.

110. Chabrot P, Cassagnes L, Alfidja A, Mballa JC, Nasser S, Guy L, et al. Revascularization of traumatic renal artery dissection by endoluminal stenting: three cases. Acta Radiol. 2010;51:21–6.

111. Lopera JE, Suri R, Kroma G, Gadani S, Dolmatch B. Traumatic occlusion and dissection of the main renal artery: endovascular treatment. J Vasc Interv Radiol. 2011;22:1570–4.

112. Agolini SF, Shah K, Jaffe J, Newcomb J, Rhodes M, Reed JF 3rd. Arterial embolization is a rapid and effective technique for controlling pelvic fracture hemorrhage. J Trauma. 1997;43:395–9.

113. Biffl WL, Smith WR, Moore EE, Gonzalez RJ, Morgan SJ, Hennessey T, et al. Evolution of a multidisciplinary clinical pathway for the management of unstable patients with pelvic fractures. Ann Surg. 2001;233:843–50.

114. Starr AJ, Griffin DR, Reinert CM, Frawley WH, Walker J, Whitlock SN, et al. Pelvic ring disruptions: prediction of associated injuries, transfusion requirement, pelvic arteriography, complications, and mortality. J Orthop Trauma. 2002;16:553–61.

115. Hagiwara A, Minakawa K, Fukushima H, Murata A, Masuda H, Shimazaki S. Predictors of death in patients with life-threatening pelvic hemorrhage after successful transcatheter arterial embolization. J Trauma. 2003;55:696–703.

116. Yoon W, Kim JK, Jeong YY, Seo JJ, Park JG, Kang HK. Pelvic arterial hemorrhage in patients with pelvic fractures: detection with contrast-enhanced

CT. Radiographics. 2004;24:1591–605; discussion 1605–1596.

117. Eastridge BJ, Starr A, Minei JP, O'Keefe GE, Scalea TM. The importance of fracture pattern in guiding therapeutic decision-making in patients with hemorrhagic shock and pelvic ring disruptions. J Trauma. 2002;53:446–50; discussion 450–441.

118. Miller PR, Moore PS, Mansell E, Meredith JW, Chang MC. External fixation or arteriogram in bleeding pelvic fracture: initial therapy guided by markers of arterial hemorrhage. J Trauma. 2003;54:437–43.

119. Gourlay D, Hoffer E, Routt M, Bulger E. Pelvic angiography for recurrent traumatic pelvic arterial hemorrhage. J Trauma. 2005;59:1168–73; discussion 1173–1164.

120. Metsemakers WJ, Vanderschot P, Jennes E, Nijs S, Heye S, Maleux G. Transcatheter embolotherapy after external surgical stabilization is a valuable treatment algorithm for patients with persistent haemorrhage from unstable pelvic fractures: outcomes of a single centre experience. Injury. 2013;44:964–8.

121. Shapiro M, McDonald AA, Knight D, Johannigman JA, Cuschieri J. The role of repeat angiography in the management of pelvic fractures. J Trauma. 2005;58:227–31.

122. Velmahos GC, Toutouzas KG, Vassiliu P, Sarkisyan G, Chan LS, Hanks SH, et al. A prospective study on the safety and efficacy of angiographic embolization for pelvic and visceral injuries. J Trauma. 2002;53:303–8; discussion 308.

123. Wong YC, Wang LJ, Ng CJ, Tseng IC, See LC. Mortality after successful transcatheter arterial embolization in patients with unstable pelvic fractures: rate of blood transfusion as a predictive factor. J Trauma. 2000;49:71–5.

124. Cullinane DC, Schiller HJ, Zielinski MD, Bilaniuk JW, Collier BR, Como J, et al. Eastern Association for the Surgery of Trauma practice management guidelines for hemorrhage in pelvic fracture--update and systematic review. J Trauma. 2011;71:1850–68.

125. Demetriades D, Karaiskakis M, Toutouzas K, Alo K, Velmahos G, Chan L. Pelvic fractures: epidemiology and predictors of associated abdominal injuries and outcomes. J Am Coll Surg. 2002;195:1–10.

126. Blackmore CC, Jurkovich GJ, Linnau KF, Cummings P, Hoffer EK, Rivara FP. Assessment of volume of hemorrhage and outcome from pelvic fracture. Arch Surg. 2003;138:504–8; discussion 508–509.

127. Sheridan MK, Blackmore CC, Linnau KF, Hoffer EK, Lomoschitz F, Jurkovich GJ. Can CT predict the source of arterial hemorrhage in patients with pelvic fractures? Emerg Radiol. 2002;9:188–94.

128. Pereira SJ, O'Brien DP, Luchette FA, Choe KA, Lim E, Davis K Jr, et al. Dynamic helical computed tomography scan accurately detects hemorrhage in patients with pelvic fracture. Surgery. 2000;128:678–85.

129. Stephen DJ, Kreder HJ, Day AC, McKee MD, Schemitsch EH, ElMaraghy A, et al. Early detection

of arterial bleeding in acute pelvic trauma. J Trauma. 1999;47:638–42.

130. Velmahos GC, Chahwan S, Falabella A, Hanks SE, Demetriades D. Angiographic embolization for intraperitoneal and retroperitoneal injuries. World J Surg. 2000;24:539–45.

131. Totterman A, Dormagen JB, Madsen JE, Klow NE, Skaga NO, Roise O. A protocol for angiographic embolization in exsanguinating pelvic trauma: a report on 31 patients. Acta Orthop. 2006;77:462–8.

132. Takahira N, Shindo M, Tanaka K, Nishimaki H, Ohwada T, Itoman M. Gluteal muscle necrosis following transcatheter angiographic embolisation for retroperitoneal haemorrhage associated with pelvic fracture. Injury. 2001;32:27–32.

133. Ramirez JI, Velmahos GC, Best CR, Chan LS, Demetriades D. Male sexual function after bilateral internal iliac artery embolization for pelvic fracture. J Trauma. 2004;56:734–9; discussion 7 39–741.

Yooun-Joong Jung

11.1 Introduction

Patients with critical injuries or those in whom certain special injuires are identified should be considered for early transfer to a higher level trauma center. However, hemodynamically unstable patients who need to be transferred to such a center may appropriately undergo operative control for ongoing hemorrhage before transfer if a qualified surgeon is promptly available at the referring hospital.

Agreement between institutions for the transfer of trauma patients is essential; it must be determined in advance which patients will be transferred and what the process needs to be. Direct physician-to-physican contact is essential. Once the need for transfer is identified, no process, including laboratory and diagnostic procedures, should delay the transfer.

Interhospital transfer monitoring is essential for safe patient transport. To ensure patient safety during transfer, the receiving hospital should have input, feedback, and communication with the physician responsible for the transport process [1–4].

It is the responsibility of the referring physician to initiate and maintain resuscitation until the patient's arrival at the referred hospital.

> **Check Points**
> - Identify the optimal institution with the qualified trauma surgeons who accepts the patients before transfer
> - Provide appropriate transportation in a vehicle with life-support equipment and staff to maintain resuscitation during transportation
> - Send all records, test results, and radiologic studies to the referral hospital before the patient transfer begins

11.2 Approach to Transfer of Trauma Patient

The decision to transport a trauma patient, either within a hospital or to another facility, is based on an assessment of the potential benefit of transport weighed against the potential risks.

Transfer of patients to the appropriate level trauma center is based on specialty medical care needs and resources required for patients' injuries. Patients with such critical injuries should be considered for early transfer [5, 6].

Y.-J. Jung (✉)
Critical Care Nursing Team, Asan Medical Center, University of Ulsan College of Medicine, Seoul, South Korea
e-mail: joong@amc.seoul.kr

© Springer Nature Singapore Pte Ltd. 2019
S.-K. Hong et al. (eds.), *Primary Management of Polytrauma*,
https://doi.org/10.1007/978-981-10-5529-4_11

11.2.1 Indication for Transfer

11.2.1.1 Physiologic Criteria

1. Depressed or deteriorating neurologic status
2. Respiratory distress or failure
3. Requiring advanced airway management and/or ventilator support
4. Serious cardiac rhythm disturbances associated with a traumatic event
5. Status post-cardiopulmonary arrest following a traumatic event
6. Shock, uncompensated, or responding inadequately to treatment
7. Injuries requiring blood transfusion of two or more units of packed red blood cells
8. High-risk obstetrical patient following a traumatic event
9. Patients requiring any one of the following:
   - Invasive monitoring (arterial and/or central venous pressure)
   - Intracranial pressure monitoring
   - Central venous pressure or pulmonary artery monitoring
   - Unresponsive or prolonged vasopressor administrations
   - Treatment for severe hypothermia or hyperthermia
   - Treatment for renal failure, acute or chronic, requiring immediate dialysis

11.2.1.2 Anatomic Criteria

Neurotrauma

1. Head trauma [7]
   - Penetrating injury or depressed skull fracture
   - Open injury with or without CSF leak
   - GCS score <14 or GCS deterioration
2. Spinal cord injury

Key Points
- Airway can be maintained during transfer recommendation. Intubate prior to transfer if respiratory failure is likely to develop during a prolonged transfer.
- Supplemental oxygen is being administered, and ventilation is adequate whether spontaneous or assisted.
- Circulation – hemodynamically stable/secure IV access.
- Immobilization of the spine is adequate and secure recommend
  - If spinal board – with appropriate padding
  - If hard collar – in definite or suspected cervical spinal injury

Thoracic Trauma

1. Widened mediastinum or other signs suggesting great vessel injury
2. Major chest wall injury or pulmonary contusion
3. Cardiac injury (blunt or penetrating)
4. Patients who may require prolonged ventilation

Key Points
Chest tube management during transfer
- Never clamp a chest tube while transporting a patient.
- Clamps must not be used on the patient for transport because of the risk of tension pneumothorax.
- The chest tube bottles need to remain below the patient's chest at all times.
- If the patient needs to be transferred to another department or is ambulant, the suction should be disconnected and left open to air.
- If suction is required during a transfer, arrangements must be made for suction to be set up prior to transfer.
- Flutter valve systems (Pneumostat, Heimlich) may be used for patient interhospital transfer.

Abdomen/Pelvis

1. Solid organ injury
2. Pelvic fracture with shock or other evidence of continuing hemorrhage
3. Open pelvic injury

Key Points
- The patients need to undergo resuscitation and more definitive intervention prior to transfer. If this is impossible, early transfer to a trauma center may be life-saving.
- Two wide, large intravenous cannulas should be in place before transfer.
- Shock resuscitation must be managed with intravenous fluids, bloods and/or vasopressors during transfer.
- Cross-matching blood may be prepared.

Major Extremity Injuries

1. Fracture/dislocation with loss of distal pulses
2. Open long bone fractures
3. Crush injuries or prolonged extremity ischemia

Key Points
- Do not wash, rinse, scrub, or apply antiseptic to extremity. Apply dry sterile gauze or toweling (depending on size).

Partial amputation
- Placed severed part(s) in a functional position.
- Apply dry sterile dressing.
- Splint.
- Elevate extremity.
- Apply coolant bag or ice bag to the outside of the dressing.

Amputation
- Package amputated extremity in a sealed plastic bag, and place ON TOP of coolant bag or sealed bag of ice in a container.
- If possible, control bleeding with pressure. If tourniquet is necessary, place it close to the amputation site.
- Consider appropriate pain medication

11.2.2   Interfacility Transfer Algorithm

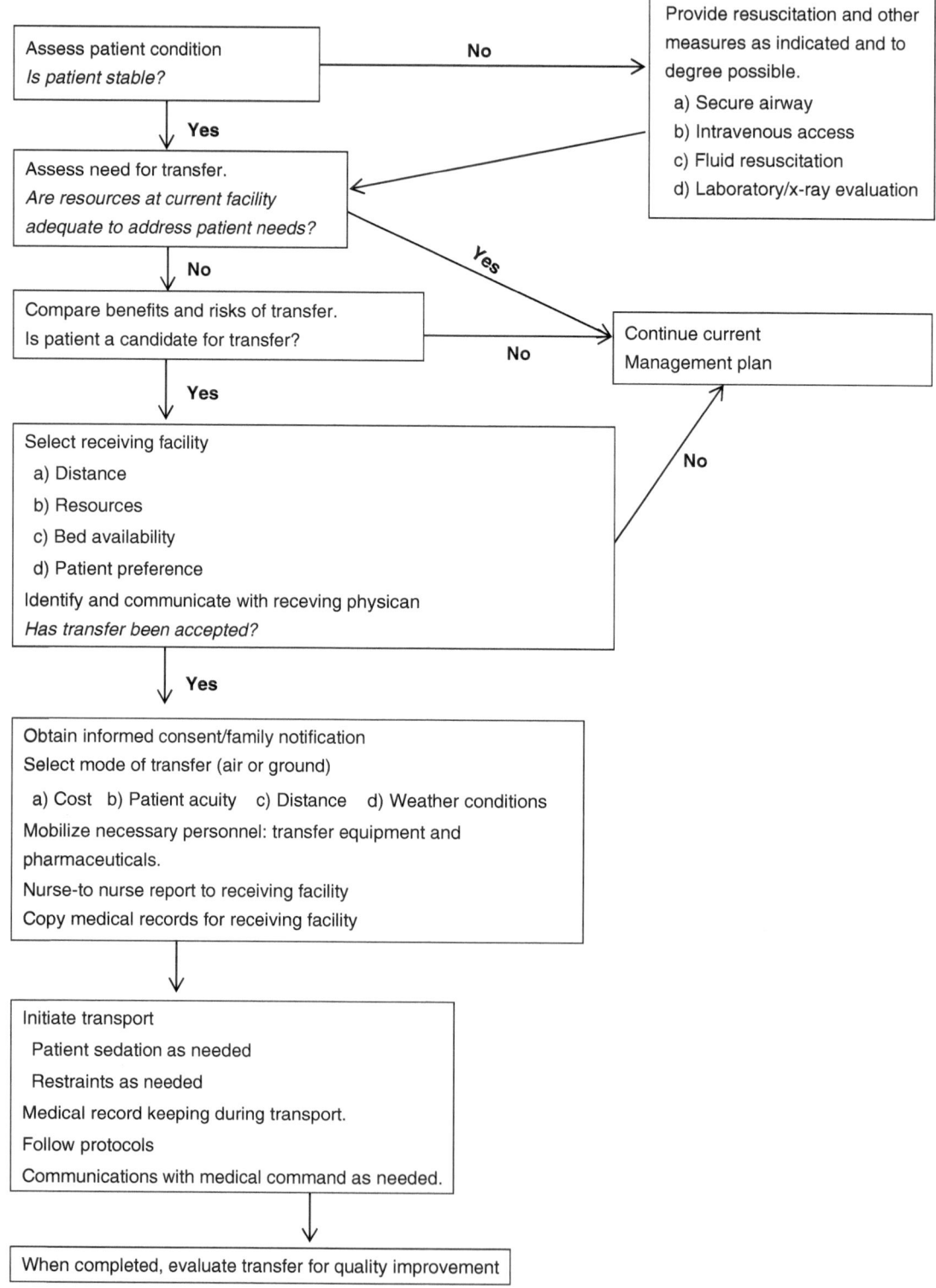

From recommendation Guidelines for the inter- and intrahospital transport of critically ill patients.2004

11.3 Planning the Transfer of Trauma Patients

11.3.1 The Transfer Team

The types of crew configuration vary as much as the types of ambulances and helicopters used in different countries. The combination of physicians, nurses, paramedics, and emergency medical technicians (EMTs) on critical care transport teams varies.

For inter-hospital (ambulance and air medical) transport, additional training is required for a physician to be able to adequately provide critical care support. It is recommended that each of the team members has the appropriate educational qualifications, because a specialized transport team provides better care, with decresed morbidity during and after transfer (Table 11.1).

11.3.1.1 Referring Staff Check

- Initiate the transfer process by direct contact with the receiving trauma surgeon
- Initiate resuscitation measures within the capabilities of the facility
- Transfer all records, test results, and radiologic evaluations to the receiving facility.
- Reassess the status of the patient prior to transfer
- Provide enough medication and medical supplies for the patient during the transfer. Consider which medications are indispensable and which may be interrupted temporarily.
- Ensure the presence of:
  - medical devices and machines according to the kind of ambulance or air transport
  - extra battery or wall sockets for use in ambulances or air transport,
  - suction device, if patient is intubated or has an inserted chest tube,
  - emergency kit to access quickly in the situation of a patient emergency.

Table 11.1 Transport team configuration recommendations

Severity	Team	Equipment	Care level
Stable with no risk of deterioration	Basic life support (BLS)	Oxygen, monitoring of vital signs, saline lock	Emergency medical technician (EMT) attending to patient;
Stable with low risk of deterioration:	Intermediate life support (ILS, if available) or advanced life support (ALS)	Patent intravenous (IV) access, use of IV medications including pain medications, pulse oximetry, increased need for assessment and interpretation skills.	EMT with IV endorsement if fluids are given without medication
Stable with medium risk of deterioration:	Advanced life support (ALS) with consideration of cirtical care transport team (CCTT)	Cardiac monitoring, basic cardiac medication, e.g., heparin or nitroglycerine. Requires advanced care such as an ALS service. An appropriate CCTT should be given consideration based on the patient's underlying medical condition and reason for transfer.	Critical care transport nurse or registered nurse (RN) with critical care and transport training.
Stable with high risk of deterioration	ALS with use of CCTT highly encouraged in patients requiring advanced airway management	Intubated, stabilized patients with potential for deterioration, based on assessment or knowledge of transferring facility.	Critical care transport nurse or RN with critical care and transport training.
Unstable	ALS with use of CCTT	Any patient who cannot be stabilized at the transferring facility, who is deteriorating or likely to deteriorate, patients requiring invasive monitoring, balloon pump, patients on multiple vasoactive medications, post-resuscitation, or those who have sustained multiple trauma-related injury require the use of a specialty transport team.	Critical care transport nurse or RN with critical care and transport training.

11.3.1.2 Receiving Staff Check

- Ensure that the resources required to care for the patient are present
- Provide consultation to the referring physician regarding the specifics of the transfer, and additional evaluation or resuscitation before transport.
- Clarify who will provide medical care, including resuscitation, during transportation.
- Identify a Performance Improvement Patient Safety (PIPS) for transportation, allowing feedback from the receiving trauma surgeon to the transport team directly, or at least allowing feedback to the medical director for the transport team and the referring hospital

11.3.2 Transfer Equipment

The minimum recommended equipment and pharmaceuticals needed for safe interhospital transfer are listed (Tables 11.2 and 11.3). Emphasis is placed on the airway, oxygenation, hemodynamic monitoring, and the pharmaceutical agents necessary for emergency resuscitation and stabilization as well as maintenance of vital functions. Very short or very long transports may necessitate deviations from the listed items, depending on the severity and nature of the patient's illness or injury.

All items are checked regularly for expiration of sterility and/or potency, especially when transports are infrequent.

- If peripheral venous access is unavailable, central venous access is established.
- All intravenous fluids and medications are to be stored in plastic (not glass) containers.
- A patient should not be transported before airway stabilization if it is judged likely that airway intervention will be needed en route

- The airway must be evaluated before transport and secured as indicated by endotracheal tube.
- For trauma victims, spinal immobilization is maintained during transport, unless the absence of significant spinal injury has been reliably verified.
- Chest decompression with a chest tube is accomplished before transport.
- A Heimlich valve or vacuum chest drainage system is employed to maintain decompression.
- Soft wrist and/or leg restraints are applied when agitation could compromise the safety of the patient or transport crew, especially with air transport (Table 11.2).

11.3.3 Transfer Medications

The drugs needed for patient transfer include muscle relaxants, sedatives, analgesics, inotropes, and resuscitation drugs. The person in charge of patient transfer should ensure that proper supplies of these emergency drugs are available. Some of these drugs may be required to be prepared in pre-filled syringes before the transfer. For drugs such as propofol for sedation, an extra syringe should be prepared before departure (Table 11.3).

Key Note

Before transporting a patient after resuscitation for hemorrhagic shock, check that red blood cells and clotting products (platelets, fresh frozen plasma or concentrated factors) are available.

However, if testing of blood takes too much time, remember that cardiovascular stabilization depends more on the amount than on the type of fluid. Do not lose precious time waiting for blood products.

Table 11.2 Essential equipment for use during transfers

Airway	Circulation
Guedel airway	Syringes
Laryneal masks	Needles
Tracheal tube	Alcohol wipes
Laryngoscopes	IV cannulae
Intubating stylet	Arterial cannulae
Gum-elastic tracheal introducer	Central venous cannulae Intraosseus infusion
Magill's forceps	Intravenous fluids
Cricothyroidotomy kit	Infusion sets/extensions
Lubricating gel	Three-way taps
Cotton tape for securing tracheal tube	Dressing and adhesive tape selection
Sterile scissors	Minor instrument/ cut-down set with sutures
Stethoscope	Fluid-warming device
Suction	Safety
Closed-suction catheter system or suction catheters	Secure container for pre-filled syringes
Nasogastric tube	Female luer-lock IV caps for drug syringes
Indwelling urinary cathether kits	Portable sharps disposal
Ventilation	
Chest tube	
Needle and surgical cricothyroidotomy supplies	
Ventilator	

Safe Transfer and Retrieval: The Practical Approach, Second Edition

Table 11.3 Recommended minimum trasport medications

Albuterol, 2.5 mg/2 mL	Lidocaine, 100 mg/10 mL
Amiodarone, 150 mg/3 mL	Lidocaine, 2 g/10 mL
Atropine, 1 mg/10 mL	Mannitol, 50 g/50 mL
Calcium chloride, 1 g/10 mL	Magnesium sulfate, 1 g/2 mL
Cetacaine/Hurricaine spray	Methylprednisolone, 125 mg/2 mL
Dextrose 25%, 10 mL	Metoprolol, 5 mg/5 mL
Dextrose 50%, 50 mL	Naloxone, 2 mg/2 mL
Digoxin, 0.5 mg/2 mL	Nitroglycerin injection, 50 mg/10 mL
Diltiazem, 25 mg/5 mL	Nitroglycerin tablets, 0.4 mg (bottle)
Diphenhydramine, 50 mg/1 mL	Nitroprusside, 50 mg/2 mL
Dopamine, 200 mg/5 mL	Normal saline, 30 mL for injection
Epinephrine, 1 mg/10 mL (1:10,000)	Phenobarbital, 65 mg/ mL or 130 mg/mL
Epinephrine, 1 mg/1 mL (1:1000) multiple-dose vial	Potassium chloride, 20 mEq/10 mL
Fosphenytoin, 750 mg/10 mL (500 PE mg/10 mL)	Procainamide, 1000 mg/10 mL
Furosemide, 100 mg/10 mL	Sodium bicarbonate, 5 mEq/10 mL
Glucagon, 1 mg vial (powder)	Sodium bicarbonate, 50 mEq/50 mL
Heparin, 1000 units/1 mL	Sterile water, 30 mL for injection
Isoproterenol, 1 mg/5 mL	Terbutaline, 1 mg/1 mL
Labetalol, 40 mg/8 mL	Verapamil, 5 mg/2 mL

From Recommendations for the intra-hospital transport of critically ill patients. *Crit Care.* 2010

PE Phenytoin equivalent

11.3.4 Transfer Checklist

The transfer trolley and equipment should be checked before and after each transfer, with a checklist to be signed for quality aduit.

Inter-Hospital Transfer Checklist

GENERAL INFORMATION

1. Transfer from _____

   Transfer to _____

2. Date of transfer _____/_____/_____

3. Patient : Name _____ DoB _____/_____/_____ Gender _____

4. Physician: Name _____ Phone _____

5. Contact person (Guardian) Name _____ Phone _____

6. Reason for transfer _____

PATIENT INFORMATION

7. Primary Diagnosis _____

8. Vital sign _____ BP _____ mmHg, PR _____ bpm, RR _____ bpm, T _____ °C

9. Consciousness   Alert _____,   Confusion _____,   Drowsy _____

                 Stupor _____,   Semicoma _____,   Coma _____

10. Pain   ☐ No   ☐ Yes (0~10: _____)

11. Restraint   ☐ No   ☐ Yes

12. Respiratory Support   ☐ No   ☐ Oxygen _____   ☐ Ventlartor _____

13. Isolation   ☐ No   ☐ MASA   ☐ VRE   ☐ ESBL   ☐ Others _____

14. Diet: ☐ No   ☐ Regular   ☐ Special   ☐ Tube Feed

15. IV access   ☐ No   ☐ PICC   ☐ CVC   ☐ Peripheral   ☐ Chemoport

16. Insertion device   ☐ Tracheostomy   ☐ Endotrachecel tube

                         ☐ Foley Catheter   ☐ Chest Tube   ☐ L-Tube   ☐ PT BD

                         ☐ JP   ☐ Hemovac   ☐ colostomy

17. Attached Documents
    ☐ Face sheet
    ☐ Medication lists
    ☐ Labs, Radiologic Data (CD)
    ☐ Operation Record

---

17. Sending facility Contact _____ Phone _____

18. From Completed By _____ Phone _____

11.4   Conduct of Transfer

11.4.1   Safety

Essential : In case of the patient's condition is deteriorate at any time during the transfer or before leaving the safe environment such as ED or ICU, make a plan to do additional therapy (i.e. medications, transfusions). Physicians and nurses should ensure the safety of the patient at all time during the transfer.

For the safety, check the initial assessment of the patient and reevaluate patient's condition prior to transfer.

Doctors and nurses should ensure the safety of the patient at all times during the transfer.

Those responsible for the care of the patient during transit must make an initial assessment of the patient, and re-evaluate prior to and during the transfer.

11.4.2   Transport Modality

The objective is to get the trauma victim to the receiving hospital quickly and safely. It is essential that the physician assesses the patients' capabilities and limitations to allow for early differentiation between those patients who can be safely cared for at the receiving hospital and those who require transfer to another hospital for definitive care. Transfer of the trauma victim must be organized by way of a transfer protocol that minimizes the risk to the patient during the transfer process.

The mode of transportation should be decided with consideration of the distance to be travelled, the geography, the weather, the patient's condition, the skill of the transport personnel, and the availability of equipment. This should be discussed between referring and receiving staff.

11.4.2.1 Ground Ambulance

In many cases, ground ambulances can be a safer mode of transporting a trauma patient than an air ambulance because they often offer more space for diagnostic or therapeutic equipment and there is less noise and vibration.

- *Basic life support*

A licensed BLS commercial ambulance is staffed at a minimum with an emergency medical responder (EMR) driver and an EMT attendant.

These ambulances are equipped with appropriate staff and monitoring devices to transport patients with non-life-threatening conditions, as these can only provide BLS services

- *Advanced life support*

A licensed ALS commercial ambulance is staffed at a minimum with an EMT driver and a Credit risk transfer (CRT) or paramedic attendant. These ambulances can provide ALS services such as endotracheal intubation, cardiac monitoring, defibrillation, and the administration of intravenous fluids or vasopressors. These vehicles are adequately staffed and equipped for transporting patients with life-threatening conditions

11.4.2.2 Air Medical Transport

The use of air transport has been on the rise in developed countries because of the advantages of rapid transport with the inclusion of specialized medical care [8].

Air medical transport advantanges include:

- Usually used for long-distance inter-hospital patient transfer for journeys of approximately more than 240 km,
- More rapid mode of transport with the provision of a pressurised cabin,
- Less noise and vibration than road ambulances.

11.4.2.3   Helicopter Transport

Helicopter transport advantanges include:

- Speed over long distances. Road transit times are halved for distances of 50-200 km.
- Access to remote areas, e.g., mountainous areas, or over large expanses of water.
- Indicated for severely ill/unstable patients.
- Enable early initiation of management by highly trained medical staff with special equipment.
- Faster mobilization than fixed-wing aircraft.
- Need smaller landing space and can land closer to or at hospitals.
- One study found that air ambulances offered distinct advantages in the management of Patients with traumatic brain injury.

Disadvantages and essential precautions may include:

- Staff training: Minimum requirements include safety training, evacuation procedures for the aircraft, and basic onboard communication skills. Staff must also have a detailed knowledge of how medical conditions can be affected by helicopter transport.

- Crashes: The risk is greatest at night and in poor weather conditions.
- Expense: Helicopters are the most expensive form of patient transport and there is continued uncertainty about their cost-effectivenss. There is, however, good evidence for their benefit in patients with serious blunt trauma.
- Noise and general stress may lead to anxiety and disorientation and hamper communication.
- Vibration may exacerbate bleeding/pain from fracture sites.

11.4.3 Treating and Monitoring the Patient during Transfer

Providing critical care support within a limited space and under difficult circumstances is considerably different from performing the same task in a hospital-based ICU. It requires—besides the usual professional skills—transfer experience. For inter-hospital (ambulance and air medical) transport, additional training is required for a physician to be able to adequately provide critical care support outside the ICU. The level of training of EMTs, registered critical care nurses, and employees of commercial air medical companies differs considerably between countries.

Critical care support requires the following features:

- Frequent monitoirng of vital signs.
- Provide ventilation and sipinal protection.
- Provide hemodynamic support and support for the central nervous system.

Keeping of records during transport, and providing them to the receiveing facility during patient handoff. Maintaining of communication with on line medical direction during transport. Monitoring of the patient's physiological status and essential equipment during transfer.

Key Points
- Oxygenation, blood pressure, consciousness.
- Adequate supply of oxygen: portable mechanical ventilator.
- Adequate supply of essential drugs: vasoactive drugs, IV fluids, blood, analgesics, hypnotics.
- Essential equipment: electrocardiogram (ECG) machine, invasive blood pressure monitoring, pulse oximeter, suction, battery-powered syringe pumps.

11.4.4 Problems During Transfer

Adverse events (e.g., desaturation, persistent hypotension) or specific transport-related events (e.g., unintended extubation, loss of intravascular access) should be handled according to standard critical care practice. If required (and possible) the transport vehicle can be stopped to facilitate the performance of any procedure required by the situation [9].

11.4.5 Documentation

All health care personnel are taught the importance of documentation. Nowhere is accurate and complete documentation more important than when dealing with a patient who is seriously ill or in a critical condition [10].

It is particularly important to record certain essential elements of every transfer. These include:

- The times of each set of vital signs and each assessment finding
- The details and times of each intervention (such as drug doses and routes of administration)
- Patient responses to all interventions
- Untoward or adverse reactions
- Communications with medical control
- Deviation from transfer orders or standing orders
- Diversion to another hospital.
- Refusal of treatment by the patient.

References

1. Patient transportation. Skills and techniques. Update 2011. Module Authors (Update 2011 and first edition).
2. Guidelines for the transport of the critically ill adult(3rd Edition 2011).
3. Interhospital Transfer Resource Manual. Maryland Institute for Emergency Medical Services systems. January 2002.
4. Warren J, Fromm RE, Orr RA, Rotello LC. Guidelines for the inter- and intrahospital transport of critically ill patients. Crit Care Med. 2004;32(1):256–62.
5. Harrahill M, Bartkus E. Preparing the trauma patient for transfer. J Emerg Nurs. 1990;16:25–8.
6. Davies G, Chesters A. Transport of the trauma patient. Br J Anaesth. 2015;115(1):33–7. https://doi.org/10.1093/bja/aev159.
7. Bekelis K, Missios S, Mackenzie TA. Prehospital helicopter transport and survival of patients with traumatic brain injury. Ann Surg. 2015;261(3):579–85.
8. Helicopter Transport, Authored by Dr Laurence Knott | Last edited 22 Mar 2010, https://patient.info/doctor/helicopter-transport.
9. Intas G, Stergiannis P. Risk factors in air transport for patients. Health Sci J. 2013;7(1):11–7.
10. Nocera N, Schoettker P. The N.E.W.S. Checklist: enhancing interhospital transfer of trauma patients. Aust Emerg Nurs J. 2002;45(1):12–4.